C01 6293250

Dr James Barry

Dr James Barry

A Woman Ahead of Her Time

MICHAEL DU PREEZ
&
JEREMY DRONFIELD

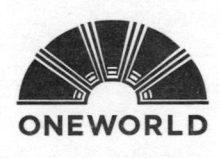

ONEWORLD

A Oneworld Book

First published in Great Britain and Australia by Oneworld Publications, 2016

Copyright © Michael du Preez and Jeremy Dronfield 2016

The moral rights of Michael du Preez and Jeremy Dronfield to be identified as the Authors of this work have been asserted by them in accordance with the Copyright, Designs, and Patents Act 1988

All rights reserved
Copyright under Berne Convention
A CIP record for this title is available from the British Library

ILLUSTRATION CREDITS

James Barry miniature: photo by Michael du Preez; James Barry commission, 1815: Museum Afrika, Johannesburg; Merchant's Quay: courtesy Cork City Libraries; Redmond Barry: public domain via Pennsylvania Hospital; James Barry RA self-portrait: Victoria & Albert Museum, London; James Barry RA's house: public domain via Yale Center for British Art, Paul Mellon Collection; Earl of Buchan: courtesy Perth Museum and Art Gallery, Perth & Kinross Council; Francisco de Miranda: public domain via wikimedia.org; St Thomas's Hospital: Library of King's College, London; RCS examination: courtesy Hunterian Museum, Royal College of Surgeons of England; James Barry portrait, 1820s: Museum Afrika, Johannesburg; James Barry portrait, 1830s: Artware Fine Art; Lord Charles Somerset: courtesy Earl of Devon; Captain Cloete: Museum Afrika, Johannesburg; Alphen: photo by Michael du Preez; The Tronk: Elliott Collection, Western Cape Archives; Newlands House: Elliott Collection, Western Cape Archives; James Barry Munnik: Rita Wiggett/The Argus; James Barry caricature, c. 1852: Army Medical Services Museum, Mytchett, Surrey; James Barry's house in St Helena: courtesy Barbara George; Kingston, Jamaica: public domain, from *A Picturesque Tour of Jamaica* by James Hakewill, via archive.org; Scutari Barracks: National Army Museum, London; James Barry commission, 1857: National Archives, London; James Barry photograph: Army Medical Services Museum, Mytchett, Surrey; RCS mural: Paul Cox, courtesy Royal College of Surgeons of England.

ISBN 978-1-78074-831-3
eISBN 978-1-78074-314-1

Typeset by Tetragon, London
Printed and bound in Great Britain by Clays Ltd, St Ives plc

Oneworld Publications
10 Bloomsbury Street
London WC1B 3SR
England

Stay up to date with the latest books,
special offers, and exclusive content from
Oneworld with our monthly newsletter

Sign up on our website
www.oneworld-publications.com

To Angela

Contents

Authors' Note   ix
Prologue   xi

Part I: 'Was I Not a Girl'
1789–1815

1	A Family at War	3
2	An Unprotected Girl	13
3	Next of Kin	23
4	A Small Fortune	31
5	A Revolutionary Plan	42
6	Sanguine Expectations	58
7	A Man of Understanding	68
8	'I Would Be a Soldier'	81
9	Qualified to Serve	94

Part II: More Than a Father
1816–1831

10	The Cape of Good Hope	115
11	'Savage Neighbours'	128
12	A Prodigy in a Physician	138
13	The Most Wayward of Mortals	150
14	A Change of Circumstances	160
15	Heaven and Earth	166
16	'If Rumour Speaks Truth'	178
17	Dr Barry's Nemesis	188
18	'Blighting My Fair Prospects'	203
19	A New Life	213
20	A Precipitate Departure	224
21	An Indefatigable Friend	229

Part III: Flagrant Breaches of Discipline
1831–1845

22   Fever Island   245
23   The Past Revisited   254
24   An Officer and a Gentleman   263
25   Homeward Bound   273
26   Friends in High Places   283

Part IV: The Most Hardened Creature
1846–1856

27   The Navel of the Mediterranean   299
28   A Question of Numbers   307
29   The Most Kind and Humane Gentleman   319
30   Prodigality and All Wickedness   329
31   The Land of Mornise   338

Part V: A Useful and Faithful Career
1857–1865

32   'This Vorld of Voe, this Wale of Tears'   349
33   This Life and No Other   363
34   A Perfect Female   375

Epilogue   383
Appendix A: James Barry and the Physical Examination   387
Appendix B: Who Discovered Dr Barry's Secret?   390
Notes   393
Bibliography   451
Acknowledgements   465
Index   471

Authors' Note

Throughout this book, the gender pronouns used for James Barry vary according to situation, depending on whether he/she is appearing in the persona of the male 'James Barry' or that of her original female identity; between those extremes, Barry is referred to as either 'he' or 'she' depending on whether the viewpoint is 'his' outer persona or 'her' inner self.

The currency in use in the United Kingdom in James Barry's lifetime comprised pounds, shillings and pence (£ s d), divided thus:

£1 = 20s
1s = 12d

In this book, sums are given according to the convention of the time – for example, £1 4s 6d (one pound, four shillings and sixpence).

The modern value of historic sums is impossible to give accurately, due to huge changes in the relative values of labour, commodities, property and retail prices. For instance, £100 in 1800 would now be equivalent to between £7000 (based on retail price inflation) and £120,000 (based on income and GDP), while the labour value (i.e. the amount of labour it could buy) would be about £106,000, and measured as a proportion of the total value of the UK economy it would be worth nearly £500,000.[1] Thus the anticipated value of the estate left by the painter James Barry RA in 1807, for which his relatives contested, would today be worth somewhere between £390,000 and £24 million.

Prologue

D r Barry was dying. He knew precisely how the end would be; in a lifetime's medical service, Dr Barry had seen it all, cured some of it, and watched hundreds leave the mortal world along the same ugly, degrading path that he was now treading.

Beyond the open window, London sweltered under a July heatwave. The traffic in Margaret Street racketed past with intolerable noise – iron-shod hoofs pulled iron-shod wheels over the stones, heading for the press of Oxford Market; passers-by and loiterers shouted to make themselves heard, and the shrieks of street-hawkers pierced the whole cacophony. It was hard for a human to bear at the best of times, but for the sick it was an exquisite hell.

The heat and the familiar symptoms of the disease awakened memories of the tropics where he'd spent so much of his working life: the hospital wards filled with groans, and lonely rooms whining with nocturnal mosquitoes. He knew how the disease would progress, like a conductor knows the movements and motifs of a concerto – and what a hideous composition, of pain, dizziness and rushing, watery efflux, as if the body were trying to eject its innards in one frantic torrent; the sagging, blue-tinged skin and sunken eyes. Soon the last dissonant chords; then the shadow must fall.

There was something he had to do before the end – something important. But in the heat and noise, with his mind wandering on the edge of delirium, it eluded his grasp.

At last the old gentleman's chest stopped rising and falling, and the fluttering of his closed eyelids ceased.

★

Sophia Bishop heated a large copper of water on the range, under the supervision of the ill-tempered charwoman. This person, old enough to be the young housemaid's mother, came in once a week to help with the laundry, but today she was here in her other capacity, as layer-out.

The water boiled, and Sophia lifted the steaming copper off the range while the charwoman gathered up cloths, soap and a calico winding-sheet. As had once been common in England, this woman earned part of her living from a dual career as a midwife and layer-out of the dead, usually working among the poorer or more parsimonious members of society (the prosperous days were long gone, the mortal end of the trade having passed into the hands of undertakers). She was a hardened creature who cared mainly for money, and like her literary counterpart Mrs Gamp she 'went to a lying-in or a laying-out with equal zest and relish'.[1]

Sophia carried the copper up to the death room. It was she who had found him dead and reported it to the authorities. That had been as much involvement as she wanted; she set down the copper and left the older woman to her business. The layer-out was an old friend to death; she'd attended the corpses of many a person in her life. One more old fellow was nothing out of the ordinary.

In the heat, the smell in the room was enough to unsettle even her strong stomach. Still, the proper obligations must be taken care of and she must get her due payment; perhaps something extra to cover the unpleasant circumstances and the lack of help.

The old man had been a slight, stooped figure, narrow-shouldered and short; in death, his large nose and pointed chin were accentuated by the sunken flesh, and the dyed red hair had been slicked back from the domed forehead by the sweat of sickness. The layer-out peeled back the bedclothes and raised the body to remove the soiled nightshirt. After dipping a cloth in hot water, she gave the corpse a melancholy glance before beginning to wash it … and paused.

Something wasn't right. She glanced again at the hollowed-out face. That was the old gentleman all right – Dr James Barry. The layer-out had seen him about the place before he took sick, and would recognise him anywhere. And yet those were certainly not a gentleman's private parts. Indeed, the gentleman's whole body, though thin and dilapidated by age, was unmistakably female in every way – the genitals, the deflated breasts and the hairless face. And there was more – distinctive striations on the skin of the belly. The layer-out had marks like those herself; they came from childbearing. Moreover, in all her experience, she had only ever seen them quite as pronounced as that in girls who'd had babies at a very early age.[2]

How could this be? She knew that Dr Barry had been an Army man, and served a long career. How was it possible for a woman to get away with being a *surgeon*, let alone in the Army? The puzzle was too great and shocking. Suppressing her amazement, she carried on with the laying out. Soon the body was cleaned and enveloped in its shroud, looking the same as any other.

She was so bewildered, she couldn't even speak of it at first; but then her native acumen told her that it might be profitable to hold on to this secret. The body, unexamined by any other person, went off to the undertaker, and it was only when a couple of weeks had gone by and Dr Barry was cold in his grave that the layer-out finally spoke of what she had seen in that deathbed.

The sensational story flew around the Empire, spreading from newspaper to newspaper, and from place to place, reaching the ears of people who'd known James Barry throughout his career and all the way back to his youth more than half a century earlier. Almost everyone seemed to recall that they'd thought him a strange fellow, and even a few claimed they'd always guessed he was female. But not a single one of them could answer the most intriguing question of all: how on earth had a woman managed to perpetrate such an audacious deception? How had she sustained it over so many decades? And if she wasn't 'James Barry' – which she manifestly wasn't – then who the devil *was* she?

PART I

'Was I Not a Girl?'

1789–1815

I

A Family at War

A little girl with red-gold hair stood on the busy quayside, wrapped up in a muffler and bonnet. She watched, hypnotised, as an elegant Royal Navy cutter eased through the morning mist towards the north channel of the River Lee, the light breeze filling the single sail. Her blue-green eyes followed the line of the bow slicing through the grey river; the cry of an order came faintly across the water, the sail started to furl, the oars came out like the petals of an opening flower and began to propel the boat towards the town quays.

Everyone knew that the cutter came from the man-of-war HMS *Bellerophon*, anchored downstream at Cobh. For two months, terrifying rumours had been reaching Cork of a French fleet that was expected to land in Ireland. Now the French had been dispersed, the threat had lifted, and here was *Bellerophon*, the leader of the English defenders, calling to take on stores before sailing for home.[1] Not every person on the quayside welcomed the sight of the cutter, or what it represented, and a few would have been quite happy to have the French liberate Ireland from British rule. But they wisely kept their silence.

Cork was the nexus of Irish trade, and the beating heart of the city was the long, spear-shaped island, crowded with busy streets, dividing the river in two. Along Merchant's Quay, the ships' masts clustered like a thicket in the mist, moored two deep on both sides of the river. They brought the wide world to Cork: the salt of the Indian Ocean in their sails and the damp of Nova Scotia in their timbers; bottoms barnacled at the Cape and slimed in jungle estuaries. In return they took Ireland to the wide world, in the form of hides and tallow, thick Kerry butter and good Irish soldiers. Cork was one of the greatest ports of the British Empire, and the British would do anything to defend it.

To the little girl, Cork was both home and the world. Her name was Margaret Anne Bulkley and she was eight years old; she'd been born in this city to parents who had also been born here, and it was all she knew. A vivid, stimulating world for a child to grow up in, a storm of sensations – the noise of carts on the cobbles and the slopping of the water under hundreds of wooden hulls, the creak of mooring ropes straining against the rise and fall of the tide, the squeal of gulls, and the strident talk of men in all the tongues on God's earth; the smells of tarred rope, river weed and brine mingled with the reek of horseflesh, sweaty linen, ripe cheeses, cooking meat and baking bread, and the astringent odours of gin, beer and grog.

Margaret turned away from the sight of the Navy cutter and hurried along the heaving quayside, past the shop windows – vintners, taverns, ironmongers, ships' chandlers, sailmakers, all bustling with trade. She turned in at the familiar doorway of the grocer's shop, with the proprietor's name painted on a board above the doorway: *Jeremiah Bulkley*.

This was Margaret's home and the centre of her universe. Its shelves were stacked, cupboards bulging and the floor piled high with victuals for the marine trade. Over it all presided Margaret's father, Jeremiah, bearing the perpetually anxious air of a man burdened with debts but hopeful for the future. *Bellerophon*'s arrival would be welcome news; in Jeremiah's world, war meant ships, and ships meant income; and war was everywhere these days.

He had borrowed heavily to set up in trade. The house belonged to his wife's family, which was a saving, but to start the business he'd borrowed hundreds of pounds,[2] which would take long years of graft to pay off. But Jeremiah was slowly building a position for himself in Cork's mercantile community; besides the grocery shop he'd acquired a post at the city's Weigh House – a mark of some distinction, especially for a Catholic in English Ireland. Here the produce of Kerry, Cork and Limerick was brought for grading and weighing. Each year hundreds of thousands of firkins of butter were scrutinised by the inspectors, weighed and branded, before being transported to the quaysides.

History has forgotten what Jeremiah Bulkley's post in the Weigh House was – probably one of the three butter inspectors, drawing a generous salary of £140 per annum.[3] Processing goods worth over a million pounds a year, the Weigh House was rich in lucre to be creamed off; producers and traders paid a fee to have their goods approved and branded, and the Committee of Merchants lapped up two or three thousand pounds' worth of revenue from it each year. Thus, as long as Jeremiah Bulkley kept his job in the Weigh House, there was reason to hope for a bright future.

His wife, Mary Anne, needed as much hope as she could get; she was an anxious, nervy sort of woman. She'd been born into the Barry family, fairly well known in Cork as decayed but respectable former gentry, with interests in several modest businesses and a handful of crumbling properties in the city. Mary Anne's parents, John and Juliana Barry, had raised five children, with Mary Anne the only girl among four wild, tempestuous older brothers. They weren't particularly nice boys, and Mary Anne's only childhood comfort had been her father (her 'only true friend').[4] By the time she reached womanhood, her brothers had moved on. John had died, Patrick and Redmond had gone to sea, while James – who had shown a prodigious talent for drawing – had become a painter. Acquiring eminent patrons, James Barry had toured Europe and settled in London, where he built up a reputation as a first-rate artist and a volatile personality. He taught at the Royal Academy of Arts, becoming a fellow and professor there. In 1782 Mary Anne Barry was wed to Jeremiah Bulkley,[5] of no particularly remarkable family, and they produced two surviving children: a son, John, and a daughter, Margaret Anne.[6]

Money would be an abiding worry throughout their marriage. Mary Anne had been left £100 by her dear, departed father, of which she'd had to give £40 to her living, not so dear, mother, in order to purchase her life interest in the house on Merchant's Quay.[7]

Jeremiah and Mary Anne raised their two children in the manner of gentlefolk, in expectation of their fortunes improving. John was earmarked for the legal profession, while Margaret's schooling was that of a young lady whose destiny would be marriage; she may have been cleverer, more literate and more industrious than her brother, but she was a girl, and little else was expected of her.

From the shop doorway, Margaret looked back the way she had come, along the teeming waterfront. A column of soldiers marched along the quayside, looking brave and splendid in their scarlet jackets and pipeclayed white crossbelts, the cockades on their hats quivering as they marched. How unfair it was that Margaret couldn't hope to be a soldier! The notion appealed to her sense of adventure, and would be an abiding daydream in the years to come.[8]

Ruin came gradually to Jeremiah Bulkley, and it began with politics. Trouble between nationalists and loyalists had been fermenting in Ireland for decades, and in 1798 it boiled over. The Society of United Irishmen launched an armed rebellion against British rule. It began in Dublin and spread to other counties. The fighting was vicious; there were rumours of atrocities and massacres on both sides, and for ordinary families like the Bulkleys it was terrifying. In August, Napoleon sent an invasion force to Ireland to help the United Irishmen; a thousand French soldiers landed in County Mayo and fought their way towards Dublin.

The rebellion was short-lived; by the end of September British troops had defeated the French and the United Irishmen. The fighting had not reached as far as Cork, but the city had played a part – the Royal Cork Militia had helped crush the rebels in Dublin with cavalry and cannon-fire.[9]

Although the rebellion was over, the grievances that had caused it remained and intensified. Catholics like the Bulkleys, regardless of whether they had nationalist sympathies or not, came under greater suspicion than ever, and their lives grew more precarious. Yet the shop ledger remained strong on the income side, the debts were secure, and Mr and Mrs Bulkley's anxieties held in check.

It couldn't last; the world was changing, and Margaret's life would be forcibly bent to fit it. The after-shocks of the 1798 rebellion rumbled on for years. Britain tightened its grip on its Irish possession, and in 1800 the Acts of Union were passed. The Parliament of Ireland, stuffed with loyal Britons who took their cue from the Parliament in London, voted itself into extinction. Ireland was absorbed formally into the United Kingdom of Great Britain, the St Patrick's cross was incorporated into the Union flag, and the Irish parliamentary seats were transferred – with their occupants – to Westminster.

They included Colonel Mountifort Longfield, MP for Cork, who happened to be the city's Weigh-Master, with authority over the Weigh House (the institution had been seized from the city corporation by the British government in 1792 and British loyalists put in charge).[10] Eager to enforce the new regime against the background of continuing raids and attacks by rebels,[11] Longfield decided to cleanse the public offices of

Catholics. Jeremiah Bulkley was dismissed from his post at the Weigh House.[12]

For a man burdened by debt, the loss of the £140 salary was a painful blow. As well as the credit that kept the grocery business running, Jeremiah had borrowed even more money in his attempt to improve the family's future prospects. In 1801 young John had been apprenticed to an attorney in Dublin, at a premium of around £400.[13] The ships of life and commerce floated on a sea of credit, but the tides were treacherous, and Jeremiah Bulkley was not a skilled navigator. He loved his only son, had faith in his prospects, and pinned the family's future on him.[14] But John was not a reliable young man; whereas Margaret was bright, imaginative, inclined to dedicate herself to a cause, her elder brother was less intelligent, lived in the moment and gave little thought to the consequences of his actions. Had their sexes been reversed, Margaret might have done well for herself, but in the world she'd been born into the best she could hope for was to marry well – and with no fortune to offer, the chances of that were remote. So off John went to Dublin, to serve, scribe and study.

In the first years of the new century, life on Merchant's Quay continued as normal. The ships' masts clustered as thickly, the wharves were as busy, and the gulls and sailors cried as raucously as ever; but Margaret's childhood would be forever altered by an experience she underwent at some unrecorded moment between 1801 and 1803. Still just a half-grown adolescent between twelve and fourteen years old, Margaret had the hardships of womanhood thrust prematurely upon her.

There had been an addition to the family. Quite how it happened is uncertain – the Bulkleys avoided recording the details, although rumours must have run along the quayside and through the town. As soon as the gravity of the situation was realised within the family, Mrs Bulkley and Margaret probably went away together for a while; when they returned, all that was known publicly was that the Bulkleys had a new baby girl.

It was hardly plausible that Jeremiah and Mary Anne would have a child now – they'd produced only two living children in two decades of marriage, and were both entering middle age. But under the law, if one took a child as one's own, then so it was. Gossips could say what they liked; publicly this infant was Margaret's sister. They called her Juliana after Mary Anne's late mother, as if to confirm the link.[15]

For the rest of her life Margaret would carry the physical marks of having borne this child. The marks left on her mind could only be guessed at. Her exact age at the time of the birth is not known,[16] but the child was in existence by 1803, when Margaret turned fourteen.

The identity of the man who raped her would never be revealed. The compass inevitably swings towards her family and their circle.[17] Her father? Her brother? Perhaps some family friend, or a teacher or local priest. There were few relatives remaining in Cork – no known grand-parents or cousins. But there was – for a short while – a single uncle on the Barry side of the family, who came to visit at about this time and then left under an extremely dark cloud.

Of Mrs Bulkley's four brothers, Redmond was the worst; he shared the volatile Barry temperament, unleavened by intelligence or talent. He and Patrick had both gone off to seek adventure. Patrick had joined the Royal Navy as a marine; he later deserted, and was believed to have died somewhere in the Orient.[18] Redmond also went to sea, and served more than four decades as an ordinary seaman aboard Royal Navy war-ships.[19] Wild and uneducated, Redmond was brutalised by life at sea. In 1781, shortly after a period in action, he wrote in his barely literate hand, 'there is no Respect of Persons on Bord of a man of war there are the greatest Vilions I suppose that Could be Found any where', and he admitted that he was one of them.[20] By 1789 – the year his mother died – Redmond was on a brief hiatus from the Navy, living with a woman in one of London's slum districts. Patrick, who had also washed up briefly in London, destitute and starving, stayed with them, and even he was dismayed by Redmond's squalid, lawless life. During Patrick's stay, Redmond and his woman got a sailor drunk and robbed him; they then absconded, leaving Patrick terrified of being charged with the crime; 'my poverty prevents me from any place of refuge in safety, so must trust to providence as I am conscious of my innocence, only being at their house to prevent lying in the street or field'.[21]

After this incident, Redmond returned to the Navy. But then, early in 1802, he reappeared in Cork – the city of his birth, which he hadn't seen for nearly thirty years – seeking charity from his sister and her husband. In middle age, Redmond Barry was lean and muscular, looking every inch the 'Vilion': a lantern-jawed face with deep, close-set eyes and an immensely long, blade-sharp nose; his thin, fair hair fell back from a knobbly, domed forehead, and a lank moustache drooped over his mouth, whose lower lip had a tendency to slump into a discontented glower.[22]

He'd always regarded himself as hard done by – his brother James had got all the success in life, while Mary Anne had received an unfair share of their parents' legacy. (Patrick was the same – he claimed that Mary Anne had 'entirely deprived me of every means of life'[23] in inheriting her portion.) And so, when Redmond, hardened and embittered, arrived in Cork in 1802, he regarded it as the bounden duty of his pampered sister and her seemingly well-off husband to give him alms and accommodation. Redmond felt sorry for himself; he had been 'hampered About in the Service of the Country Untill I am Scarcely Able to render Any degree of Labour to procure a living for Myself'.[24] Jeremiah and Mary Anne, whose financial situation was growing more precarious by the month, gave Redmond what he asked for – but grudgingly.

And then something had happened that had caused Mary Anne and Jeremiah to take against Redmond with a vehement loathing. According to Redmond they used 'every means in their power to prevent me from getting bread', until at last, in desperation, he rejoined the Navy, 'never to come to pay Ireland a visit Again, let the Consequence be as it will'.[25] Jeremiah and Mary Anne had, in effect, run Redmond out of town on a rail. When he called on James in London that summer, he was rebuffed, and suspected that James had heard damning reports from their 'Infernal Sister' about what had happened in Cork. Redmond asked James to 'look back and Consider if you weare in My Situation and I in yours how you would Approve of my behaviour'.[26]

It is more than possible that the 'behaviour' that had caused his expulsion was the rape of his niece, Margaret. The Bulkleys had no choice but to bear the burden and the social shame with which they'd been left.

Trouble is a faithful companion, and rarely content with visiting only once. Between them, Jeremiah Bulkley and his beloved son brought about the family's downfall with a reckless precision that could hardly have been exceeded.

Two years into his legal apprenticeship, John's prospects must have seemed fair. He had met a Miss Ward, 'a young Lady of genteel connexions', who fell in love with him.[27] She had a small fortune of her own amounting to some £1200, which would more than enable John to complete his training, and her family connections would become priceless when he set out on his own account as an attorney. But there was an obstacle. Although Miss Ward's parents were dead, she was protected by 'an infamous set of Brothers'[28] who wouldn't agree to a marriage settlement unless John could match her fortune. As neither he nor his father had anything approaching £1200, the engagement seemed doomed. John wrote that he would be 'very unhappy … if all the family would be distressed on my acct',[29] but the emotional pressure he applied was great – if he didn't obtain Miss Ward's advantages, his hopes of being an attorney would be shattered.

Jeremiah didn't have the cash, but he did own some valuable properties. A marriage settlement was drawn up, under which Jeremiah signed over to John a farm (presumably tenanted), a dwelling house and offices in which he had previously invested £1200. He topped off this gift with £300 in cash.[30] The matter was settled, and the couple were married. Jeremiah had, in effect, wagered the family's financial security on John's future career.

Word soon spread among the traders and money-men of Cork that Jeremiah Bulkley had disposed of the properties that secured his debts, which stood at £700. His creditors 'immediately became importunate', and he had to cease paying his instalments;[31] thereafter, demands for repayment in full began to arrive at the shop. This clatter of small stones turned into a landslide, and soon creditors were hammering at Jeremiah's door. When that failed to elicit payment, they pursued legal recourse. Jeremiah still had goods and property worth more than his debts, and he offered to turn them over to his creditors, but they refused – they wanted cash. Given the impossibility of selling anything for a fair price in the circumstances (for what sensible person would pay the going rate to a man desperate to sell?), the Bulkleys were doomed. Jeremiah considered sailing for the West Indies (where great fortunes could be made) and sending back his earnings. Meanwhile, he prolonged negotiations with his creditors, hoping to gain time to raise the money.

Trouble took up residence in Mrs Bulkley's home; always a nervous, highly strung woman, she grew ill with worry. In theory, the females of the family should be safe; John's marriage carried the condition that the properties he acquired must be used for the assistance of Mrs Bulkley, Margaret and Juliana 'if Ocasion required his doing so'.[32] By early 1804, occasion required it urgently, and Mrs Bulkley wrote to her son to tell him so. In April she received a letter from him that bewildered and wounded her; she didn't preserve it, nor describe what John had done, but whatever

it was, she attributed it to 'his youth and want of experience', as well as
to bad advice. Given Mrs Bulkley's distress and the events that followed,
it seems that John had sold the properties and invested (or spent) the
money. He had left his mother, Margaret and Juliana without a lifeline;
if Jeremiah fell, they would be destitute.

Mary Anne had only one person left to whom she might turn for
help – her eldest brother, James Barry. As a famous painter, a professor
at the Royal Academy, celebrated in London society, he must undoubtedly be wealthy. And he must, with equal certainty, be willing to help
his unfortunate sister. Mary Anne hadn't seen James since he left Ireland,
when she was a young girl and he was a keen, ambitious man in his early
twenties. He'd always had a mercurial spirit, but was as intelligent and
talented as his brothers were wayward and reckless. And in his youth,
James had kept his family in his thoughts, hoping to make up for the lack
of a legacy from their father:

> I have that reliance on God, my profession, and my friends, that in such
> a place as London is, where art is so caressed, I shall bring such a portion
> of it with me there, as will not only put me out of the want of any
> thing else, but will further enable me on my own part to make some
> little additions to any thing my father may have to leave them. I am
> then, thank God … provided for, and the greatest part of my anxiety
> is only how I may provide still better for the poor people at home.[33]

Thirty-five years had passed since then, but Mary Anne hoped the generous sentiment still held. She couldn't write the letter herself; the distress
she'd been through had caused a constant tremor in her hands, so Margaret
wrote for her, and no doubt helped with the composition. She was
growing up – at fifteen, adulthood and responsibility were encroaching
on what was left of her adolescence. Yet the prospect of communicating
with her famous uncle – whom she had neither met nor seen, but of
whom she had heard much – must have been exciting.

Looking across the table at her daughter, quill in hand, the implements
of writing laid out – fresh white paper, penknife for repairing the nib,
pot of ink, the bar of sealing wax beside the candle – Mary Anne might
have recalled her last memories of James, when he was a young man and
she a child. His features were discernible in Margaret's maturing face; she
was most certainly a Barry rather than a Bulkley.[34] She had the same fine,

fair, reddish hair as the young James, the same large blue-green eyes and arched eyebrows; she was developing the long, curved nose of the Barrys (the one feature James did not share) and the protruding chin; and last of all Margaret had the Barry mouth, with a plump underlip that could give an impression of sullenness, and the Cupid's bow that had prettified the face of James in his youth.

'My Dear brother,' Mary Anne commenced; Margaret's goose quill twitched as she carefully inscribed her mother's words in her best hand-writing. 'I have been always very unwilling to trouble you, knowing the multiplicity of your avocations, or you shou'd have oftener heard from me, while things were going on prosperously with me.'[35] She related her tale of woe in detail: John's marriage, the ruinous settlement, the loss of Jeremiah's job at the Weigh House, and the onslaught of the creditors. She delicately refrained from asking outright for help, or even hinting at it; it was plain enough from the story she told that she was in need. She concluded her dictation: 'With the greatest deference I remain Most truly & sincerely your most Affectionate &ca &ca Sister', and trusted to her brother to do his duty.

Looking over what she'd written in her neat but unsophisticated hand, Margaret quickly added a postscript of her own: 'Sir, My Mother is not able to write legible on account of a tremour in her hand, desired me to write for her, My inexperience and so much unaccustomed to letter writing I hope will be accepted by you as an Apology [for] the length, the many faults & Errors in this letter by Sir, by yours Most Affectionate &ca &ca &ca ~~Marg~~ᵗ Margaret Anne Bulkley.'[36] Evidently Margaret's education had been neither as full nor as thorough as her wit deserved.

They were unable to find out his address, and simply directed it to 'James Barry Esq., R.A. & Professor of Painting to the Royal Academy'.[37] The letter was sealed and sent. April passed into May, June approached and still no reply came; the situation grew more tense by the week. The creditors were threatening to seize the premises on Merchant's Quay, and Jeremiah was intending to protect it by putting it in John's name – a sure way to lose it entirely. Mary Anne was indignant. The legal right to occupy the house had been hers – acquired from her mother – and had become Jeremiah's when she married him, but full title to the property still belonged to James Barry. Only he, by asserting his legal rights, could now save Mary Anne, Margaret and Juliana from eviction. There was nothing for it but to go and seek him out in London.

2

An Unprotected Girl

Little Castle Street, London: June 1804

London exceeded all imagination; a true metropolis; teeming, lurking, cacophonous, it was like a multitude of cities conjoined. Every corner one turned, there were more streets, more winding alleys, more dank yards and mansions. It seemed that one could walk forever and never find its end.

Margaret and her mother had arrived in London by stagecoach from Bristol, after the shortest possible voyage from Cork. It was perilous to be at sea: the previous year, after a peace lasting just fourteen months, war with France had broken out again, the nations were fighting for ascendancy in the seas around Europe, and any vessel was a legitimate prize of war. But if the female Bulkleys were to save themselves from the follies of their male relations, there was no option but to brave the seas and come to England.[1]

They had discovered James Barry's address and taken lodgings nearby, in Little Titchfield Street. It was decided that Margaret should go alone to visit him. Perhaps Mary Anne believed that his protective instinct would be aroused by a young girl who might remind him of his own youth and the promise he had made. Margaret, a bright and bold girl, was willing to take up the challenge. So, with a hired servant as a chaperone, she set off into the warren of West London.[2]

The noise and density of the traffic assailed the senses, as did the press of people – the passers-by, the hawkers, the barrow-women in yellow blouses and scarlet cloaks, the street-side stallholders and carters, and everywhere the strident accent that was much harder on the ear than the fluid speech of Ireland. She crossed a wide thoroughfare named Margaret Street – an auspicious coincidence. A little further on was the bustling open square of Oxford Market, leading to Little Castle Street* lined with tall, handsome townhouses – not marked by wealth, but respectable. Number 36 was a slender townhouse like the others, but there the resemblance ceased. Margaret's astonished eyes ranged from the windows, their panes grimy and cracked, some broken, to the dilapidated portico over the street door, whose pillars and pediment tilted precariously to one side. The whole house had the appearance of a drunkard, slumped and leaning against his two stiff, embarrassed neighbours. The railings were rusted, and the steps down to the servants' entrance were clogged with litter, including several skeletons of stray dogs and cats.[3] James Barry RA evidently did not live in the manner implied by his stature.

In fact, Mr Barry's place in society was not what it had been. Always volatile, he was reputed to have grown ever more irascible in his old age; he was no longer a member of the Royal Academy, and had been dismissed from his professorship some five years earlier.[4] The inhabitants of the streets around Oxford Market regarded his house with suspicion and even terror. It was said to be 'occupied by an old wizard, or necromancer, or Jew' – they couldn't make up their minds which, but were agreed that 'whatever he was, he lived there in unholy solitude, that he might the better dedicate himself unobserved to some unrighteous mysteries'.[5]

The huge door knocker made a loud, dismal boom. After a long wait, there came sounds of bolts being withdrawn and a key turning in the lock. The door opened a crack, and a single eye peered out with wary hostility. Seeing a respectable young girl on the step, the owner of the eye opened the door wider, revealing himself to be an elderly, thickset man.

Margaret's mother would scarcely have recognised him. His appearance had changed in almost every way; the eyes were still bright hazel, but were set among such an arrangement of lines, bags and thick, heavy brows that they seemed small and beady; the jaw and jutting chin had grown heavy, almost ape-like, and the Cupid's bow had receded from his upper lip, so that the protruding, sulky underlip was the only Barry feature still recognisable. One acquaintance described his face as 'coarse and angry ... rugged, austere, and passion-beaten; but the passions traced there were those of aspiring thought and unconquerable energy ... sullenly exulting in its resources'.[6] His clothes were oddly matched and almost as dilapidated as his house. The poet Robert Southey, who knew

---

* now Market Place and Eastcastle Street

him 'in his worst (that is to say, his maddest) days', recalled that Barry habitually wore 'an old coat of green baize, but from which time had taken all the green that incrustations of paint and dirt had not covered. His wig was one which you might suppose he had borrowed from a scarecrow; all round it there projected a fringe of his own grey hair.'[7] The rest of his dress included a black waistcoat, grey worsted stockings, and 'coarse unpolished shoes with leathern thongs'. However, 'His shirt was not only perfectly clean, but equally genteel in point of texture, with even a touch of dandyism in the elaborate plaiting of the ruffles.'[8] On his head, when not wearing his wig, he would put an old peaked hunting cap, its velvet all worn off, which doubled as an eye-shade when he worked on his engravings at night.

This was the celebrated James Barry, the only hope of the female Bulkleys. He eyed Margaret suspiciously, and demanded – in an accent still redolent of Cork – what the devil she wanted.

As Margaret introduced herself, her uncle's stony expression softened somewhat. She didn't belong to any of the categories he abhorred: mischievous neighbours; thieving servants (he had dismissed his last maid in the belief that she'd tried to steal engravings from him, and refused to have another servant under his roof); and the most feared and loathed group of all, the artistic rivals and Royal Academicians he believed were conspiring against him, and to whom he traced all his troubles. Even the abuse he experienced in the neighbourhood was instigated by them, he believed. This young girl was visibly a Barry, and she was Irish. The Irish – of whom a few lived hereabouts – were among the handful of groups with whom James Barry was still disposed to be civil.[9]

The door opened fully, and Margaret stepped into the gloomy, musty house. Without servants the painter was reduced to taking care of himself, and had neither the aptitude nor the inclination; he took his dinner each day at a chop-house in Wardour Street, and let his house go uncleaned. Dust clung to every surface, and the corners and doorways were draped with cobwebs. He led Margaret upstairs to a chamber on the first floor that doubled as living room and engraving studio (his painting studio was on the ground floor). Another visitor who came that year described this room:

He opened the door ... and entered first to clear away the cobwebs before us. The place was full of engravings, sketches and casts, confusedly heaped together, and clotted with damp and dust. The latter he every now and then removed by a vigorous slap with the skirt of his coat. There were some engravings there that he valued highly … I perfectly recollect the ardour, and the occasional delicacy and tenderness of manner with which he explained their beauties.[10]

Although Barry was civil to his niece, he wasn't prepared to be charitable. He had received the letter written by Margaret and her mother, so knew of his relations' plight,[11] but he was visibly impoverished himself. His other recent visitor, Irish lawyer William Henry Curran, had been shown some of the pictures in Barry's bed chamber but forbore from describing the room in detail – 'For the honour of genius, I would forget the miserable truckle upon which a man whose powers were venerated by Edmund Burke lay down to forget his privations and his pride.'[12] Southey described it as a bare bedstead with no linen and just a single blanket nailed to one side[13] ('poor fellow! he is too mad and too miserable to laugh at').[14]

Margaret explained that they didn't want money, but a resolution over the house in Cork. Mary Anne possessed a letter that James had written at the time of her marriage, handing over his claim on the house to an uncle of theirs, on condition that it pass to Mary Anne when the uncle died. She hadn't made the letter public because it was worse than useless – the moment she acquired title to the house, it would become Jeremiah's and therefore be forfeited either to John or to the creditors. Therefore, Mary Anne wanted James to arrange for the house to pass directly to Margaret.

James seemed to understand none of this. He had the impression that his sister had sent her daughter to beg from him, and it vexed him just as it had when his brothers, Patrick and Redmond, had done the same. It was impossible to make him see reason – all he could discern was another pair of impoverished relations expecting him to support them. Two years earlier, Redmond had received such a rebuff that he'd protested, 'your Undeserved Cruel treatment to me Almost has broke my heart'.[15] Margaret – who had considerable charm and was manifestly enthralled by her uncle James's artistic genius – did not receive such a callous, hostile dismissal. Nonetheless, she went away from that eerie, dishevelled house empty-handed.

*   *   *

They took the long journey back to Ireland in a despondent mood. Margaret's visit to her uncle's house, unrewarding as it had been financially, had given her a glimpse of a vista beyond the confines of Cork and its mercantile life: a life in which a gifted mind and hand could extend the bounds of human achievement. To Margaret's mind, in his prime James Barry had conquered nature itself through his art.[16]

Jeremiah had gone ahead and signed over their rights in the house to John. It was a useless gambit – the house was seized and, although it couldn't be disposed of because of the difficulties over title (Mary Anne kept James Barry's old letter hidden), the Bulkleys were forced to leave.[17] The shop was finished, and their entire livelihood with it.

Abandoning Jeremiah to his fate, the female members of the family sought refuge with Cooper Penrose, James's rich patron and a generous, longstanding friend of the Barry family with a reputation for giving shelter to waifs and fugitives.[18] Margaret and her mother (and presumably little Juliana, who must have been about two or three years old) were taken into the Penrose fold while Jeremiah Bulkley took to the streets and tried to vanish; his family lost sight of him, but his creditors didn't.[19]

Margaret and her mother had to try to earn a living. There they faced the problem of Margaret's inadequate education, her mother lamenting that she had 'not been brought up to think of Labor and, Alas! whose Education is not finished to put her in a way to get Decent Bread for herself'. Nor could Mary Anne work, because 'the fruit of my Labor would be seized on by Bulkley's Creditors'.[20]

Her thoughts kept returning to the house, now standing empty. Persuading James to sign it over to Margaret, to be held in trust for her until she came of age, was the only way to preserve it. Writing to him was futile; another attempt would have to be made to persuade him in person. So, after just a few months, Margaret and her mother set out again for London.

Little Castle Street, London: Monday 14 January 1805

The metropolis hadn't been congenial even in summer, but now the ground was all ice and muddy slush, everyone's clothes were permeated by damp, and the air was thick with the smoke and smuts of a hundred thousand chimneys.

On this freezing morning, Margaret found herself again standing by the rusted railings outside the dilapidated house. It was in an even worse condition now. The superstitious locals, in their fear of the old 'necromancer', had erupted in violence. Brickbats and dirt had been hurled at the house, the steps were even more clogged with rubbish, the bricks were splattered with mud, and the windows had scarcely a whole pane of glass among them.

A few weeks earlier, in December 1804, the *Morning Chronicle* had reported:

> A series of outrages have been recently committed upon the residence of that celebrated artist, Mr Barry. This respectable Gentleman's house ... has been attacked in the dead of night several times within the last two months. His door has been battered, his windows broken, and the whole of the front of the house covered with filth ... It would be a national disgrace to allow to pass unnoticed or unpunished such wanton outrage against a man whose character and talents have rendered him uniformly and universally the object of respect and regard among the great and the good.[21]

This was over-egging it enormously; although he still had a few devoted friends and admirers in high places, James Barry had alienated most others. The house appeared empty; indeed it looked quite uninhabitable. A dead cat lay on the ledge of the parlour window, and most of the broken panes had been filled in with sheets of parchment, which on closer inspection proved to be old etchings, turned upside down. One sheet, next to the dead cat, contained a notice in James's handwriting: a proclamation that 'a dark conspiracy' was responsible for the violent campaign against him. It concluded with an offer of a reward to anyone providing information leading to the detection of the offenders.[22]

At Margaret's knock, an upstairs window flew up and a familiar head jutted out, staring angrily and demanding – with a bouquet of curses – to know who was disturbing him.[23] He recognised his niece; the window slammed down (dislodging a few shards of glass) and after a pause there came the sounds of the street door being unbarred and unlocked.

James Barry's appearance was the same as ever, the green baize coat replaced by 'a loose, thread-bare, claret-coloured great coat that reached to his heels'.[24] Letting Margaret in, he double-locked the door behind her. He scarcely went out at all these days; Robert Southey had tried to persuade James to visit him, but he refused, stating that 'if he went out in the evening the Academicians would waylay him and murder him'.[25] In James Barry's mind the hostility of the neighbourhood and all the woes of his life had been instigated by the Royal Academy. Their 'brutal persecutions', he told his friend and patron the Earl of Buchan, were 'unceasingly contrived to distract & misoccupy my attention':

> 'Tis a great hardship to be obliged to contend with such desperate opponents, who regardless of all honourable pursuit are even dead to the sense of shame & infamy & provided they can keep clear of pub-lick detection & legal punishment, would stick at nothing to compass their ends.[26]

He was a little friendlier to Margaret this time; perhaps because she took an interest in his work. Indeed, as Southey recalled, although Barry could be irascible and surly and 'interlarded his conversation with oaths as expletives', with people who took his art seriously 'it was pleasant to converse with him; there was a frankness and animation about him which won good will as much as his vigorous intellect commanded respect'.[27]

Worthy visitors were treated to a view of the large canvases in his main studio at the back of the house. In winter it was disused – too cold and dark to work in, the skylights covered with snow.[28] Propped against one wall was his new masterwork, completed after thirteen long years of work. *The Birth of Pandora* was a vast canvas nine feet high and seventeen wide. It was dominated by a mighty, muscular Zeus seated among a gathering of gods and goddesses, handing Pandora the fateful jar on a platter.[29] The subject had gripped James Barry for decades, and he saw this as the culmination of his career as a painter.[30] The Earl of Buchan, Barry's keenest supporter (who had recently contributed to 'an exemplary annuity of ten pounds' for him), declared it 'a picture with which I was more captivated than with any thing I have ever seen'.[31]

By the time Margaret left the house, her uncle had thawed a little. She took away a message for her mother; although James had declined to settle the Cork house on Margaret, he would be willing to give Mary Anne a letter of attorney that would empower her to sell it on his behalf (and presumably to keep the money).[32]

Mary Anne was exasperated. Was this man completely obtuse? Could he not see that this would be of no use at all? She sat Margaret down immediately and dictated a letter. 'Sir,' she began (he was no longer 'my Dear Brother'). 'From the message you sent to day by Margaret … I have been induced to write to you to explain my Reasons for soliciting you for the Deed.'[33] She went on at length about her situation, and the certainty that if she were to own or sell the house, 'Bulkley's Creditors could fall on it'; therefore, only a deed of settlement in favour of Margaret would do. Margaret being only fifteen years old, a trust would be set up; Mrs Bulkley had arranged for a London attorney to manage it if only James would sign the deed over. If he would not, then the property would 'remain with my son for Ever'.[34] She went on:

> You ask why I came to London, Sure Sir you could not Deceive yourself so much as to think I came *to Beg from you*.
>
> If indeed you did think so I am convinced this will alter your opinion, give me leave to propose a single Question to you – What did you give my Child when she was here last June, did you Ask her to Dinner, in short did you act as an Uncle or a Christian to a poor unprotected, unprovided for Girl … whose share has been given to a Brother –

Mrs Bulkley broke off there, refraining from elaborating on what she thought of her son. She went on angrily:

> I must indeed have lost my Reason if I came to you for Support – No Sir, I left Ireland because I have been Ill, very Ill treated there …
>
> I had no Choice left but to starve or come here to try to Get Bread – often had I been importuned by my friends to come and see you but I would not, nor would I come here now if I knew any other Country. I forget I am speaking to a disinterested person … I shall no longer intrude on your time[35]

She added sadly that she had hoped to see him after thirty years apart, and wished that there might be 'one Relation of whom I may ask advice in the World but Disappointment has attended that & many others of the undertakings of … Mary Anne Bulkley'.

Having delivered this flourish, she added that James would 'greatly oblidge' her 'if you will sign the Deed, it is my last request. Adieu.'[36]

It was a hopeless request. He did not sign it.

Margaret and her mother stuck it out in London for some time, facing the choice of either eking out what little capital they had in the hope of finding a livelihood, or spending it on the expensive journey by stage and ship back to Ireland. Reluctant to slip into absolute penury, they gave up their lodgings and travelled back to Cork.

Again they were taken in by the Penrose family. It would be futile for Mary Anne to work, and Margaret was unsuited to employment; she had no trade skills, and her education was insufficient for a governess's position; she wrote a good hand, but her grammar was imperfect, and her command of languages and the arts was not of the standard expected by wealthy families.[37]

Jeremiah had fled Cork. Nobody knew for certain where he'd gone, or even whether he was living or dead. Eventually news filtered through that he was in Dublin, 'in very indigent Circumstances'. His creditors had caught up with him; he'd been arrested for debt and imprisoned in the Four Courts Marshalsea.[38]

There were two debtors' gaols in Dublin. The City Marshalsea – by far the more miserable of the two – housed prisoners whose debts were under £10. The Four Courts Marshalsea, which stood behind a high brick wall on Marshalsea Lane, was for prisoners 'whose health has been injured by confinement in the unwholesome air of the Sheriff's prison'.[39] They could also take advantage of the periodic Acts for the Relief of Insolvent Debtors passed by Parliament – a precursor to bankruptcy that forced creditors to come to an arrangement over repayment. To benefit, an imprisoned debtor had to lodge a petition with the authorities. Jeremiah Bulkley had done so.

He would be in gaol a long time – three Acts of Insolvency would pass without fully liberating him from his burden of debt. Indeed, his gulli-bility drove him further into trouble within the Marshalsea's walls. He was taken into the confidence of a fellow prisoner, the Reverend Doctor Stafford. This indebted clergyman had a fortune of £400 a year, implying that his debts must have been vast, since he was a 'tenant for life' with no hope of relief or release. He seemed a kindly man and was 'very civil',[40] and when he asked Jeremiah to act as guarantor on two credit notes worth

£36, Jeremiah found it impossible to refuse. The money was borrowed and spent, upon which the Reverend Doctor promptly died, leaving Jeremiah saddled with the debt.

Mary Anne and Margaret knew nothing of what was happening to Jeremiah, and showed little sign of caring. The female Bulkleys had, in the course of the past five years, been variously betrayed, (probably) raped, ruined and made homeless by their male relations. Mary Anne was bitter and unforgiving, while Margaret acted as if her father and brother were dead.

But for the kindness of the Penrose family – which must have its limits – all that Margaret's future seemed to hold was a downward road towards poverty, drudgery and debasement. Then, early in 1806, as another winter was beginning to give way to spring, news came from London. James Barry was dead.

3

Next of Kin

On a bitter morning in winter, for the first time in many years, the damp, cobwebbed, crumbling house in Little Castle Street was alive with visitors. A small party of well-dressed gentlemen – all friends of the late occupant – had gathered by arrangement to secure the ramshackle house and its contents against vandals and plunderers.[1] The Saturday just gone, James Barry, painter, former Royal Academician and eccentric of great repute, had met his end after a brief, sudden and (from a medical point of view) most interesting illness.

The previous year, after the visit from Margaret, the old painter had fallen into an even worse state of self-neglect than usual, and his health had failed. According to Robert Southey, he fell ill from sheer lack of nourishment.[2] He lay shivering beneath the single blanket on his squalid bed for several days; then, summoning the last of his strength, he crawled downstairs, opened the street door, and lay on the threshold, clutching a note requesting that he be carried to the house of Anthony Carlisle in Soho Square.

Carlisle, a famously gifted surgeon, revived and treated him. His response to treatment was remarkable – 'the danger from which he had thus escaped seems to have cured his mental hallucinations. He cast his slough afterwards; appeared decently drest and in his own grey hair, and mixed in such society as he liked.'[3] But his home remained in its run-down state, and his eccentric habits continued. One day in the middle of February 1806, he attended a meeting at the Society of Arts – an organisation to which he had devoted his energies for many decades, especially following his expulsion from the Royal Academy. After the meeting he walked from the Society's headquarters near the Strand to the eating house in Wardour Street where he regularly ate his dinner. Despite the frigid weather, he'd come out without the thick Spencer he normally wore.[4] Customers at the eating house noticed that Mr Barry seemed unwell, and were startled when he was gripped by some kind of fit.

An Irish friend who happened to be present – a Mr Clinch – put the semi-conscious artist in a coach and accompanied him to Little Castle Street. Arriving there, they found that the key wouldn't go into the lock – Barry's local persecutors had filled up the keyhole with dirt and stones. Thinking quickly, Mr Clinch took him to a lodging house above a shop in Mortimer Street.[5] James was given a room and put to bed. He quickly grew alarmingly worse; after sleeping for a day and two nights he began bleeding from the nose so profusely that the bed linen was ruined and the landlady – having charged 36 shillings for the damage – insisted on his being moved elsewhere. He was taken to the nearby house of Joseph Bonomi, an Italian architect, at the invitation of Bonomi's wife, Rosa.

By this time, Barry had rallied sufficiently to go and visit a friend, but on his return to the Bonomi house his condition deteriorated rapidly – 'it appeared that violent humours had been floating in his constitution which at one time seemed to produce an effect like appoplexy, but ... the disorder which became positive was *in his Chest*.'[6] His friend Dr Edward Fryer was summoned, and concluded that James's condition was terminal. The patient was informed, and advised that a priest should be called. James Barry RA passed away in a state of sublime forgiveness.

Carlisle performed an autopsy, and declared the cause of death to be 'an inflammation of the lungs'.[7] (In fact, Barry's condition was probably pituitary apoplexy related to a pituitary tumour – hence the profuse bleeding from the nose – with complications and subsequent bronchopneumonia.)

James Barry's body was laid in state in the Great Room of the Society of Arts, beneath the encircling mural he had painted three decades earlier, when he was in his prime: *The Progress of Human Knowledge and Culture*, a triumphant work intended to repudiate the Continental European view of art and mark England as the centre of future progress.[8]

Before the death was even announced publicly, a group of the late painter's friends, along with a representative from the local police office, met at Barry's house.[9] As well as securing the building, they searched for a will; Barry was not known to have lodged one with an attorney, and after an extensive search of the house, none was found.

This was a serious matter. For all his apparent poverty, James Barry's estate was of considerable value. Only the previous year, several of his wealthiest friends had raised an annuity for him; and he had ready money, which he treated with characteristic eccentricity; while he was dying in Bonomi's house, his carers discovered over £40 in coins and banknotes about his person (it was taken for safekeeping, and despite his terminal condition Barry noticed the absence and managed to crawl downstairs to inquire after it). They also found bank receipts for the deposit of £163,[10] and a search among his papers revealed that he had money invested in British and American government stocks.[11] He had £400 at Wrights bank, another £500 in bank stock, and £1500 in American government stocks,[12] not to mention his effects and artworks, which were reckoned to be worth thousands at auction. For a man who had lived for so long in a condition of abject squalor, James Barry had left a substantial estate.*

Without a will, his friends had no option but to attempt to find his next of kin, whoever and wherever they might be.

Portsmouth: May 1806

Lopsided, rank and rotting, the prison ship HMS *Suffolk* towered above the water like a slum mansion; her gun ports were heavily barred and her upper works covered in a shambling assortment of wooden gantries and hutments, shingle-roofed and pierced by smoking chimneys. Her masts had been reduced to stubs, and where sails and signal flags had once fluttered and cracked in the ocean winds, there now hung a drapery of motley laundry.[13] Within the hulk's rotten innards were crowded hundreds of prisoners: the dangerous and the wretched, the lost and the damned. A platoon of invalid marines were their gaolers and a handful of broken-down seamen maintained the ship, preventing it from crumbling altogether into the murky waters of the harbour.

One of these old sailors sat now in a wooden hut that overhung the forecastle rail. Illuminated by the flicker of a reeking tallow candle, Redmond Barry was peering at two pieces of paper. One was a letter from

---

* Including the anticipated worth of Barry's art at the time, the economic value of the estate in 2016 terms would be about £6.5 million, while in terms of standard of living it would be about £390,000 (see 'Note on money' above).

a London attorney informing him of the death of his brother James; the second was a cutting from *The Times* giving an account of the funeral. Amidst the noise and stink of the hulk, the reprobate seaman learned how his brother's coffin, having lain in state for three weeks, had been taken to St Paul's Cathedral, borne by pall bearers including Sir Robert Peel, the satirist Caleb Whitefoord and the Chamberlain of London. 'A great number of Artists and Members of the Society [of Arts] attended on foot, and fell into the ranks of the procession,' reported *The Times*.[14] James Barry RA was laid to rest in a place of honour within the cathedral, close to the graves of its builder, Sir Christopher Wren, and Barry's old friend, rival, and founder of the Royal Academy, Sir Joshua Reynolds (who, perhaps fortunately, hadn't lived to see Barry's disgrace).

It was an astonishing report. He must have been much richer than he seemed; indeed, the piece referred to annuities totalling £120 that had just been raised for him, founded on over £1000 in capital. And there must be more in his estate than that – more than enough to set an old sailor right after years of suffering. According to the attorney's letter, the old devil had died intestate, and his leavings would go to the next of kin.[15] It was only by chance that Redmond knew of it – he'd just happened to write one of his pleading letters to James, and had received the attorney's letter in reply.[16]

Redmond seized his chance. He wrote immediately to the attorney, explaining his situation and confirming his identity, and also to James's friend Mr Bonomi, asking for more particulars about his late brother's affairs.[17] Then he waited impatiently for his turn to go ashore (the hulks were lashed together out on the water, and the only way on and off was by boat); when his time came, Redmond sought out an attorney in Portsea and began the arrangements for staking his claim to the estate.[18]

Margaret and her mother picked their way through the press of pedestrians and traffic on Gracechurch Street, one of the main thoroughfares of the ancient City of London (still regarded with some disdain by the more fashionable City of Westminster). Opposite the sprawling warren of Leadenhall Market was the entrance to a narrow alley, whose small, grimy sign admitted confidentially that it was Corbet Court. The alley opened into a tiny courtyard fronted by six small buildings, jammed up against the houses in the alleys on either side.[19] At number 2 was the office of Daniel Reardon, attorney at law.

Mr Reardon was a man of Cork and apparently connected to the Barry family.[20] Mrs Bulkley had consulted him on her previous visit to London. Now her business was even more urgent and many times more important. The news of James Barry's demise had taken months to reach Cork. Hearing that he had died intestate and that the estate might be substantial, Mrs Bulkley had arranged for proof of her identity to be provided by William Edward Penrose, who went before the Mayor of Cork on 6 May and made a sworn statement that he knew Mary Anne Bulkley and 'verily believed' her to be the 'Naturall and lawful Sister' of the late James Barry. He also affirmed that she was separated from her husband and that he was believed to be in prison for debt.[21] In law, this signed, witnessed statement was as good a proof of her entitlement to her brother's legacy as Mary Anne could hope for.

Thus armed, she and Margaret – who was now seventeen and all but a woman – set out on another long and hopeful journey to London.[22] (Little Juliana was apparently left behind – possibly in the care of the Penroses.) On arriving, Mary Anne applied to be recognised as the heir to the Barry estate. Only now did she make the shocking discovery that she'd been forestalled. The tarry fingers of brother Redmond were reaching out to grasp the estate. He already had a London attorney, and appeared to have been accepted as a bona fide claimant by the lawyers handling the estate: 'Redmond Barry the Brother,' they recorded, 'has applied for Administration to his Brother's Effects & Messrs Shelton & Poulden are his sureties that he will administer the Effects according to Law.'[23]

Appalled, Mary Anne presented her credentials, and watched in dismay as her claim was laid alongside Redmond's. For the time being, neither was given administration. It disgusted Mary Anne that this wastrel who'd brought nothing but trouble to his family should have any share at all in James's estate – it wasn't huge, and she would surely need all of it if she were to save herself and give Margaret a future.

In fact Mary Anne expressed doubt that her rival – who hadn't been able to come to London in person – was really her brother. Paying a call on Joseph Bonomi, in whose house James had died, Mary Anne was shown a letter from 'the Man who stiles himself Redmond Barry', and declared that the writing was not her brother's.[24] (She might have been correct; Redmond's hand was inconsistent, possibly because his semi-literacy forced him to rely on others to write his letters for him.) The lawyers disagreed, and it was judged that the brother and sister should have joint administration.

And so Mary Anne and Margaret made their way through the heaving City to Corbet Court to consult Mrs Bulkley's old friend and legal adviser.

Daniel Reardon was in the prime of his life, and stood high, despite the shabby situation of his offices.[25] An attorney at law and a solicitor in the High Court of Chancery, he practised both Law and Equity, and was eminently qualified for Mrs Bulkley's purpose.[26] She was a demanding, temperamental client, but Mr Reardon was a forbearing gentleman, and as the case unfolded, he would take a fatherly interest in Margaret. Mr Reardon was a widower who had recently remarried a younger woman and was about to start a family.[27] His position in life must have given Mrs Bulkley many reminders of how bitterly her own son had disappointed her. Reardon had a young clerk called Philip Davis who was close in age to John Bulkley and had nearly completed his training as an attorney: the very model of what John might have been had he applied himself to his work and his studies rather than romance.[28] (Where John was now, they had scarcely any idea, but time would prove that he hadn't exhausted his talent for disaster.)

And so negotiations began between Mary Anne in London and Redmond in the gloomy hulk at Portsmouth, while their lawyers' quills scratched away in their City offices, and their fees began steadily to mount.

Meanwhile, there was Margaret's education to be attended to. Mother and daughter – apparently now living on monies advanced by Daniel Reardon against their expectations – began making friends with some of the more genteel members of James Barry's social circle, a few of whom took a charitable interest in the unfortunate women. Joseph Bonomi was friendly, but foremost was Dr Edward Fryer, perhaps the most devoted of Barry's friends, who had overseen the care of the painter's possessions after his death. Like Bonomi, Dr Fryer lived in Marylebone, just around the corner from Little Castle Street, at 76 Newman Street. He had in his care many of James Barry's pictures (including the vast *Pandora*); some others were with Carlisle, while the other effects were being looked after by James Christie at his auction house in Pall Mall.[29]

Edward Fryer was a physician by training, a polymath by inclination, and a gentleman by nature. Born into an obscure Somerset family in

1761, he'd been apprenticed to a medical man in Wiltshire, then studied medicine at the universities of Edinburgh, Leiden and Göttingen. He developed a line in light poetry, publishing 'Ode to the Genius of Patriotism' and 'Ode to Health', the latter in honour of George III's sixth son, Prince Augustus Frederick, whose personal physician he became.[30] Although medicine was Edward Fryer's profession, literature and books were his love; he took a keen interest in the Prince's library and had a role in its curation. He was well known in London literary society, and as a member of the Society of Arts he had been close to James Barry.

Since the artist's death, Fryer had begun work on an edition of Barry's writings. Mary Anne Bulkley, as joint heir to the copyright, supported this project, keen to enhance her brother's stature (and thereby the saleroom value of his estate). At the same time she began putting together a book of the etchings Barry had made of his Society of Arts paintings, for which Dr Fryer had offered to furnish a dedication.[31]

Meanwhile, Dr Fryer took upon himself the task of extending Margaret's education. He must have found her capabilities sorely lacking in a young lady seeking a career as a governess. Her command of written English needed polish and she would also require excellent French (and ideally Italian), geography, history, a reasonable proficiency at the pianoforte, and skill in drawing.[32] It wasn't a path that required a wide scope of learning; it contained no science or mathematics beyond basic arithmetic, no philosophy, no classical languages or literature. Girls and their governesses were not thought to require a broad or deep education; they needed only to conduct themselves domestically and socially with grace, good manners, taste, piety and the appearance of intellectual refinement. Mary Somerville, who had a prodigious gift for mathematics, recalled: 'From my earliest years my mind revolted against oppression and tyranny, and I resented the injustices of the world in denying all those privileges of education to my sex which were so lavishly bestowed upon men.'[33] Of one young lady Somerville believed that 'the consciousness that she might have done something better, had female education been less frivolous, gave her a characteristic melancholy which lasted through life'.[34]

In encountering Edward Fryer, Margaret had been fortunate; besides being a well-connected gentleman, he was respected for his 'various and extensive knowledge', his 'strict probity' and his 'unsullied honour', and was noted for his dedication and generosity; he also possessed 'the most engaging and gentlemanly manners', all of which 'combined to render him beloved and admired by all who knew him'.[35]

Margaret's tuition was probably confined at first to the requirements for a governess. Many progressive voices had been raised in favour of extending women's education into the areas of science and scholarship. Dr Fryer himself, as a free-thinker, must have been sympathetic to this movement. Barry's sponsor, the Earl of Buchan (whom Margaret had not yet met), was a vocal advocate of female advancement.[36] Yet the idea of educating a young lady in the classics and the sciences was still seen as deeply eccentric. Margaret's studies would be limited by the needs of her inevitable future career teaching the offspring of the wealthy.

While her mother fretted and haggled and badgered Daniel Reardon over the settlement of the Barry estate, Margaret practised her penmanship and grammar, studied French and learned the globe. And while her fingers traced the lines of the continents and islands, and the growing British Empire, on the far side of the earth, in Spanish America, a conflict was going on – a conflict that was insensibly reaching out to draw her in. One of its great protagonists, an extraordinary gentleman of vision and learning, was setting sail; another of James Barry's friends, a man who was an even more passionate bibliophile and far more of an eccentric than Dr Fryer, an adventurer who'd been abroad for two years, attempting to liberate his homeland from Spanish rule. His heroic venture had ended in disaster, and he was now on his way back to England.

4

A Small Fortune

Portsmouth: New Year's Day 1808

The frigate *Alexandria* had dropped anchor in Portsmouth harbour on the last day of 1807, after a long and stormy voyage from Tortola in the Virgin Islands. General Don Francisco de Miranda gazed out at England, the land he had left nearly two years earlier, the land that had been his place of exile for most of the past decade.[1] His young English wife was here, and his two infant sons. At the age of fifty-seven, General Miranda had now spent more of his life wandering the world than he had in his native Venezuela. He had left England in 1806 to raise an army and liberate his homeland from Spanish rule, but having embarked with high hopes and fair plans, he had come back defeated. Miranda needed to reach London with all speed to resume his diplomacy with the British government and ensure that his standing wasn't diminished.

Before this expedition, his position in London had been good, but was dependent on Britain's long enmity with Spain, and tarnished by his having once briefly served in the French Revolution (before becoming one of its victims). People were fascinated by General Miranda, and statesmen were drawn by the possibilities his campaign presented for staking a profitable British claim in Spanish America. Even in metropolitan London, an imperial capital embroiled in global war and steeped in intrigue, he was a man of note; soldier, itinerant revolutionary and self-styled statesman, he had led a life of extraordinary political and military adventure.

Sebastián Francisco de Miranda y Rodríguez de Espinosa had been born in 1750 into a wealthy Venezuelan family of Canarian Spanish and Caracas Criollo* lineages – a precarious mix, given the tension between

---

* colonial-born people of Spanish descent

the Spanish colonial rulers and the Criollo caste.[2] As a young man he
had crossed the ocean to Cádiz, where he joined the Spanish army and
served in several of its campaigns. He was more a scholar than a soldier,
however, and read voraciously, becoming fascinated by the politics of
rebellion. Everywhere he went he was an outsider, even in his homeland;
in Venezuela he was seen as more Spanish than Criollo, while in the
Spanish army he was too Criollo. This sense of otherness, coupled with
his innate self-confidence (which many found indistinguishable from
arrogance), coloured his outlook on life. He developed a liberal turn of
mind, determined to champion the oppressed; but as far as his Spanish
masters were concerned, his faults were his scholarship, fondness for the
English and willingness to serve their interests. Miranda was accused of
being 'a traitor, an Anglophile … a disloyal intriguer', as well as a bibliophile who possessed books banned by the Inquisition.[3]

Giving his accusers the slip, Miranda travelled to the newly independent United States of America, where he met George Washington and
Thomas Paine, and made friends with Madison and Jefferson. In 1785 he
travelled to Europe; becoming entangled with the French Revolution,
he was charged by the new republic with treachery, imprisoned and
twice sentenced to death. By 1798 he'd extricated himself and made for
England. Deciding once and for all that the British were his best friends,
he settled down in London to dream his dreams and nurture his plans
for Venezuelan liberation.

Now well into middle age, Miranda believed he could free not only
Venezuela but the whole of South America from Spanish rule. With the
outbreak of a new Anglo-Spanish war in 1796 and the British capture
of Trinidad, he'd begun to acquire advocates in the British armed forces;
eventually he gained support within the government, and there was talk
of giving him assistance for a military expedition to the Spanish Main,
the vast Spanish possessions stretching from southern North America to
the northern coast of South America. The whole region was prodigiously
rich in trade; hence the endemic piracy associated with it and Britain's
strategic interest in gaining territory and influence there.[4]

By 1803 Miranda had settled in a fine four-storey townhouse at 27
Grafton Street, between Fitzroy Square and Tottenham Court Road on
the northern outskirts of the city.[5] It became a meeting place for radicals
and intellectuals of all nationalities: British, Irish and Spanish-Americans
among them. Miranda's political circle crossed over with the arts and

sciences, and men such as Dr Edward Fryer and James Barry became acquainted with him.

At the end of 1805, with France and Spain's maritime power critically weakened by the Battle of Trafalgar, the long-term trade benefits of a British incursion in the Spanish Main became ever more attractive. But by that time, Miranda had already embarked on his own doomed expedition. Perhaps his heart was no longer wholly in it. He'd been travelling for decades, his home was in London now, and he had a young family. Two years before, he'd met Sarah Andrews, niece of London portrait painter Stephen Hewson and an affectionate friend of James Barry. She and Miranda had married – or at least set up home together – and had a son, Leander. When Miranda departed for the Americas in 1805 (travelling covertly as 'George Martin') Sarah was pregnant again.[6] He named his expedition's flagship *Leander* – a mark of hope in the future of his lineage.

The expedition was a shambles from beginning to end. It was secretly equipped by the United States government, manned by a handful of idealists and mercenaries, and commanded by a leader who had vision and ambition but lacked military skill – as one of his followers put it, 'more learning than wisdom; more theoretical knowledge than practical talent; too sanguine and too opinionated to distinguish between the vigour of enterprise and the hardiness of infatuation'.[7] Along with a few hundred survivors, Miranda was forced to take refuge with the British on the island of Trinidad. And yet his spirit was unbroken. An American officer who'd served with him noted that when General Miranda sailed for England, 'His enthusiasm, after all the dampers it has received, was not extinguished. He said that he expected to be in Caracas in the following summer.'[8]

With that hope still burning, Francisco de Miranda hurried from Portsmouth to London to resume his diplomacy. Waiting to meet him was a young woman who needed his help.

Although Margaret's education had advanced considerably, she still had little experience as a teacher and lacked references from respectable parents. Dr Fryer was unmarried, and Daniel Reardon and his wife had only just produced their first child, a girl called Ellen, in October 1807.[9] Margaret, who'd become a close friend of the Reardons in the past two years, would grow deeply attached to Ellen (probably missing her own child, Juliana), but she was still a baby; besides, Mr Reardon,

as a professional man and not a born gentleman, might not suffice as a
character reference.

However, one child with whom Margaret was familiar was Leander
Miranda, four years old, an attractive and precocious boy who displayed
a bold, intelligent temperament similar to his father's.[10] Margaret had
never met the General, but she'd become acquainted with Leander's
mother. Besides being an old friend of James Barry, Sarah Andrews was a
kind-hearted soul who was particularly struck by the plight of Margaret
Bulkley and her mother. They'd first met during a visit to Mr Bonomi
in September 1806. Sarah had adored James Barry – an unusual trait in
a young woman. In the first few months after Miranda had departed for
the Americas, she had relied on him for personal advice; the General
admired the painter and regarded him as preferable to Sarah's relatives
('Take advice from Mr Barry if you want it; don't let your brother come
near the house.').[11] Sarah regarded Barry as 'the Best friend I ever had';
he loved Leander, and Sarah believed that 'he gave me the Best of Advice
at all times'.[12] (If this was so, he must have been better at giving advice
than living by it.)

His death almost broke Sarah's heart; 'in him I have lost the senser-
est and most disintrested friend in the world'.[13] (Sarah's education was
limited and her spelling echoed her Yorkshire speech.) Learning that his
paintings were to be auctioned for the benefit of his 'power Relations',
Sarah wrote to Miranda suggesting that he order the paintings to be
purchased on his account immediately.[14] Nothing was done – he had
problems of his own, and wasn't about to borrow money to purchase an
unwanted art collection.

With no income of his own, Miranda relied on donations and loans
to maintain his gentlemanly lifestyle as well as his political campaigning
and military expeditions. Much of his personal expenditure had been
ploughed into his fabulous library, which contained thousands of precious
volumes. By 1807 it was estimated that he owed up to £5000 to London
booksellers,[15] and while he was away on his doomed expedition, moves
were made by the creditors to seize his books. It was an abiding anxiety
for Sarah, who fretted constantly over a plan to box them up and hide
them in a friend's house.

Meanwhile, Sarah lived from week to week, eking out her allowance
and pleading fruitlessly for more. Four-year-old Leander, a bright boy
who was already half-literate, was reaching an age where his personality

was asserting itself and needed guidance from a tutor. In early 1807 Sarah wrote to Miranda that 'some people wonder I daunt send him to school, such a great Boy, but if it was posable I had much rather he had a lesson at home, I should be afrade of him going least he shoud catch some complant or other a mong so meny childron'.[16] In the same letter she complained that her allowance barely covered feeding Leander and his infant brother Francisco *hijo*.* Under such circumstances, she could hardly do better than employ Margaret; she was a friend, and Sarah trusted her friends.[17]

The library must have been an attraction for Margaret; her appetite for education was keen, and Miranda's collection contained riches that Edward Fryer would not have been able to supply. Most of the books had been boxed ready to be spirited away, but with the General's imminent return, they could be brought out again.

By the time Miranda returned to London, Margaret's need to pursue her career had grown urgent. During the past year, the Barry estate had at last been settled, and divided equally between Mary Anne and Redmond. Mary Anne's share would be placed in an investment trust administered by Cooper Penrose and Daniel Reardon; she would receive the interest and at her death Margaret would inherit the principal.[18] She also gained possession of the house in Cork, which was let out. Supplemented by whatever Margaret could earn as a governess, this should have provided her with a small fortune that would enable her to find a respectable husband.

But after what they had been through, Mrs Bulkley had craved something better. What had followed was a surprising act of skilful manipulation – probably on advice from Daniel Reardon. By December 1806 James Barry's artworks – which were expected to realise the bulk of the estate's value – had still been in storage, most of his money locked up in investments, and only a small proportion was in cash.[19] Redmond, having bought himself out of the Navy and come to live with his wretched wife in London, had grown impatient. Small sums were advanced to him by Daniel Reardon, who, in common with most family solicitors of that period, had taken on the role of estate banker,[20] but it wasn't enough.

Sensing Redmond's impatience, Mary Anne made him an offer. After discussion with James Christie the auctioneer, she obtained an advance of £300 from Mr Reardon in order to purchase outright Redmond's share in

---

* *hijo*: son, or 'junior'

the artworks.[21] If he took the offer, he would be giving up a much larger sum in the future – possibly running to many thousands. His hunger proved greater than his patience, and by February 1807, Redmond had signed away his share of the art to Mary Anne.[22]

Convinced that she had secured a magnificent bargain, Mary Anne had anticipated a huge return. In April 1807 the artworks and library of the late James Barry RA went under the hammer at Christie's auction room in Pall Mall. The catalogue proclaimed with expectant grandeur that the sale would include:

ALL THE ORIGINAL FINISHED AND UNFINISHED
Paintings, Drawings & Sketches
Of that great Genius and distinguished Artist,
JAMES BARRY, ESQ. R.A.
DECEASED:
Including his grand and justly celebrated chef d'Œuvre,
Pandora receiving her Presents from the Gods[23]

Mrs Bulkley had listened to her brother's admirers, studied the going prices, and talked it over with James Christie himself, and anticipated that the bidding for *Pandora* alone might run as high as £3000 (it had never before been seen in public, and there had been a good deal of speculation about it).

She and Margaret attended the sale with high hopes. It took place within the pale-green walls of Christie's Great Room, under floods of sunlight from the glazed roof, with the chattering rows of ladies and gentlemen crammed onto the long green upholstered benches, with Barry's works displayed around them. Mother and daughter sat down to watch their fortune and security mount up.[24]

There were many lots in the sale, and it was through a long and exacting process that the Bulkley ladies' expectations were dashed and trampled. It gradually became apparent that James Barry RA was no longer the admired and sought-after painter that his sister, Dr Fryer and James Christie had imagined him to be.[25] Portrait painter Sir Nathaniel Dance-Holland claimed that Barry had 'talked & bullied people into a belief of His being a great artist'.[26] Now he was gone, the illusion had apparently fallen away. It was heartbreaking. When the *Pandora* came under the hammer, the bidding was sparse and slow, petering out at a paltry 230 guineas. *Adam Tempted by Eve* reached a mere 105 guineas before halting, while *Venus Rising from the Sea* did little better. Sarah Andrews, who attended the auction, was distraught as 'power Mr Barry's' paintings were knocked down for prices that were not merely disappointing but insulting – 'if he could have forseen thare end,' she wrote, 'he would sooner have destroyed them'.[27]

As the final lots came under the hammer, it looked as if Redmond might have got the better half of the deal. Yet the sale itself was not the end of the humiliation; the anonymous gentleman who had purchased the *Pandora* suffered buyer's remorse and never collected the painting.[28] Another gentleman who'd purchased a set of plates had the same experience and returned them, paying a small penalty fee.[29] As the takings of the two-day sale were totted up, it was far from certain that Mary Anne would recoup her £300 payoff.

In all, after paying the auctioneer's fees, the sale raised £1416 and some shillings. Taking the payoff into account, that left Mary Anne with £408 over the half-share she would have received.[30] So it had been worthwhile after all – but still a dreadful, embarrassing disappointment. When all the estate's accounts were rendered, the monies shared and the lawyers paid, Mary Anne and Margaret were left with £2075 2s 4d.*

They moved from noisy, teeming Little Titchfield Street to lodgings in a house at 27 Charles Street,† just north of Fitzroy Square, which had views of open fields from the rear windows.[31] Margaret's future appeared more modest than her mother had hoped, but secure; as long as General Miranda returned to London and furnished her with a reference (if he was willing), she would be fit for a governess's position and in due course could attract a tolerably respectable husband.

Meanwhile, Redmond Barry, newly released from His Majesty's Navy, began disposing of his lesser share.[32] He hung around London for a while, pestering his sister and Mr Reardon for any stray bits and pieces of the estate that might have escaped notice – he became fixated upon the late James's clothes, and made a point of taking a fine pair of gloves, which he wore with pride at a meeting with his sister and their lawyers at Mr Bonomi's house.[33]

---

* Equivalent to 2016 values between £148,000 (standard of living) and £2.5 million (economic status relative to the population).
† now Drummond Street

When Redmond and his wife walked away replete with wealth, Margaret and her mother dearly hoped they'd seen the last of him.

27 Grafton Street, London: January 1808

Margaret approached General Miranda's house with her nerves on edge. Meeting him was intimidating enough, but her future depended on his giving her a good reference. Nine months had passed since the Christie's auction, and steady employment was both necessary and urgent.

The house was quite similar to James Barry's – a genteel, lofty town-house on a long terrace – but a storey taller and an entire world more salubrious, with its unpretentious mahogany furniture, paintings of religious scenes and prints of Raphael, plaster busts of Apollo, Cervantes and Homer in the front drawing room, prints of Chinese costumes, and a few pieces of decorative silver.[34] Nonetheless, it contained a similarly intimidating inhabitant who, in the wake of his failed expedition to Venezuela, had reason to be in a foul temper. At least she already knew the house and had allies in Sarah and the two boys – particularly Leander. And whereas before her only company had been a maidservant, today she had Dr Fryer to speak for her, and her kinship with James Barry would stand in her favour.

A first encounter with General Francisco de Miranda would be an anxious one for any young woman; his radicalism was well known, and his reputation as a seducer was as great as his renown (or infamy) as a revolutionary. He was quite beyond all Margaret's experience of men. Yet her life had changed significantly in the last eighteen months, and she was no longer quite the timorous creature who had once shyly begged her uncle's pardon for 'the many faults & Errors' in a letter.[35] Under Dr Fryer's tutelage, she had begun to show real learning and promise.

The General was in his beloved library on the second floor. Since returning to London, he had immersed himself in a programme of diplomatic overtures, and was making good progress. The British government was coming around to the view, expressed by the Governor of Trinidad, that General Miranda felt a 'zeal and anxiety ... for the honour and success of His Majesty's arms, as well as for the welfare, prosperity, and glory, of the British Empire, towards which both his heart and mind are as strongly bent as those of the most loyal and faithful of his Majesty's subjects'.[36]

Opinion was that opening up the Spanish Main to British trade would produce 'such a commercial intercourse with our country as would enable us to view with indifference any attempt on the part of France against England'.[37] General Miranda, blaming the failure of his expedition on the duplicity or the faint-heartedness of his American and English allies and the machinations of politicians, asked for firmer support.[38]

He had consulted with the two men who were most apt to help his cause: Viscount Castlereagh, Secretary of State for War, and Major General Sir Arthur Wellesley, who was acquiring a reputation as a great military commander. Both men were Anglo-Irish and had some sympathy with repressed peoples – although neither let it interfere with the interests of the Empire. General Miranda's proposals appealed to both liberty and profit. In the opinion of *The Times*, 'though the object of General Miranda is difficult, it is desirable. Bonaparte has got the Continent of Europe in his hand; he squeezes it at pleasure: when its resources are thus dried up, they may be again replenished from the foreign settlements of the vassal States. To divert this source of wealth, is an object worth attempting.'[39]

Wellesley agreed that it was desirable to keep Venezuela out of French hands: 'through General Miranda the British government have the means of communicating with the people of that country, and have reason to believe, as far as his judgment can be depended upon, that they are inclined to a revolution.'[40] Miranda wanted to found a republic, but Wellesley believed that a constitutional monarchy would better serve Britain's interests; for the sake of diplomacy, Miranda agreed.[41] Wellesley drew up a plan for an invasion force, commanded by him, comprising a corps of ten thousand British, German and colonial troops, plus artillery and engineers. They would assemble on the island of Grenada and then begin their assault on the Spanish Main at Caracas.[42]

It was in the midst of these negotiations, which dominated the early months of 1808, that Miss Margaret Bulkley came into General Miranda's view. He always had time for young ladies – especially if they were personable – and so he tore himself away from his work to take a look at her. She was shown up to the library. There were two rooms, plainly furnished but richly stuffed with scholarship. Here the General kept not only his thousands of books but also the numerous cases of letters, diaries and documents relating to his travels and campaigning. It was in the 'little library' at the rear of the house that the General spent much of his time, often with his secretary, Tómas Molini. Within its walls, lined with books and maps of South America, stood a desk, a deal table and a plain rush-bottomed chair. When his visitors entered, General Miranda put aside his work and rose to his feet.

He was a man who made an impression – tall, sturdily built, and his features were dark, florid and instantly striking. His silver-grey hair – which he whitened with powder – was worn long and combed back severely, with the ends plaited into a queue tied with a black ribbon, and he wore a small gold ring in his left ear. But it was his eyes that caught one's attention. They were hazel, 'piercing, quick and intelligent, expressing more of the severe than the mild feelings',[43] and overarched by the most remarkable eyebrows – thick, jet black and exquisitely curved, as if they'd been drawn on by a calligrapher. His nose was long, sharp and tilted up as if catching a scent, giving the impression that in 'the contour of his visage you plainly perceive an expression of pertinaciousness and suspicion'.[44] Miranda was known as 'a courtier and gentleman in his manners. Dignity and grace preside in his movements. Unless when angry, he has a great command of his feelings; and can assume what looks and tones he pleases.'[45] With women, his hauteur and distance would fade, and his warmth and gallantry came out.

Dr Fryer explained the reason for the visit, and Margaret's career plans. As an illustration of her talents, he presented copies of two poems she'd composed on James Barry, both intended as candidates for her uncle's epitaph:

> Thy Spirit fled and here thy Ashes lie
> But thy immortal Fame can never die
> This Tomb indeed will hide thy human frame
> But after Ages will tell Barry's Name
> His vivid colours made the Canvas glow
> With forms of Gods above and Men below
> Arcadia's Shepherds in their Savage State
> Britannia's Heroes Learned, Good and Great
> He on the Canvas shew'd the difference vast
> Between the Present and the Ages past
> Nature with Barry Vy'd; She lost the Day
> Then in revenge she snatch'd his life away
> But great Pandora, was design'd before
> He painted, finish'd Man cou'd do no more.[46]

The second poem used less legendary imagery but was even more fulsome in its appreciation of James Barry's stature:

> Who e'er thou art that Chance shall lead this way
> Stop and behold the fate of human Clay
> Beneath this marble lies the mortal part
> Of him whose Paintings & whose Works of Art
> Obtain'd the Name upon the World's great stage
> Barry the Micha'l Ang'lo of the Age
> His Works are Gems which even Time can't rust
> Tho' he that wrought them moulders here to dust
> Let gen'rous Pity drop a silent tear
> For Virtue, Genius, Taste entomb'd lie here.[47]

Had he been living, Barry would have thought this nothing more than his due. General Miranda was sufficiently impressed by the poems – or by their author – to preserve them among his personal papers. He took them as evidence that this strangely attractive girl was brighter and bolder than most, and condescended to provide her with a 'character' for any application she made.

5

A Revolutionary Plan

Southwark: early 1808

The King's Bench Prison loomed like a monster over the surrounding streets, its brick flanks blackened by their chimneys. It was a bewildering creature; from the outside, it appeared as if a small collection of begrimed but otherwise handsome townhouses were being slowly consumed from behind by a vast mass of dirty brick, thirty feet high and topped with a fearsome rail of spikes. Within lived the renegades and cast-offs of London: its bankrupts, slanderers and a great share of its debtors. It was filthy, overcrowded, and disease ran rampant.

Margaret loathed the man incarcerated within, but had come anyway, forced by obligation. The last time she had seen Redmond, he'd been in possession of more than £1250, with which he could have purchased enough grog to float a man-of-war, and more women than a broken-down tar could have coped with. But he'd apparently done worse than that; equipped with a fortune that was scarcely imaginable for an old sailor who'd never possessed more than a few shillings, in the course of less than a year Redmond had lost it all, every last farthing.

Precisely what he'd done with it was never recorded, but he must have had help. London was filled with sharp and unscrupulous financiers, merchants and attorneys who had a fine nose for 'gulls' with fortunes they didn't know how to handle. Complicated investment bubbles sucked the sovereigns out of their hands and into the pockets of the money-men. As Charles Dickens would put it: 'A mania prevailed, a bubble burst, four stock-brokers took villa residences at Florence, four hundred nobodies were ruined.'[1] Few nobodies would be more liable to the ignorance and greed that such schemes depended on than Redmond Barry.

Poor Redmond, some of James's former friends must have said. And so to poor Redmond Margaret was obliged to go.[2] Redmond was habitually abject and pitiable, and was an experienced and articulate pleader; accordingly, when Margaret entered the prison and was conducted by a turnkey through its dismal corridors, and saw Redmond in his wretched state, he had little trouble wheedling a promise from her that she would do what she could to help.[3] In due course, Redmond's debts – which must have been quite petty – were paid, and he was released. Deciding that London wasn't friendly, he left and, following his seaman's nose, shuffled off to Bristol.

Margaret might have guessed by now that she still hadn't heard the last of him.

Life wasn't settling into the assured security that Mrs Bulkley longed for. She and Margaret moved from lodging to lodging, never staying more than a few months. They had left the green fields of Charles Street for Soho, then back to Marylebone, and by February 1808 were living at 12 Brook Street, Fitzroy Square.[4]

These frequent moves may have been caused by a search for better or cheaper lodgings or fresher air. Or, since Mrs Bulkley was an enthusiastic student of the pianoforte (although probably not very able, given the tremor in her hands), it may have been necessary to find lodgings where the landlady was tolerant (or deaf) enough to put up with her. Despite the modesty of her fortune and continual stern advice from Daniel Reardon that she should economise, Mrs Bulkley insisted on living in a genteel manner, taking more rooms than necessary, and riding in hackney coaches rather than walking.[5] She worried about money, but the shadows of the King's Bench and the Marshalsea apparently didn't haunt her as they ought.

Sitting in the parlour at Brook Street, surrounded by unfolded newspapers, Margaret must have reviewed her career prospects with despondency. There were frequent advertisements for governesses, but they were usually outnumbered by notices from young ladies seeking appointments. And the requirements were rarely amenable: 'Wanted, to live entirely in the country' ... 'not less than 30 years of age' ... 'a middle aged experienced Person, who is perfectly qualified'. Some required a governess to double as a nursemaid or servant ('willing to make herself useful').[6] The ladies offering their services always sounded so impossibly skilled and experienced, and a few even had their own premises and worked as 'daily' governesses. There was also an unspoken assumption from prospective employers that the young ladies must be of genteel birth ('respectably connected').

> A YOUNG LADY, of very respectable connections, wishes for a SITU-ATION as GOVERNESS in a genteel family.[7]

> A LADY, very respectably connected, who has been accustomed to the Education of Young Ladies, is desirous of meeting with a Situation as GOVERNESS in a Gentleman's Family. She is fully capable of teaching English, French, Writing, Arithmetic, Geography, &c. and can give the most satisfactory references.[8]

How could a girl from Cork, of no particular birth, no experience and a Catholic to boot, compete with that? A few wealthy families were not prejudiced against governesses from the lower social ranks ('No objection to a Person that has not been out'), but they were few. More depressing still, some inexperienced girls offered their services for free ('No salary will be required for her first year' … 'Salary is not an object'). Some even offered to pay a premium, which could run to 60 guineas.

There were also employment agencies, including one run by a lady from a house just around the corner from General Miranda:

> ORIGINAL FEMALE AGENCY.— To the Nobility and Gentry.— Families are provided with Governesses, Ladies with Companions, Ladies Boarding Schools with Partners, Teachers, Apprentices … and Young Ladies wishing for Situations, recommended to the first Houses in Town and Country … Mrs BURNE attends from Ten to Five o'Clock, every Day, No. 7, Fitzroy-street, Fitzroy-square.[9]

Margaret's best hope was for a personal connection, an acquaintance of an acquaintance who might take her on. She'd heard through Daniel Reardon of a lady in Camden Town who might employ her, and grew frustrated with his apparent inaction, writing him a note tinged with impatience – a measure of her fading timidity. Addressing him in the third person, she wrote that she 'would be glad to know' if Mr Reardon had taken any steps to put her forward for the position, and remarked pointedly that he 'will himself perceive the sooner that Miss B. could be placed there would be better'.[10] The new suburb of Camden Town – an outlier protruding into the countryside – was an odd mix of light industrial and rustic with genteel pretensions, and not at all fashionable; its 'beau monde' were said to 'never approach nearer to fashionable life than the one shilling gallery is to the boxes'.[11] But it would be a start.

If Margaret did get the position, she must have found it irksome, because in July a rather desperate advertisement appeared in the *Morning Post*, possibly placed by Margaret:

> WANTS a Situation in a Private Family, a Young Person, as GOVERNESS, who has from her infancy been used to Children, has no objection to be Companion to a Lady, or teacher in a School, but would prefer the first occupation and has no objection to any part of the Kingdom.—Letters addressed to M. B. at Mr. Carter's, No. 15, Vere-street, Oxford-street.[12]

What a dismal prospect for a young lady of such talent and learning; to be a governess would be bad, but to be a companion could be worse – and would certainly be less stimulating. Writing two years before Margaret's birth, Mary Wollstonecraft – who had personal experience of such a career – felt that the few occupations open to educated young women were humiliating:

> It is impossible to enumerate the many hours of anguish such a person must spend. Above the servants, yet considered by them as a spy, and ever reminded of her inferiority when in conversation with the superiors ...
>
> The children treat them with disrespect, and often with insolence. In the mean time life glides away, and the spirits with it.[13]

A few years after writing those words, Wollstonecraft returned to the subject with a far greater degree of righteous indignation, and wrote as if foreseeing Margaret's destiny:

> But what have women to do in society? ... surely you would not condemn them all to suckle fools and chronicle small beer! No. Women might certainly study the art of healing, and be physicians as well as nurses ...

It is a melancholy truth; yet such is the blessed effect of civilization! the most respectable women are the most oppressed; and, unless they have understandings far superiour to the common run of understandings ... they must, from being treated like contemptible beings, become contemptible. How many women thus waste life away the prey of discontent, who might have practised as physicians, regulated a farm, managed a shop, and stood erect, supported by their own industry, instead of hanging their heads surcharged with the dew of sensibility, that consumes the beauty to which it at first gave lustre.[14]

With Mrs Bulkley's nervous condition deteriorating, she and Margaret went for a spell of sea air at Margate. Sea-bathing was a popular cure, and for the members of London society, Margate was the place to go, where there were bathing-rooms on the waterside, and even a Royal Sea-Bathing Infirmary. During the fashionable season the town bustled with the arrival of vessels at the pier, the cries of porters, chatter of shoppers and sightseers, and the to-and-fro of bathing machines on the sands.[15]

Although June was the height of the season, Margate was not doing well in 1808, still recovering from a freak winter storm in January, when the sea had risen violently, crashing through the harbour, smashing ships and wrecking the landing pier and most of the sea-front.[16] There were a few sour individuals who believed that the gentry's loose holiday living and 'prophanation of the Sabbath' had brought divine-retribution on the town.[17] When Margaret and her mother arrived, the place was still in a sorry state, with much of the sea-front closed off by barriers, and a constant hammering and sawing as tradesmen worked to repair or replace the ruined buildings and labourers laid the new High Street.[18]

They stayed at Mr Peel's lodging house in New Street, a narrow thoroughfare leading back from the High Street and sea-front.[19] It wasn't quite Merchant's Quay, but the maritime air was reminiscent of home and childhood. The effect on Mrs Bulkley was remarkable; within a very short while she was able, for the first time in years, to hold a quill sufficiently well to write her own signature on the letters she dictated to Margaret; it was rather palsied, but it was an improvement.[20]

Mrs Bulkley and Dr Fryer were making good progress with both of their books – this very month saw the publication by the estimable Colnaghi of Cockspur Street of a giant folio titled *A Series Of Etchings By James Barry, Esq. From His Original And Justly Celebrated Paintings, In The*

Great Room Of The Society Of Arts (the self-justifying title was probably Mrs Bulkley's idea). Copies were already in shop windows across the West End of London.[21] Meanwhile, Fryer's edition of *The Works of James Barry*, a two-volume illustrated compilation of Barry's letters and writings, was approaching completion. The publishers Cadell and Davies were interested, and Fryer had assured Mrs Bulkley that she might expect to receive as much as £500 for the copyright. Indeed, General Miranda, who lent his moral support to the venture (along with an engraving from his own collection to be used as a frontispiece),[22] had told her that 'not only from his Knowledge of Books, but even from his observations on the Arts & Sciences in general in the course of his Travels' that the copyright in the prints should be worth £1000.[23]

Mrs Bulkley glowed at the thought of extending her fortunes, and placed her faith in the judgement of these learned men.

Changes were afoot in Margaret's world that year. The first to be affected was General Miranda. By June 1808 his and Sir Arthur Wellesley's plans for the liberation of Spanish America had been wrecked by a sudden gale that had blown up in Spain.

In May 1808 Napoleon, seeking to impose his will on the unruly nation, had forced King Charles IV and his son to abdicate, and in June gave the Spanish throne to his own brother, Joseph Bonaparte. Overnight, without a shot being fired, Spain had ceased being an autonomous French ally and became a conquered territory, split between the Napoleonic state and the royalist Bourbon faction. For better or worse, Bourbon Spain, as an enemy of France, became the natural ally of Britain.

The British high command made hasty plans for an intervention in the Iberian Peninsula, and General Sir Arthur Wellesley was given command. Immediately, the bulk of the force that had been earmarked for the Venezuelan expedition was redirected to Portugal. Not only was General Miranda deprived of the aid he had counted on for his revolution, he had also lost the support of the key ally he had so carefully cultivated for so many years; Britain, now allied to Spain, would not make war upon Spanish colonial possessions.

However, all was not lost. France had possessions in the West Indies and the Spanish Main, and Britain was still willing to send a force there to fight for those territories. Also, Miranda still had personal allies in the Navy and in the British West Indies. With his unfailing confidence in his own destiny, he continued laying his plans and practising his diplomacy. Those grand plans would eventually encompass Margaret Bulkley and fix her future.

With an insensible logic, the fates of the people connected with Margaret were either converging on one another or coming full circle – as if they were being organised and guided by the hand of an author. As summer faded and Margaret and her mother settled again into London life, two items of news reached them. The first, all too predictably, concerned Redmond Barry.

After being freed from the King's Bench and leaving London, Redmond had drifted to Bristol, where he had run into trouble almost immediately. He took up thieving, and proved no more successful at it than he'd been at handling a fortune. On 25 April 1808 he was convicted of grand larceny and sentenced to seven years 'beyond the seas'. His crime was probably slight; grand larceny (as opposed to petty larceny) was defined as 'a felonious and wrongful taking away, by any person, of the mere personal goods of another not from the person nor out of his house, above the value of 12d'.[24] *One shilling*. At least it hadn't been burglary, for which a man could swing. Redmond was put into Bristol's ramshackle Newgate Prison, then sent with a batch of other convicts to Portsmouth, where they were put aboard the prison hulk HMS *Captivity* to await transfer to a convict vessel outward bound.[25]

The circle was complete; having bought his way out of the crew of one hulk and gone to London a wealthy man, Redmond had returned to another as one of its inmates. He was never transported, and would remain at Portsmouth in the dark, brutal hell-hole of *Captivity* for the next six years.[26]

A second piece of news reached Margaret and her mother at almost the same time, in the form of a grubby and much-travelled letter. It had been addressed, barely legibly, to Mrs Bulkley in care of 'Grand Room Adelphy Which was Painted by Jas. Barry Esq. London'. Forwarded to their former lodgings at Brook Street, it had eventually made its way round the corner to Charles Street. The letter had come from Portsmouth, but it wasn't from Redmond. It was a scarcely coherent, pleading message from John Bulkley, Margaret's errant brother.

Little or nothing had been heard of John for some years. He'd left his legal training far behind him, along with his once-rich and now presumably ruined wife, and was now in the Army, a lowly private in a regiment about to depart for active service overseas. The Royal York Rangers was a penal regiment, one of a handful raised for the duration of the war. Most of its recruits came from the prison hulks and gaols; some were even fugitives from the gallows, pardoned on condition that they join the Army. The remainder of the Rangers were convicted deserters from other regiments.

Which of those paths had brought John Bulkley from his clerkship in Dublin to the ranks of such a regiment is unknown, but his regret was bitter and his despair all-consuming. The penal regiments, containing so many lawless and violent-tempered men, were difficult to control, and the rule of their officers (many of whom were former sergeants and corporals from line regiments) was savage. One observer recalled that discipline was 'enforced by terror and punishment, not by mind and prevention',[27] and a former commanding officer stated, 'There was no corps I ever saw, in which corporal punishment was so often obliged to be resorted to ... for there were many whom the civil power could not control, and it required a very coercive military power to keep them in subordination.'[28] The Rangers were tough, aggressive and highly expendable, and could therefore be given the most dangerous postings imaginable.

At the beginning of September 1808, John was crammed with hundreds of other men in the hold of the armed transport *Adriatic*, which lay loading up at Spithead. Once the loading was complete, the convoy would set sail for the West Indies.[29] As if conforming to a contrived pattern of connections, the Rangers had been part of the force originally intended for General Miranda and General Wellesley's expedition to Spanish America. Now that the cream of that force had gone to the Peninsula, just the Rangers and a few other regiments were slated to go and attack French outposts in the Caribbean, a sweltering, fever-ridden posting that claimed lives by the hundreds even in peacetime.

John Bulkley scavenged a scrap of dirty paper and scribbled a letter to his mother, the incoherent lines running at an angle across the page, spattered with inkblots. 'Dear mother for the love of God try and do something to promote me,' he wrote:

> For God sake direct a letter to me ... Give my love to my Dear Sister Margaret we are going to the West Indies we expect every day write to me immediately. Perhaps I may never hear from you again it will

be a great consolation to me … I remain my Dear Mother your unfortunate Son

> John Bulkley
> Private Royal York Rangers
> on board the Adriatic
> Spithead – or else where[30]

He added a postscript: 'Let a penny be put in with the Letter and then
it will come free.'

It never came at all. Mary Anne had been resolute in cutting herself
off from the husband and son who had ruined her and blighted Margaret's
life; she felt for him, but she hardened her heart and never wrote back.

But Margaret did. She penned him a letter brimming with ironic
good cheer; assuming a tone of encouragement, she twisted the knife in
his side. In her view, as a man he ought to take the consequences of the
privileged choices he'd been given – choices that had been denied to her:

> By this time I dare say you have experienced the wisdom or folly
> resulting from your substituting a musquet for a goosequill – either
> (in the opinion of a girl) may reflect honor on a man if used with spirit
> in a Good cause. Indeed my dear John a soldier fighting for his King,
> his country & his rights as a Brittain or Hiber* in my mind acts nobly,
> honorably & Gloriously, and the old phrase 'there is a reward in Heaven
> for all who die fighting for their Country' is an article in my Creed &
> I most firmly believe in it.[31]

With a relentless ardour that must have appalled her brother when he
read it, she reminded him of Horace's dictum: *Dulce et decorum est pro
patria mori*. 'Was I not a girl I would be a Soldier!' she wrote. 'However
I must honestly confess I would prefer a sword to a musquet & I should
like a pair of Colours† at least.'

She added: 'We must see what can be done for you. Write therefore an
acct. of your situation & the names of some of the principal Officers, John
write like a Gentleman or Margaret will blush for you.' She reported that
she had heard two days earlier from her father, Jeremiah, who was now

---

* Irish person
† national and regimental flags (colours) carried by a regiment; shorthand for an
officer's commission

out of debtors' prison and living in lodgings in Dublin. He claimed (she said) to have been in touch with Colonel Mountifort Longfield, who'd promised to do something to help John. This was unlikely, and possibly a fabrication on Margaret's part, designed to taunt John, who must realise how improbable it was that someone like Longfield would really help the dishonoured and possibly criminal son of a bankrupt Catholic.

Concluding, Margaret struggled to express her antipathy towards her brother without stating it outright. She began to write 'Mamma joins me ...' but crossed out 'joins me' and instead wrote, 'Mamma prays for you (and to use her own words) Desires you to take care of yourself.' Adding the cryptic remark, 'without any comment on the past', she signed herself coolly, 'I am your Sister, Margt A Bulkley.'

Even the most urgent help could not have saved John from his fate. The Royal York Rangers sailed from Spithead for Trinidad in late September – twelve hundred men crammed into armed merchant ships for the long ocean voyage to hell.[32] By the time they joined the other regiments mustering in Barbados, reports were already reaching Britain that the tropical 'sickly season' was producing 'an unusual mortality in the army'.[33] And by December the force was thrown into a bloody campaign to seize the French-held islands of Martinique and Guadeloupe. The Royal York Rangers distinguished themselves by their courage, suffering heavy casualties. No certain word reached England as to whether John Bulkley was among the dead.

Would Margaret really have swapped places with John? Perhaps not if she'd known the kind of regiment he was in. But to be a soldier – she certainly would, provided she could have her sword and spurs; Margaret was clever and daring and craved a release from the life that lay ahead of her.

In the meantime, she got to know General Miranda better. His enthusiasm for revolution was unquenched and he intended to set out on another expedition to Caracas in due course. Margaret found herself at the centre of a small circle of male friends and mentors, each of whom took a paternal interest in her. She had become a close friend of the Reardon family, and deeply fond of little Ellen, now nearly two years old. In February 1809 Elizabeth Reardon gave birth to a second baby daughter, who was christened Margaret.[34] It was in the society of the Miranda family, Dr Fryer and Reardon that a plan was first concocted.

Precisely when it first arose is not known, nor who suggested it; but it was a plan that was altogether revolutionary.

Margaret had been particularly fortunate in stumbling into this little circle; these men's minds were not closed to the idea of female achievement. They'd grown up in the age of the Blue Stocking movement – the informal societies of intellectual women who mingled with artists and writers to converse with them on an equal footing. Samuel Johnson and Edmund Burke had been among the participants, as had James Barry – indeed it was said that Barry had been responsible for the group's colourful name, having turned up to meetings in the clothes he wore to paint in, including his blue worsted stockings (white silk was normally worn for social occasions).[35] Barry had included a portrait of Elizabeth Montagu, one of the founders of the Blue Stockings, in his *Progress of Human Knowledge and Culture*; he described her as 'a distinguished example of female excellence' and depicted her 'earnestly recommending the ingenuity and industry of a young female'.[36] He had also been a good friend of the radical thinker William Godwin, the husband of Mary Wollstonecraft.[37] Barry, who had been sympathetic to rebellion and the rights of the oppressed, had participated in a subculture that welcomed women. When the Royal Academy began in 1768, two of its founder members had been women: Angelica Kauffman and Mary Moser, who exhibited at the Academy and the Society of Arts alongside their male peers.[38]

By 1809 that era was already passing away; Mary Wollstonecraft had turned feminism into a political campaign for real equality – including the freedom for women to enter the trades and professions – and the reactionary element in society was turning against it; within decades, 'bluestocking' would become a term of derision for dowdy females who devoted themselves to intellectual pursuits and denied themselves the virtuous joys of marriage and family. Although the spirit hadn't gone out entirely, and there were a few middle-aged men who were still sympathetic, the movement was dying.

The mere idea of a woman pursuing masculine paths – especially into the educated professions – was unthinkable. Yet Margaret Bulkley thought it, and had settled on an ambition. Since the summer months of 1806 she'd been surrounded by practitioners of medicine and surgery. Dr Edward Fryer was a physician of note, with royalty among his patients, and in the early days of their friendship, whenever Margaret walked to his house in Newman Street she would pass the gates of the Middlesex Hospital in Mortimer Street, an important medical school. Hundreds of medical students and surgical apprentices lodged in the district and were a common sight in the streets – young men, hollow-eyed with study, carrying books or wooden cases of precious instruments. Some of these youths might one day be among the wealthiest of England's citizens – men with riches to rival the most successful merchants. Dr Fryer's friend Anthony Carlisle estimated his own income from his patients at 70 guineas or more a week, or at least £3822 a year – a vast income for a professional man.[39] One of the country's most eminent surgeons, Astley Cooper, was said to earn £15,000 a year – even as much as £21,000.[40] Medicine and anatomy were part of the intellectual and artistic ferment of the time; as a painter, James Barry had studied anatomy 'with great attention, more than many Surgeons do',[41] just as his friend Dr Fryer had studied art. And Miranda's famous library included a collection of books 'such as might be considered to form a tolerably complete Medical Library for a private gentleman who is not of the Profession'.[42] Brilliant physicians and surgeons were on pedestals, science was in the ascendant, and the prospect of studying medicine was considerably more attractive to a bright young person than tutoring the infants of the wealthy or keeping old ladies company.

Could the revolutionary idea have come from Dr Fryer? He was known to be a free-thinker, but was also a man of 'strict probity'.[43] The thought of educating a young woman in subjects as intensely masculine as medicine or surgery would have appealed to Fryer's intellect, but he might have hesitated to go through with it. The problem was that private tuition could hardly cover the requisite knowledge, let alone the practical study involved.

There were two ways into the profession. To train as a surgeon, one must become an apprentice to an established practitioner, often at one of the great teaching hospitals; the apprenticeship lasted seven years. To become a physician, one must study medicine, which could only be done at one of the universities. Physicians learned surgery, but not very thoroughly, and rarely practised it. There was a pronounced distinction of prestige also; qualified physicians were Doctors of Medicine, whereas a surgeon was a plain 'Mr' and was a member of a profession only recently risen above barbarism. Needless to say, both pathways were firmly closed to women.

Daniel Reardon, as a particularly scrupulous member of the legal profession, probably didn't suggest the solution to this problem, and Mrs Bulkley – nervous and risk averse at the best of times – most certainly did not.

Then there was Francisco de Miranda. A born revolutionary, adventurer and radical thinker, he was also an enthusiastic amateur in medical science. He was also capable of persuading his companions that an impossible dream might be achievable. He would undoubtedly have encouraged, if not originally conceived, the idea of Margaret studying medicine by disguising herself as a man.

It had been done before, quite recently – albeit not in England. Margaret King, Lady Mount Cashell was a radical former pupil of Mary Wollstonecraft; in 1806, during a tour of Bonaparte's Europe with her lover, she disguised herself as a Frenchman in order to attend lectures in medicine and surgery at the University of Jena (which at the time was at the centre of a savage war between France and Prussia).[44] Gossip about her love affair and acrimonious separation from Lord Mount Cashell (who cut her off with nothing) would almost certainly have reached the ears of General Miranda, and might have planted the idea. However, Margaret King's disguise had only needed to endure for a few months, and she hadn't studied for a full degree; the plan being hatched in the house in Grafton Street was much more ambitious. Between them, Miranda and Margaret, with advice from Reardon and Fryer, lined it out.

Miranda was a man fizzing with more energy than an ordinary person could have borne. Even in repose he was always agitated. As one of his followers observed: 'When sitting he is never perfectly still; his foot or hand must be moving to keep time with his mind which is always in exercise.'[45] Many people found him difficult and unapproachable, but those who were seduced by his charisma found him moving and hypnotic:

In general his demeanour is marked by hauteur and distance. When he is angry he loses discretion … He appears conversant on all subjects. His iron memory prevents his ever being at a loss for names, dates and authorities.

He used his mental resources and colloquial powers with great address to recommend himself to his followers. He assumed the manners of a father and instructor to the young men … He appeared the master of languages, of science and literature. In his conversations he carried his hearers to the scenes of great actions and introduced them to the distinguished characters of every age.[46]

The plan they conceived went beyond study. In Miranda's dream of a liberated Venezuela, women would not suffer the same restrictions as they did now. If Margaret should succeed in gaining a degree, she would accompany him on his next expedition and live an altogether new life as a participant in the fight for freedom. The idea appealed to Margaret's natural courage and to the sense of adventure she had alluded to in her letter to John – '*Was I not a girl*', forsooth.

For the time being at least, the idea was kept secret. It would need the consent of Margaret's mother, who held the purse strings; studying medicine was expensive, and would mean spending their inheritance. Mrs Bulkley could not have borne the anxiety. She had enough to try her with the dismal fate of Barry's *Etchings*. Her inquiries in January 1809 had brought a sad little flurry of notes from the booksellers. Joseph Booker, a prominent Catholic with a shop in New Bond Street, wrote that he had 'not had much success' with it; blaming it on the dullness of the season, he'd tried placing it in the window and enticed several people to look at it, but his hopes were dashed;[47] other sellers reported the same.[48] James Barry was simply no longer a fashionable artist.

By March 1809 Dr Fryer was on the brink of publishing *The Works of James Barry*. Mrs Bulkley thought the publisher, Cadell and Davies, might also like to purchase all the unsold copies of the *Etchings*. They expressed an interest, and Mrs Bulkley convinced herself that they would make a success of both books. She urged Daniel Reardon to appoint a meeting; 'I am *exceedingly anxious* to have the purchase finally concluded,' she wrote.[49] She had pinned so many hopes on the book, and was driven to distraction by delays. (How much Cadell and Davies had paid for the copyright in the *Works* is unclear, but it was probably a long way short of the £1000 predicted by the ever-sanguine General Miranda.)[50]

Mr Reardon arranged the meeting, and the publishers considered the matter – taking four more agonising months over it. Then, in July, a huge package arrived at the Bulkleys' lodgings at 12 Brook Street (they'd moved yet again). Inside was a copy of the *Etchings*, accompanied by a politely terse note that told her, in the timeless spirit of publishers throughout the ages:

Messrs Cadell & Davies present Comp'ts to Mrs Bulkeley; and finding, after due consideration, that it is not in their power to dispose of the Copies of the late Mr Barry's Etchings, beg leave to decline the purchase of them, and return herewith the Copy which Mrs Bulkeley was so good as [to] send to them.[51]

The effect wrought in the little household was cataclysmic. At a stroke, with only occasional placements as a tutor and no permanent employ-ment,[52] Margaret had had her future fortune reduced to whatever remained of the £2000 from the Barry estate. It was enough for survival but not for security. Mrs Bulkley fell into a steep and dangerous decline; her fragile health failed, and she took to her bed. Within a month her condition had deteriorated so badly that she was persuaded to make her will.

The document was drawn up and witnessed by Reardon's clerk, Philip, and Rosa, the widow of Joseph Bonomi (who had died the previous year). Mrs Bulkley bequeathed her a mourning ring and three more for Daniel Reardon and his wife and Philip. Everything else would go to Margaret, as had always been intended.[53] Mary Anne signed the will with a hand that could barely hold the pen, in a wandering staccato of jagged strokes. The end seemed very near.

In fact, Mary Anne Bulkley was made of more resilient stuff than she seemed. The crisis didn't kill her, but it did leave her even more jittery than before – and possibly wandering a little in her wits. In this state, she might have consented to any idea, however mad, if she could be convinced that it would give her daughter a prosperous future.

The plan was quickly put in train and each of the conspirators sworn to secrecy. Money would be needed – every penny of the James Barry fortune. As an amateur of anatomy and a free-thinker, he would probably have approved of his old friends' plan. Indeed, as it would turn out, James Barry's fortune would not be the only thing Margaret would inherit.

That autumn, two letters arrived in London. In October, Redmond wrote to Daniel Reardon from the prison ship *Captivity*, complaining of his desperate circumstances, his poverty, his failing health, and pleading 'for God sake go to Margrett and Shew her this letter and I am Confident from her former Promise to me when I was in the Kings bench, she will be persuaded by you to help me'.[54]

A month later a second letter came, this one from Jeremiah Bulkley and addressed directly to Margaret. Jeremiah was full of his own woes; still living in poverty in Dublin, he felt bereft, knowing nothing of his son's whereabouts nor the situation of his wife and daughter. He invited Margaret and her mother to return to Ireland; he would share his last shillings with them, and assured them, 'I have made up my mind to forgive – and be at peace with the world.'[55] (Why he imagined that he should be the forgiver in this scenario, he didn't specify; presumably he felt abandoned.)

Jeremiah did mention one thing that might have tugged at Margaret's heart – he was thinking of Juliana (who must be about six years old now), and hoping that something might be done for her.[56] But Margaret had parted from her child, and, as far as can be determined, never saw her again. She had cut herself off from her former life. In fact, she was no longer in London; she had embarked on a great adventure, and had turned her back not only on her relations, but on her very person. Miss Margaret Anne Bulkley had vanished.

6

Sanguine Expectations

Miller's Wharf, Wapping, London: Thursday 30 November 1809

It was an improbable vessel in which to set out on a life's adventure. Bluff, plain, diminutive, and smelling unmistakably of fish, the Leith smack lay moored by creaking ropes to the busy quay. Despite the bleak dawn hour and the icy damp, a fair-haired young man stood on deck, gazing down at the oily water. He cut an odd figure: slight, elegantly poised despite his somewhat ill-fitting clothes, a small, pale hand resting on the rail. Lost in thought, he stared down past the black-slimed stones at the river, rank with yellow foam and litter, heaving slowly with the ebbing tide, clucking glutinously under the hull.

Labouring by the glow of lanterns and the breaking dawn, the crew were preparing for departure, hauling up the staysail while a shorehand made ready to cast off the mooring warps.[1] Beyond the grimy blocks of the wharf buildings, the sailmakers and the storehouses were the sagging cottages, chandlers' shops and taverns, cowering before the brick cliffs of the warehouse buildings of the new London Dock. The waterfront woke early, and the quayside lanes were already rattling with vehicles and foot-passengers – seamen and labourers, hawkers and merchants and thieves.

He'd passed through that teeming hive the evening before, shrinking beside his aunt in the recesses of a shuttered hackney carriage. The journey across the metropolis had been his first time out in public since the transformation, and it was as if every eye was on him as the carriage deposited its two passengers and their hillock of luggage on the wharf-side cobbles.

The transformation had been in train for weeks, and brought to completion in the last few days. First had come the apparel. It being impossible to visit a tailor, they had called at every slop-seller within walking distance of Brook Street, searching for garments that were styled for a gentleman (and in a decent state, in the case of second-hand items) yet small enough to fit. Margaret tried them on in the privacy of their rooms – an amusing game at first, seeing the odd reflection in the glass as the garments were pinned and pulled and tacked until they more or less fitted. When the linens went on for the first time, the humour paled: compared with those to which she was accustomed, the undergarments were baggy around the chest where they ought to be snug, while below the hips they clung insolently where they should be loose. (Corsets had gone out of fashion when Margaret was a child, replaced by short stays supporting the bust, so she'd never known their painful constriction and didn't benefit from a sense of release now.)

Then came the shears. Her red-gold hair was unpinned, unplaited and shorn, ropes of hair falling around her shoulders and slumping to the hearth rug. The game was now utterly serious. Margaret might have called a halt then, but shrinking from a task once she'd set herself to it was not in her nature. Mrs Bulkley snipped and combed until the remaining locks were fashioned in the modern Caesar style. Or at least an approximation of it; her hands were shakier than ever, and she was weak from the illness that had nearly carried her off in the summer. Now when she looked in the glass, Margaret saw a stranger who had stolen her face.

On the day of departure, she had put on her disguise. She didn't know it yet, but she had seen her last dawn as a woman. Yesterday's dress was packed away, to await either her triumphant return or her exposure and shame – whichever came sooner. Had she known that the dress was the last she would ever wear, she would surely have rethought her plans. Margaret was extremely particular about her clothes and always would be; she followed fashion keenly, and her identity as a girl, a woman and a person was bound up with the clothes she wore. At this moment, on the brink of an adventure, she could hardly imagine how painfully that dress, and others like it, would tug at her heart in the years to come.[2] By the time her mother joined her, the disguise was complete, and Mrs Bulkley gazed at the person standing where her daughter ought to be; for the first time, she saw the new-minted man, her instant nephew – Mr James Barry.

It had been determined that this should be her new identity. Young James, so the reasoning went, would be the son of one of Mrs Bulkley's

brothers. The brother was unspecified, but if they were pressed, Patrick –
believed to have died some years ago on the far side of the world – would
best serve the purpose. The boy had, of course, been named after his
renowned uncle James, a name that would have the double advantage of
conferring a degree of recognition and a sliver of verisimilitude.

It was a long and winding journey down through Clerkenwell and
Whitechapel, passing through ever poorer districts. As the prosperity
of the streets declined, they grew darker and grimmer: the new gas
lighting in the better streets gave way to dingier oil lights. Descending
at last towards the river, the carriage grumbled through the parish of
St Katharine by the Tower, an unsanitary slum that had accreted like
mould around the ancient church and hospital. The stink of rot and
the odour of stale yeast from the brewhouses penetrated the coach
windows. Margaret gazed at scenes of poverty beyond anything she
had ever seen. It was among the worst London had to offer – as bad
as the Rookeries around St Giles or the Devil's Acre in Westminster.
There was no street lighting here: just the glow of tallow dips in the
hovels and run-down gin shops, and here and there a rushlight fixed to
a bracket or a fire burning on a patch of waste ground, with demonic
silhouettes gathered round it. Every crooked building was smutted and
grimed, with weeds growing in the cracks, rags and papers stuffed in
broken windows and walls dripping with slime; the beasts in human
form that thronged the streets looked fierce and despairing, ragged
and vicious, many of them staggering full of Cuckold's Comfort and
Knock-Me-Down.[3]

Signs of disease, malnourishment and deformity were everywhere.
Margaret's budding medical sensibility – untutored but hungry for
understanding – must have been enthralled by it and, despite the stom-
ach-turning squalor, she must have felt for these pitiable creatures. Once
the persona of James Barry had served his purpose and Margaret had
become a doctor, she would strive to alleviate misery – not here, but in
liberated Venezuela, which must offer sights of suffering just like this,
but under a sweltering tropical sun.

The Wapping waterfront was vastly greater than Merchant's Quay in Cork. The cries of gulls and carousing seamen, the slams and rattles of doors and iron-shod wheels on the cobbles, the creaking of ropes and timbers, all made a familiar cacophonous music in Margaret's ears, and the smells of drink, tar and timber were old companions too. While their luggage was taken aboard, Margaret and her mother retreated to a dockside inn for the night.

When they emerged again before dawn, aching after a night spent dozing and fidgeting on settles in the common room of the inn, the little smack was already preparing to sail with the tide, her lanterns glowing and her deck alive with activity.

Once aboard, Mrs Bulkley retreated from the freezing November wind,[4] seeking refuge in the women's quarters – advertised as commodious and comfortable, but consisting of little more than a cramped cabin below the afterdeck, with half a dozen closed-off bunks around the four sides. Still, it would be more comfortable than the Edinburgh coach – unbearable days of sitting upright, jammed among strangers in a jolting stagecoach. The sea voyage was cheaper too, at 3 guineas each, including three barrels' bulk of luggage. True, there was a war on, with the risk of attack by French privateers (it was not unknown for the Leith and Berwick smacks to be obliged to defend themselves), but the pecuniary saving and relative comfort made it worthwhile in Mrs Bulkley's estimation.[5]

On deck, London was emerging in the dawn. Now that the pungent odour of the great brewery had faded overnight, a new smell was revealed. The huge, filth-laden Thames, passing through the great reaches of Westminster and the City, whose numberless sewers spilled their effluvia into it, gave off a deep, malignant reek. Every item Margaret wore irritated the senses: the woollen stockings chafed, the heavy tailcoat and surtout weighed the shoulders down, the high collar and tightly knotted cravat constricted the throat, and as for the breeches ... well, if the underclothes seemed uncomfortably clinging, the breeches were quite unspeakable.

If the disguise was to work, Margaret must stop thinking of men as a breed apart, and learn to think and act like one of them. The model that came clearest to mind was General Miranda – a fine, upright gentleman of heroic bearing. The left hand tucked behind, making a fist in the small of the back; the spine straight, shoulders back and chin raised ... it was hard to sustain, and would take a good deal of getting used to – if it could ever be done. (In fact, Margaret would always struggle to master this.) And there were other telling details – her voice, her smooth skin, her diminutive height and build – that could not be altered.

The smack was ready to get under way, and passengers weren't welcome on deck. The slight young gentleman stepped away from the rail and retreated. Gathering her courage, Margaret entered the men's cabin – the first small step into the exclusive masculine world. It would be a difficult and unsettling voyage, in such close proximity with several men, in a cramped space filled with sights (and odours) that Margaret had never experienced before. How would she fare in Edinburgh, where she would chance all – fortune, future and perhaps even liberty – on this thin gauze of masculinity? She would be under the eyes of brilliant men: sharp, observant, trained in anatomy – quite unlike the ordinary males with whom she would share this poor little cabin.

Above Margaret's head, the planks thumped with the feet of the crew hauling in the warps and hoisting the mainsail. The staysail caught the breeze, and the smack bore away from the quay, her bow catching the ebbing tide and turning downriver. As she moved out into midstream, the mainsail was sheeted in, filling with wind. The bluff-bowed little vessel began her journey towards the rising sun and the open sea.

6 Lothian Street, Edinburgh: Thursday 14 December 1809

From Mrs Mary Anne Bulkley to Mr Daniel Reardon, attorney at law, London:

Dear Sir,
    After a voyage of 5 days we arrived safe at Leith and as soon as possible took Lodgings at Edinburgh, where I find everything (almost) cheaper than at London ... I only pay £30 per ann. for 4 very good rooms and the use of the Servant and cooking &ca ... I could wish you would consider what can be best done to purchase an Annuity for me & to insure the principal, it is a great pity that nothing is done about the house in Ireland. Surely it would fetch something <u>handsome</u> if sold, for although it is now let at great disadvantage it produces a profit Rent of 34£ per annum but I am confident you will manage these affairs in the most advantageous manner for me. I will trouble

you to call or send to Mr. Moltino in Pall Mall for the price of a set of Mr. Barry's Etchings which remains with him, five guineas is the price but a discount is to be deducted.[6]

Mrs Bulkley paused in her dictation. Money was the abiding concern of her life, and the insufficiency of their fortune loomed over her. Even the warmth of the fire in the grate was a worry as much as a comfort. It consumed an unconscionable quantity of coals in this weather; there was snow on the ground outside,[7] four rooms to heat, and they were down to their last bit of cash. Mrs Bulkley went on:

> I request you will send me Thirty Pounds either by a Bank Post Bill or order as soon as possible, I have been oblidged to pay some necessary expenses here and to remain at an Inn till I could suit myself with Lodgings — We unite in Best Respects to Mrs. Reardon & family & I remain Dr. Sir
> Your Sincerely Oblgd
> Mary A. Bulkley

Since her collapse in the summer, she had again regained the ability to write her signature, but Margaret wrote the letter for her. That is to say – her *nephew*, James, wrote for her; it was hard to keep up, even though a fortnight had passed since the transformation. And what changes in circumstances and habits had occurred since then. Of her daughter there was rarely any clear sight nowadays, even when they were both at home; the disguise was growing into her, obscuring without ever fully concealing the girl beneath.

Mr James Barry had enrolled at the university, and now studied all hours of the morning, evening and night. Mrs Bulkley might catch a glimpse of Margaret, nose buried in a book, cravat loosened and tossed aside, ink-stained fingers poring over pages of notes and sketches; then the femininity was clear, in the tilt of her head or turn of a hand. And when she rose and stretched, the shadow that the candle threw on the wall was as sinuously feminine as ever.

Despite all her months of tuition with Dr Fryer and her reading in General Miranda's library, Margaret had never worked so hard in her life – and she gloried in it: 'I have my hands full of delightfull business,' she wrote to Mr Reardon (signing as 'James Barry'), '& work from seven o'clock in the Morning till two the next.'[8] Her mood was euphoric, triumphant – and not only with the joy of learning and of a clear goal. She'd been through tests that had inspired dread from the moment she assumed her costume and the smack heaved its slow way to Leith. After arriving, James had had to sign the Matriculation Album, declaring the courses he intended to take and paying a fee of half a crown towards the expansion of the library; this was followed by a visit to each of the professors to purchase tickets for admission to the lecture courses he intended to take.[9] They would surely detect the imposture, wouldn't they, all those brilliant, sharp-witted men? But no, for once Margaret benefited from the world's colossal, cold indifference. So far as the university and its professors were concerned, James Barry was a mere name on a roll, a face – admittedly a rather smooth, dainty one – among the many that massed before their teachers in the theatres of instruction. James Barry was an effeminate-looking young man, slightly built and small – by what possible reason should they bother to look beyond this simple fact? As the nephew of a famous painter and the protégé of a celebrated revolutionary, he caused one or two eyebrows to be raised in interest, but beyond that … nothing. And so James Barry signed the book, paid his half-crown, and purchased his tickets for courses in anatomy, chemistry, natural philosophy and Greek, at 3 guineas each.[10] He'd joined the university a month late, and had a lot of catching up to do.

Margaret had barely had a chance to get used to the initial success of her disguise when another test arose that she would have to face without the shield of obscurity: James Barry was introduced formally to his eminent sponsor, His Lordship the Earl of Buchan, who'd been told of the young man's ambition to become a doctor, and whose interest had been piqued.

In his late sixties, David Steuart Erskine, 11th Earl of Buchan, was a notable eccentric. Taking a keen and provident interest in the education of the young, he had agreed to lend the light of his countenance and the gravity of his rank in support of the late painter's nephew. He'd admired Barry greatly, and was more than willing to help his heir. Lord Buchan was a man of progressive, sometimes radical, views, a participant in the intellectual life of the country, and influential in the university. He fancied himself a man of the arts, and patronised both Robert Burns and Walter Scott; the latter described him as 'a person whose immense vanity, bordering upon insanity, obscured, or rather eclipsed, very considerable talents'.[11] The previous year, it was said, he'd been so angered by an edition of the *Edinburgh Review*, he'd had a footman open his front door and place it on the threshold, then personally kicked it out into the street, expecting that this show of displeasure would bring down the publication (it didn't). Buchan's family seat was at Dryburgh Abbey near Selkirk, some forty-five miles from Edinburgh, but he kept a house in the city too, in the fashionable new thoroughfare of George Street, at the heart of the wealthy New Town.

His Lordship was a kindly-looking man, with heavy, fleshy features and large, gentle eyes, but he could be quixotic and high-tempered. He warmed immediately to young Barry, who had a natural charm, and as their acquaintance grew, he even began to acquire a paternal regard for him. Once again, Margaret's disguise had triumphed, and James Barry had won support that would pay off handsomely in the years to come.

Thus far, Margaret wrote happily to Mr Reardon, 'every thing has far exceeded my most sanguine expectations and Mr Barry's Nephew is well received by the Professors'.[12] Thoroughly satisfied now with the disguise, she noted complacently that it had been 'very usefull for Mrs Bulkley (my Aunt) to have a Gentleman to take care of her on Board Ship and to have one in a strange country'. Having been admitted to the scholarly and intellectual life of men, and having acquired another influential friend, she added that she hoped 'in due time to perfect all my plans'.[13]

There was a long way to go yet. She would have to carry on the charade for three years, but when she finally travelled to Venezuela, Margaret could re-emerge, casting off the shell of James Barry. So confident did she feel, indeed, that it amused her to imagine keeping him alive – she joked about James introducing himself to little Ellen Reardon, who would be five years old by then and wouldn't remember Margaret. It didn't occur to her that her satisfaction and optimism might be premature.

The weeks of December passed in an endless round of lectures and studying. Margaret discovered one of the delights of being a man – unfettered walking. The ability to stride out, without the encumbrance of skirts or a chaperone, opened up a world of liberty. There was a good deal of walking to do. The lodgings at 6 Lothian Street stood right beside the university's new buildings (still only half-finished, the work having been suspended nearly twenty years earlier due to the wars against France, which had caused funds to dry up), and just a little way from the Royal Infirmary, where medical students attended many of their classes and other duties; but the sheer number of journeys from class to lecture to home and back again tested every student's stamina.

Growing in confidence, young Barry began to attract the notice of his teachers. James wrote to General Miranda that 'the celebrated Professor of Anatomy' Dr Monro had singled him out for attention. He 'speaks of you whom he knows by Fame & of Dr Fryer whose correspondence with Lord B[uchan] – his particular friend, he has read with Enthusiasm'.[14]

Lord Buchan was already proving a good friend to James. On Christmas Day he condescended to visit him and his aunt at their humble lodgings,[15] which threw Mrs Bulkley into a state of delight and alarm; Mr Reardon had neglected to send the £30 she had asked for – she hadn't a shilling left and their circumstances were wretched. But Lord Buchan was the spirit of Yuletide generosity; he offered there and then not merely to patronise the book of Barry prints, but in the New Year would find a seller for them. All their troubles were being resolved.

On New Year's Eve, James was invited to dine with Buchan at his house on George Street. Once again the meeting was a success. They conversed about General Miranda, to whom Buchan had once been introduced upon the General's arrival in England, and James told His Lordship about the General's elegant and extensive library. They drank the health of Dr Fryer, the mutual friend who had furnished young James so admirably with a liberal education.[16]

It seemed that Lord Buchan had begun to identify young James with his late uncle. He'd promoted James Barry RA far and wide as one of the great painters of the age, as well as purchasing pictures from him and encouraging his artistic vision. But his enthusiastic endeavours had been curtailed by Barry's sudden death. Buchan had been shocked – he loved to be in control of events and the destinies of men, especially those he singled out for patronage, and to have one snatched away, even by God, was an affront.[17] For Lord Buchan, whose relationship with reality was sometimes a little vague, taking 'poor James Barry' (as he habitually called the young man) under his wing was a continuation of his unfinished patronage of the uncle. Sir Walter Scott considered Buchan a fantasist, inclined to believe in his own fictions;[18] perhaps this predisposed him to believe in the false persona of young James Barry.

Whatever motivations and fancies were at work, the fiction was held to be true. Mr James Barry had arrived. The university authorities, the professors and now the Earl of Buchan had between them conjured him into existence more fully than any amount of pretence could achieve. Margaret had moulded him, and they had placed the guinea's stamp upon him.

Concluding the letter to General Miranda, James wrote happily, 'I could not deny myself the pleasure of wishing you very many happy returns of the new year', a sentiment in which 'Mrs. Bulkley (my Aunt) joins with me'. It was a new year that was to bring new challenges, and leave Margaret's womanhood ever further behind – a mere memory in James Barry's past.

While James Barry came into his own in Edinburgh, in London letters continued to reach Daniel Reardon from Margaret's male relations. Her father wrote several times pleading for news of her and her mother, believing the worst.[19] 'The death or some misfortune of a Wife & Daughter Racking my mind day and night,' he said of himself, with questionable sincerity, adding that until he heard news from Mr Reardon, 'I will remain in suspence and the greatest Anxiety &c &c &c.'[20]

Redmond Barry, even more wretched, wrote from the prison hulk *Captivity*, having sold his daily allowance of bread for a penny to buy the paper. He too begged for news of his sister and his niece, and pleaded with Mr Reardon, 'my Only friend, do not cast me Away'.[21]

Acting on instructions, Mr Reardon replied to none of these letters; neither did he forward them, or any information about them, to Edinburgh; Mrs Bulkley didn't want to hear from any friends, 'English or Irish, as I do not like to be harrassed with letters'.[22] In particular, neither she nor Margaret were willing to be exposed any longer to the clutches of the men from their past.

7

A Man of Understanding

Shortly before six o'clock in the evening, a small group of nervous young men gathered in the gloomy, malodorous hallway of a run-down house in Horse Wynd, a little alley off the Canongate. They'd come in ones and twos, each carrying papers, pencils and an air of furtive circumspection. Each had descended the dingy cobbled alley, knocked on the door and been discreetly admitted. An ignorant observer might have supposed it to be a house of fornication or illicit gambling, but in fact it was something that the populace might consider even worse. The house belonged to Mr Andrew Fyfe, anatomist and prosector* in the University School of Anatomy. The nervous young men, all students of medicine, had gathered for the first class in one of Mr Fyfe's private courses on practical anatomy: the dissection of a human subject.[1]

Some of the young men were finely dressed, the sort whose pocket-books could shed as much as £500 in a year without distress, and who took a casual approach to study; and at the other extreme, those whose coats showed signs of repair and whose eyes were feverish with lost sleep. One was shorter and fairer than most, and smoother-skinned, and if he was more nervous than his fellows, he had reason to be. James Barry, done up against the cold in a baggy surtout, did not invite conversation with any of his fellows. Margaret was growing used to her male skin, but wasn't confident enough to let James socialise with his peers – acquaintances were safe enough, but chums couldn't be relied on to keep a respectful distance.

Like the others, James had been attending the course of lectures given by Dr Alexander Monro, Professor of Anatomy. Besides having a

---

* a professor's dissector, employed to conduct demonstrations during lectures

month's work to catch up on due to his having arrived late the previous
term, James had been forced to contend with the course's several negative
aspects – not the least of which was Dr Monro himself. James had been
flattered by the personal recognition he'd received from Professor Monro,
and tried to appreciate his teaching, but it was hard. Monro, known as
Monro *tertius* (his father and grandfather having previously held the
post), was middle-aged, with a jutting underlip and small black eyes like
a vole's; his thick crop of russet hair had prematurely thinned to sparse
wisps, inadequately concealed by a combed-forward Caesar coiffure.
Although a fine anatomist, as a lecturer he had an intolerably tedious
style; on and on he would drone, in the most wearisome, pedantic and
spiritless manner, through the endless litany of bones, ligaments, viscera
and muscles, in all their various aspects and connections. Charles Darwin,
who studied medicine at Edinburgh a decade after James Barry, recalled
of Monro, 'I dislike him and his lectures so much, that I cannot speak
with decency about them';[2] he 'made his lectures on human anatomy as
dull as he was himself, and the subject disgusted me'.[3]

If listening was bad enough, seeing was even harder. Monro lectured
in the early afternoon, so that the light would be optimal for the demonstrations by his prosector: in the centre of the octagonal amphitheatre,
flooded with light from the glazed roof, stood the dissecting table, at
the base of a pit formed by steep ranks of seating, where the diminutive
James had to vie with hundreds of other students and the many interested
members of the public (mainly artists and legal men) who had paid to
attend, all trying to gain a view of the proceeding. Even for the tall it was
difficult to witness the details of the dissection properly. In conjunction
with the insufferable prosing of Monro, the experience was an exercise
in frustration.[4] Any student who desired a proper education in anatomy
had to take one of the private practical classes offered by the school's
anatomists and prosectors. For a fee of 3 guineas for a course of three
months, a man could learn the subject at close quarters, with the scalpel
in his own hand.[5]

A clock somewhere within the house chimed six, a door opened, an
aroma of cooking mingled with the unpleasant odour of decay, and a
man made his entrance, encumbered by a stack of books and a candlestick.
He was a tall, thin fellow in late middle age, wearing an old-fashioned
periwig and an anxious expression. He peered warily into the faces of
the young men, recognising them as typical specimens of the medical

student genus, and spoke in a halting, nervous manner: 'Err, yes … er, gentlemen,' he mumbled. 'This way, er, yes … this way …' Mr Andrew Fyfe, prosector to two generations of Monros, had finished his dinner and was ready to instruct.[6]

He opened a door and ushered the young men through a room in which a woman and several children of various ages were seated at desks, busy with coloured inks and brushes, carefully shading fine anatomical diagrams – Mr Fyfe's wife and offspring were active in the family trade, and these were the plates for his next textbook.

The young men were led through a back passage and into a spacious room, lit by a good number of tallow candles. The putrid smell permeating the house had its origin here. Even in daytime it would need artificial light, for the window panes were whitewashed over to keep out inquisitive eyes (Mr Fyfe was cagey about his trade, and tended to give out publicly that he was a surgeon).[7] Two walls were lined with shelves laden with books and glass jars of preserved specimens. A variety of hand-pumps and syringes lay on one shelf, ranging in size from little glass tubes to great brass cylinders with handles and plungers, used for injecting waxes, varnishes and other compounds into the blood vessels of specimens dissected for display. Pails and butts stood about the floor, along with heaps of muslin and rags. The fireplace was empty, and the room was bitterly cold.[8] In the centre stood two plain deal tables surrounded by low stools. Upon both lay unmistakable forms draped with sheets. The young gentlemen's air of nervous anticipation abruptly heightened, and all talk ceased.

Mr Fyfe approached the nearer of the two tables and flung aside the sheet, then gestured for the students to approach. In sombre silence they gathered round and looked upon the corpse.

Legally, the bodies of executed murderers were permitted to be dissected – not as a favour to anatomists but as a deterrent to would-be murderers, who shared the universal horror of post-mortem dissection. But however this young woman had died, it had not been by the gallows. She'd been pulled nefariously from her grave within hours of being laid in it.[9] The grave had not been nearby: the surface of the corpse bore traces of the salt used to pack it and fend off putrefaction during transit. There had been a time when the subjects required for dissection by the anatomists of Edinburgh had been supplied from the city's own graveyards and mortuaries by the local resurrectionists – the reviled sack-'em-up gangs – but demand had long outstripped supply in this small town, and bodies had to be sought elsewhere. London and Liverpool were the richest sources; the resurrectionists in those cities packed up stolen corpses in casks, salted like herring, and shipped them to a receiver in Leith. It was a lucrative trade; a skilled sack-'em-up gang could lift half a dozen corpses in a night, and got good prices for them: about 4 guineas for an adult, 1 guinea for a child; even a foetus could fetch 10 shillings.[10]

Under Mr Fyfe's guidance, the young men donned sleeve protectors and aprons that were stiff with soiling. James found himself holding an old octavo copy of *A Compendium of the Anatomy of the Human Body*, authored by Mr Fyfe himself, bound in oilskin and unpleasantly stained from long service, the pages crinkled with damp, browned at the edges, and spotted here and there with flecks and sprays of bodily fluids. The entire volume was visibly rotting away.[11] The implements – a fine-tooth saw, forceps, scissors, a thin knife and a wooden-handled scalpel – were worn and speckled with rust. The students were sorted into pairs, and each pair assigned a quarter of the subject. James and his partner were given the right thorax.

How this young woman had died, James couldn't begin to guess. As for who she had been, he could never know – just a lost body; she might have been a pauper, a prostitute or the daughter of any well-to-do family. She was no longer a woman, merely a corpse, a subject, her identity and personhood immaterial. The body was lifted and a wooden block placed under the shoulders, raising the thorax and letting the head drop. James picked up the knife while his partner held the book open at the appropriate place.

Holding the implement in the proper manner, like a pencil, James laid the point of the knife on the notch at the top of the breastbone; he began to cut ... and succeeded only in incising a groove in the pale flesh. The skin was tougher than one would expect, and the blade dull. Pressing harder and resisting the trembling in his fingers (a universal thing, this), he began again, and made an incision, more or less straight, from the top to the bottom of the sternum, cutting right to the bone. Then, following the Edinburgh method, while his partner extended the subject's arm (warily, as if it might come to life and strike him), a second incision from the middle of the first one, diagonally to the upper arm.[12] Grasping the edge of the incision with the forceps and swallowing to suppress his nausea, James worked the back of the knife between the skin and the subcutaneous tissues, carefully separating them. Gradually he folded back the upper triangle of skin, laying bare the superficial tissue. Then came the grimmest part – working his bare fingers under the fatty layer and lifting it away from the glistening surface of the pectoral muscle.

All the while, Mr Fyfe, holding a naked candle, oblivious to the molten wax running onto his hand, tutted and hummed and offered comments and advice, dividing his time among the pairs of students who were cutting away at their allotted portions, poring over their books and sketching what they saw.

Making a third incision, James began to lift the skin of the lower part of the dissection. The lateral incisions ran above and below the woman's breast.

Mr Fyfe's voice piped harshly in his ear. 'Indeed, err, the *mammae* add much to the, er, ornament of the person, do they not?' Fyfe gestured eagerly, splashing candle-wax onto his sleeve. 'But the, er, the gland serves in particular, yes, most particularly, for furnishing nourishment to the child – conveyed, you see, through the medium of the, er, nipple – here.' Mr Fyfe's stained finger indicated the dark, puckered point of flesh, and he smirked knowingly. 'When you are older, young man, you may find that a woman's nipple is capable of, er, distension – yes, distension, from titillation, or when influenced by the *passions of the mind*.'[13]

The hillock of white skin lay under James's hand. It was a mere organ, a formation of tissue; the passions of the mind had no place here, nor indeed its frailties. He lowered the blade, and began to cut.

At the end of the class, James found himself back out in Horse Wynd, older by an hour and wiser by years. The air in the alley, damp and acrid with coal-smoke, now seemed like the very breath of wholesomeness. As the minutes of that first hour had ticked away, layer by layer the dead woman's muscles had been separated from their attachments, and the upper arm laid bare. Every blood vessel, every ligament, tendon and nerve was examined, matched to the book and sketched.

This ordeal was just the beginning. All that week, at the same time every evening, James made the journey back to the house in Horse Wynd, where he and his partner resumed their morbid exercise. The axilla was dissected – an awkward procedure, with sticky fat obscuring the major vessels and nerves. The costal cartilages were cut, the sternum removed, the ribs sawn through and turned back, exposing the organs. Having been studied, the muscles, fat, vessels, bones and viscera were dropped into the pails standing by. Each evening the task grew a little harder, the students competing with the process of putrefaction, which always threatened to reduce the corpse faster than they could. Despite the cold, the tissues darkened, softened, turned slimy and slippery, and the air in the room became ever more choking.

It was depressing work for new students – a brutal introduction to the fragility and fleetingness of man's mortal frame. Their hands were never free of the odour of it. 'Every one who has been engaged in post-mortem examination,' wrote a contemporary, 'must be aware of the very disagreeable smell, which it is impossible to get rid of, even by the most careful washing.' It became 'more penetrating and more lasting the more dissections have been made'.[14]

The work was painstaking but also hurried and sometimes crude. And in such unclean conditions, it could be a risky business; bare hands, sharp blades, putrefying flesh, fatigue and haste made a dangerous combination; and the danger was hidden, because nobody knew about bacterial infection. There was also risk from any communicable diseases (usually unidentified) from which the subjects might have died. It was not unknown for practical anatomy to become a fatal pursuit.[15]

Gradually the chest cavity was explored and hollowed out, and James worked his way down to the very heart of the woman on the table, annihilating her body, transmuting it into knowledge. At the same time, Margaret receded a little further. But she did not die, didn't even go to sleep; she looked out on the world and waited patiently until she could return to it.

As the weeks of the Winter Session passed, James worked harder than ever and his femininity was assailed constantly. Like all girls brought up respectably according to the values of her era, Margaret had been conditioned to feel that the merest mention of intimate bodily facts was shameful to the point of impossibility; but James was now experiencing a scientific world in which every part of the body, female and male, within and without, was frankly mentioned, discussed, examined and opened up for study. The emotional effect, at least initially, must have been profound – much greater than for someone brought up a boy. The professors, demonstrators and dissectors would have been utterly mortified if they'd known that a young lady was hearing and seeing all this.

While Mr Fyfe's practical classes continued (with fresh subjects supplied, and the students taking their turns at the body's various parts),
James purchased tickets for more courses, and his daily timetable filled
up. Anatomy, natural philosophy, chemistry and Greek were joined by
moral philosophy and medical jurisprudence. Determined to perfect
his understanding, James attended an additional private lecture course
in anatomy given by Dr John Barclay at his house in Surgeons' Square,
near the Royal Infirmary, a splendid colonnaded building equipped with
a purpose-built anatomy theatre on the upper floor. Barclay was a genial,
humorous man who claimed to have no sense of taste or smell and gave
lively lectures, punctuated by frequent doses of snuff (which he took
without bothering to wipe the debris of dissection off his fingers).[16]

Summer came and went, and in James's second year, yet more subjects were added to his list: practice of physic (clinical medicine), theory
of medicine, *materia medica* (pharmacy), morbid anatomy (pathology),
surgical anatomy, military surgery, midwifery, clinical surgery and
botany.[17] Having been toughened by his experience of dissection, he faced
the ordeal of taking a blade to a living person – a fully conscious being
whose blood pumped and whose body tensed and twitched and shrieked
in pain, restrained by the muscular arms of the theatre assistants. It was
a formidably difficult hurdle to surmount. Seeing living flesh cut for the
first time, and a surgeon's saw rasping into living bone, every student
experienced the dark, dizzy haze, the sudden numbness and inevitable
slide to the floor. Like the others, James overcame it, and passed through
the harrowing vale of darkness into the enlightened land of Surgery.

Besides lectures, students had to attend the wards of the Royal
Infirmary, following the doctors on their rounds, as well as at the Public
Dispensary and the Lying-in Hospital, a maternity facility founded in
1793 'for the purpose of affording relief to the wives of indigent tradesmen'.[18] James's days, from dawn to the toll of midnight and beyond, were
packed with work. Rising about seven, he would read until the first lecture at eight or nine. He might snatch some breakfast between lectures, if
he had time to spare from transcribing lecture notes. Dr Barclay's private
anatomy lectures were in the late morning, and Monro's official ones
in the afternoon, with rounds at the infirmary in between. A swift bite
of lunch could be had at about two or three in the afternoon, and then
there were more lectures until five. Some dinner might follow, combined
with reading and note-making, and in the evening came private classes

and more studying. Supper about ten, then writing-up until he could bear no more and fell into bed, exhausted, sometimes as late as two in the morning.[19]

James was better off than some, having his 'aunt' and a servant to look after him. But financially he was poorer than many of his peers, and what with the cost of living and of taking so many courses, Mrs Bulkley's financial worries never ceased. She plagued Mr Reardon with queries about money, and travelled to London twice in her bid to sell her brother's remaining prints and paintings; she pursued several potential buyers of the *Pandora*, but none ever took it. Despite these circumstances, Mrs Bulkley managed to find the cash to have her piano refurbished by a firm in Soho and shipped all the way from London to Leith.[20] It was as if the mind of a miser had been melded with that of an impulsive spend-thrift, and the result was not a happy one. Yet the money was always there for James's education, which came first.

As the months grew slowly into years, Margaret's male pose became more assured. But she never quite lost her fear of discovery, and James Barry caused amusement among the other students by spurning the fash-ion for shooting-coats and sticking with his all-embracing, all-concealing surtout, even in warm weather.[21]

Margaret had an outgoing, sociable personality; but balancing the desire for friends against the risks of intimacy, James played it safe and avoided the society of his peers. Only one fellow student got close to him during his time in Edinburgh. James's friendship with John Jobson grew up quickly; James took him home to meet his aunt (a slip-up was made in the introductions, and Jobson came away with the impression that the lady was James's mother). Like James, John was a small man, but athletically inclined, and became something of a protector to his vulner-able friend. He tried to teach him to box, but although James went along with the endeavour, stripping down to his shirt-sleeves, he wouldn't raise his hands properly to fight, stubbornly and inexplicably holding them in front of his chest all the while.[22]

Despite his general effeminacy, neither Jobson nor any other student or professor had the least suspicion of James Barry's sex, and when his disguise eventually faltered, it was in a most unexpected way, threatening to undo all his carefully laid and arduously executed plans. Whispers began to circulate among the students about the peculiar, unsociable Barry. It was put about that 'Mr' James Barry was not a man at all — he was very obviously *a young boy*. Not merely a youth, but a veritable *child*, not even past puberty. The evidence was abundant and unambiguous: his short stature, his slightness of build, his unbroken voice, his delicate features and smooth skin. And consider his domestic circumstances – he'd been accompanied to Edinburgh by his *mother*! Or was she his aunt? Whatever the lady's precise relation to the boy, she was clearly *in loco parentis*. On the occasions when she went away, young James was placed into the care of others.

Perhaps there was a strand of envy in the gossip about James Barry, and a dislike of his stand-offishness. In her previous life, Margaret had been friendly and charming – people warmed to her quickly and easily – but James wasn't, at least not with students. Moreover, he was proving himself a gifted student and was highly favoured by Lord Buchan – a recipe for jealousy. Any gossip was worrying; but in believing that they'd detected James in a minor imposture, it didn't occur to his peers to perceive a major one. Still, it could lead to closer scrutiny and serious trouble.

Lord Buchan remained a rock. While Mrs Bulkley was in London on a money-raising trip in July 1810, James boarded with Dr Robert Anderson, the Edinburgh biographer and publisher. He was a friend of Buchan, who wrote to thank him for 'the expression of yr kindness to poor Barry & yr willingness to take him under yr care as a Boarder'. Buchan explained: 'Considering the friendship which subsisted between Barry's Uncle and myself & other circumstances, I have taken the liberty of recommending him more particularly to yr Attention as you will see by the two Billets which I send inclosed to yr care.'[23] The 'billets' would be instruments of payment for James's keep; this was remarkable, as Buchan was notoriously parsimonious.[24]

In the early autumn of 1811, in advance of his final year of study, James spent five weeks as Buchan's guest at his country seat, Dryburgh Abbey, where he 'employed himself in my library very busily in usefull reading of Books connected with his professional views'.[25] James was preparing his dissertation, which had to be written in Latin. This was still the language of scholarship, and no man could be a doctor without a solid command of it. Margaret had been given a firm grounding in classics by Dr Fryer, but despite doing well at Greek (which she loved and continued to pursue at Edinburgh), her Latin was less than perfect. This concerned Lord Buchan, who asked Dr Anderson 'to look at the Latinity of his Thesis'.[26]

By the beginning of James's final year, the allegations about his age had become universally believed. Lord Buchan himself accepted it as true, writing that 'tho he is much younger than is usual to take his Degrees in Medicine & Surgery, yet from what I have observed [is] likely to entitle himself to them by his attainments'.[27] The University Senate disagreed. Having become convinced that he might be as young as twelve, they declared that he was too young to take a degree and declined to enter him for the final examinations.[28]

After all the study, the work, the indignity of the disguise, it seemed the plan would come to nothing. At the same time, the cost of studying and living in Edinburgh was becoming unsustainable, and Mrs Bulkley was growing frantic: by April she had debts of £80, and a planned trip to London had to be postponed because her creditors wouldn't allow her to leave Edinburgh. She pleaded with Mr Reardon for an advance on the sale of her late brother's works, and prayed to God for James's graduation, which would 'put an end to all my extraordinary expences'.[29] If the graduation didn't take place, it would be a disaster in every conceivable way; no money, mounting debts, no qualification, no prospects.

The Earl of Buchan would not allow such a thing. With incontrovertible logic, he pointed out to the Senate that there was nothing in Edinburgh University's statutes to prevent a boy of any age from being examined and awarded his degree. The professors conferred, and were forced to admit that His Lordship was perfectly correct. They reversed their decree.[30]

So, in July 1812 James Barry began the ordeal that, it was hoped, would bring all his plans to perfection. Three weeks prior to the examination, he presented the certificates of attendance for all the courses he'd taken, and paid the £10 examination fee. The first stage of the exam was an oral interrogation – like all exams, conducted entirely in Latin – held at the house of one of the professors. Having passed this, James proceeded to the next stage: a series of further written and oral exams held in the University Library, on all aspects of his studies. The centrepiece of the process was the oral examination on his *Disputatio Medica Inauguralis* – his inaugural dissertation – which was conducted in the university's public hall in front of all the other MD candidates (of whom there were fifty-eight that year).[31]

James had been working on the dissertation since the end of the previous summer, and its Latinity had been duly inspected by Dr Anderson.

Significantly, James had taken as his subject the condition known as *mer-ocele*, or femoral hernia, a relatively rare type almost entirely confined to women.[32] In the introduction, he remarked that one of the reasons for this (aside from anatomy) was the practice of wearing corsets – 'now, happily, less common'. Margaret's generation had been spared, but unfortunately for women everywhere, corsets would make a huge comeback in the 1820s, tighter than ever and causing a world of discomfort, damage and illness.

His dissertation gave no hint as to why a young boy should be so interested in a female condition. He'd also studied midwifery to a more advanced level than most students. This might have been a side effect of his choice of curriculum, which included military surgery (for the purpose of serving General Miranda); midwifery was a requirement for military doctors, who typically had officers' wives to care for (students were also advised to study eye diseases and 'mental derangement', both chronic problems in the Army).[33]

De Merocele vel Hernia Crurali, by Jacobus Barry, *Anglus*,* expensively printed and bound, was dedicated jointly to the author's benefactors: to General Francisco de Miranda, 'exalted and most celebrated leader ... on account of his fatherly care and the very many favours bestowed on James Barry and his family'; and secondly to 'that best and most worthy of men', David Steuart Erskine, 11th Earl of Buchan. Still smarting from the Senate's earlier ban, James inserted a Greek epigraph taken from Menander: 'Do not consider whether what I say is a young man speaking, but whether my discussion with you is that of a man of understanding.'[34]

The Principal consulted the professors, who declared that James Barry and his peers had merited their doctorates. On payment of yet another fee – the enormous sum of £24 3s – James was awarded his degree and the coveted 'MD' after his name.

Dr James Barry had been officially conjured into existence. Three years of planning, of studying, of financial anxiety and of dangerous deception had come to fruition. The professors had been prevailed upon, or so they believed, to confer the precious doctorate upon a mere boy; it never crossed their minds that they'd given it to a woman.

As for whether that 'best and most worthy of men' Lord Buchan had any suspicions about his protégé, perhaps it is significant that he chose

---

* Englishman

the year of James Barry's graduation to republish a collection of his essays and polemics, including a piece first written in 1793 – shortly after the publication of Mary Wollstonecraft's *Vindication* – on the education of women. The female sex, Buchan argued, 'in the present state of civilised society, should have, in almost every respect, an as truly learned institution as men'. Women should be entitled to 'an education no way differing from that of men, in all things relating to the cultivation of the rational powers' and 'every instruction in the sciences and fine arts'.[35] Perhaps Buchan knew James's secret – perhaps he had guessed, or perhaps Margaret had loved and respected him enough to confess. If he found out, he kept the secret.

(Buchan's essay made no difference to the world. As Sir Walter Scott and many other contemporaries often noted, David Steuart Erskine was a man clearly not right in the head, and society took no notice of his eccentric views.)

James was looking to the future; he had discussed his plans – which weren't at all secret – with Buchan, who just a few months earlier had mentioned to a friend that young Barry meant 'to go by invitation of General Miranda to the Caracas'.[36] The charade was as good as over. With all her plans perfected, the time was coming for Margaret to cross the ocean and fight for revolution, putting aside the shell of James Barry, casting off the surtout, the cravat, the breeches and hat, the posture and imposture. Margaret Bulkley would emerge again, bringing her dresses out of storage, saved forever from the doom of drudgery as a governess or a man's possession. In the new revolutionary utopia of Venezuela, all that would matter would be her hard-won skills and knowledge. Margaret had come a long way in the three years since embarking on the voyage to Leith; now it was time to sail back in triumph, then on to a new, bright future.

Things had progressed while Margaret had been in Edinburgh. A coup had occurred in Venezuela in 1810, without Francisco de Miranda's involvement, and the new government had sent a small delegation to London to meet the British government and bring back Miranda. Among them was a youthful revolutionary called Simón Bolívar, who looked up to Miranda as a mentor and recognised that the revolutionary government's diplomacy depended on his network of connections. He'd returned with Bolívar to Caracas, where he received a mixed reception – many Venezuelans distrusted him due to his long absence.[37] Also, it was a struggle to sustain an independent republic in a land marked by turmoil, and Miranda's idealism was at odds with Bolívar's authoritarianism. The situation rapidly devolved into war.

Exactly when the bad news reached Margaret is not recorded. In July 1812, while James Barry was going through his final exams, General Miranda's fortunes suffered a terrible reversal. Following a year of violent turmoil and political intrigue, he was betrayed by Bolívar. Accused of treason, Miranda was handed over to the Spanish royalist authorities and taken back to Spain, where he was thrown into a dungeon in the Arsenal de la Carraca in Cádiz. He never saw freedom again.

There would be no Venezuelan dawn for Margaret Bulkley. Without her principal benefactor and the unique escape route he had offered, she had no choice but to remain in Britain, no more able to escape her male persona than Miranda could free himself from his Spanish gaol. Whatever the future held, Dr James Barry was not yet done with, and the trunk of dresses and petticoats would remain shut.

8

'I Would Be a Soldier'

Southwark: Friday 6 November 1812

A little before ten o'clock in the morning, opposite the Boar's Head tavern on the Borough High Street, a young man looked to cross the road, which was filled with the press of vehicles coming down from London Bridge: hackney coaches, carriages, dozens of carts and wains filled the carriageway in both directions, grinding along between the tightly packed rows of shops and inns. He had the appearance of a gentleman, but one short of cash; carefully but not expensively dressed, he wasn't at all out of place in this district, which was far from fashionable. Southwark had an odd character, as if it couldn't decide what kind of place it ought to be; parts were almost genteel, but there were industrial works, riverfront wharves, and dark, dangerous areas of poverty like the notorious 'Mint', a festering rookery west of the High Street filled with dens of thieves.[1]

The young man, carrying a black leather bag, dodged nimbly across the road between the vehicles, walked a little way among the crush of foot-passengers, then turned in at the great iron gateway of St Thomas's Hospital, which was just being unlocked by the head porter.[2] Within the hospital gates was a courtyard surrounded by three-storey colonnaded buildings housing the female wards. Scarcely glancing about, Dr James Barry hurried through the next archway and up the steps to the second courtyard, fronted by the chapel in which the elderly hospitaller,* Reverend Servington Savery, gave morning prayers four times a week (all walking patients were obliged to attend). Dr Barry passed on to the third and final courtyard, Clayton's Square; here were the male wards,

---

* chaplain

and on one side the admissions rooms and the shop of St Thomas's apothecary, Richard Whitfield, to whom Dr Barry was a pupil. Despite his
qualification, James was only a student of the hospital, albeit one who
was uncommonly highly trained.

After coming down from Edinburgh, Margaret had had to remain in
the guise of James Barry; he had a real existence in the world now, and
only through him could she make use of the knowledge and skills she
had so painstakingly acquired. Margaret might have defied society and
hoped to be taken seriously as a female practitioner, perhaps abroad. It
wouldn't be wholly unthinkable; Margaret King, Lady Mount Cashell,
who had disguised herself to study medicine at Jena, now practised without disguise in Pisa.[3] But her case, even if Margaret knew about it, was
different; although Lady Mount Cashell had studied, she hadn't qualified; her practice was confined mainly to children and was homely and
unorthodox. She was not by any means a professional doctor. Moreover,
she was an aristocrat, and therefore permitted a degree of eccentricity.

For the time being, Margaret put Dr James Barry to work in the only
way she knew – as a student. There was always more learning to acquire,
and skills to be perfected.

It was an expensive choice – the Barry inheritance was long gone,
and everything had to be paid for by borrowing. On 17 October 1812,
James had signed on as a pupil to Richard Whitfield for a period of six
months, paying £20 for the privilege.[4] He was the only MD to do so;
Whitfield's pupils were normally surgical apprentices or trainee apothecaries. He also signed up for lecture courses in anatomy and surgery,
which cost another 10 guineas;[5] his Edinburgh training had equipped
him well in these subjects, but in London he would have the advantage
of learning from the great Astley Cooper, the surgeon at Guy's Hospital,
who ran the course in collaboration with St Thomas's surgeon, Henry
Cline. And unlike the Middlesex or Bart's, Southwark was far removed
from the districts where Margaret and her mother had previously lived,
and where the risk that she might be recognised and unmasked hardly
bore thinking about.

St Thomas's was an ancient institution, founded in Southwark in the
Middle Ages. Guy's, which had been constructed amidst the warren of
backstreets and inn-yards behind St Thomas's, was much newer, founded
in 1721 by the rich bookseller whose name it bore. They'd become partner

institutions (known as the United Hospitals) and, as a pupil, Dr Barry would be able to attend at both. He'd enrolled somewhat late (again); Cooper and Cline's course had begun on the first of the month,[6] and James would retake the entire course again when it had its winter run in January, extending his knowledge of surgery and taking the opportunity to walk the wards of a London hospital as part of a great surgeon's retinue.

Today, being Friday, Astley Cooper would make his ward rounds. In the meantime, there was dispensing work to do in the apothecary's shop, and patients to attend. Up to 450 could be accommodated at St Thomas's, all from London's poorer classes.[7] The hospital's motto was *miseratione non mercede* ('for compassion, not for gain'), and it was declared that all the sick 'without distinction, or regard to any other consideration than the extent and degree of their sufferings, are humanely received'.[8] In fact, compassion required a small donation; an admission fee of 3s 6d was charged, which was increased to 10s 6d if the patient's condition was of a 'foul' or 'unclean' kind (meaning venereal). This made it virtually impossible for the very poorest to get into hospital, and they had to take their chances or go to the dreaded workhouse infirmary.

Despite the hospital's 'come all' principle, each case depended on several factors. In addition to the entry fee, the would-be patient had to provide a sponsor (typically a churchwarden) who undertook to supply clean body linen once a week and pay a guinea deposit to cover the expense of burial in the event of death (or swear to dispose of the body himself). A personal recommendation from one of the hospital governors was also required. These hurdles ensured that would-be patients were winnowed down to those considered morally worthy and unlikely to be an excessive burden. There were medical restrictions too – St Thomas's wouldn't admit anyone who was 'visited, or suspected to be visited, with the plague, itch,* scald-head,† or other infectious diseases',[9] nor anyone with an incurable condition. Other hospitals (such as Guy's) took incurable and chronic illnesses, while St Thomas's specialised in treating injuries, hernias, ulcers, stones, inflammations, aneurysms, tumours, some infections and a variety of acute conditions.

If the petitioner passed all the requirements and was deemed suitable, he or she would pay the admission fee and be taken to the appropriate

---

* scabies
† ringworm of the scalp (*tinea capitis*)

ward.[10] In return for that nominal few shillings, the patient would be cared for, treated, and provided with food and clean bed linen until either cured or dead, whichever came sooner. (There was a limit of six months, after which the illness would be officially deemed incurable, and the patient would be discharged.)

Treatment was the best of its day – that is to say, a blend of exquisite skill and diabolical crudeness; blood-letting, leeches and amputation of limbs were among the commonest treatments, along with sophisticated, specialised surgery and efficacious remedies. General hygiene was limited, and its importance poorly understood, but St Thomas's was better than many London hospitals, which were generally damp, infested with rats and fungus, and where unwashed patients could lie untended for days at a time, with operations carried out on the ward, in sight of other patients.[11]

Discipline at St Thomas's was strict; patients were expected to be compliant, sober and orderly, religiously devout, and adhere meticulously to the segregation of sexes. They could be ejected from the hospital if they didn't conform. Until lately the governors had had the power to physically punish unruly patients, and there had been a whipping post and stocks in the hospital grounds – at the time of James Barry's arrival, the stocks had only recently been removed.[12]

As well as treatment, the patients were provided with diets designed for their health. The full diet was twelve ounces of bread per day on top of a breakfast of gruel, dinner of beef or boiled mutton and butter or cheese, and a supper of broth. For some there was a milk diet (recommended for gout and tuberculosis), consisting of two or three pints a day, and rice pudding for dinner. Then there were reduced 'dry' and 'fever' diets. Most patients had two pints a day of a special beer brewed in the hospital, 'deemed an excellent common beverage for the patients', but if a stronger drink such as porter or wine was thought necessary, it was provided and 'of the very best kind',[13] all paid for by the hospital charity on the grounds of proven medicinal efficacy. There were absolutely no vegetables in any of the diets, as they were not believed to have any beneficial properties.[14] St Thomas's was proud of its attention to diet, and found that in some cases the regimen was almost sufficient in itself to effect a cure.

Care was given to the moral and spiritual well-being of the patients, in the expectation that sobriety and virtue were good for their health, diverting them from 'those excesses from which it is so difficult for the lower classes to be weaned'.[15] To this end, scriptural and theological literature was provided by the hospitaller (much of it on the subject of preparing one's soul: 'As sickness is the usual forerunner of death … reflect on your behaviour in life, and carefully examine yourselves how far prepared you are for that great change').[16] Unsurprisingly, some patients abused their periodic leaves of absence by getting drunk.

Three times a week the physicians and surgeons gathered to variously admit in-patients, see out-patients and make rounds of the wards, with individual rounds twice a week. Between those times, the job of tending to patients' general needs fell to the nurses, while their medical needs were handled by the apothecary, Mr Whitfield. As was common in most trades, Richard Whitfield had inherited his post at St Thomas's from his father, and in due course would hand it on to his son. He was more highly salaried than the surgeons and physicians (who worked part-time), and took a sizeable remuneration from the fees paid by students and pupils.[17] He worked hard for his money; whereas his colleagues attended the hospital a few times a week, the apothecary was there every day, working long hours. Besides dispensing, he made a round of the wards twice a day, advising, observing and prescribing. James had chosen wisely in attaching himself to him, there being no better way of learning the hospital and its workings inside-out; he saw more of the wards than a surgical apprentice would, and polished up his *materia medica*, spending long hours in the dispensary or in the garret above St Thomas's church, a long, airy space accessed from the hospital and used for storing herbs. James took a particular interest in medicinal botany, and there was much to fascinate him among the bundles, sprigs and jars stored under the dusty rafters.[18]

That Friday morning, James had only a short time in the dispensary before joining Mr Whitfield on his morning round, which began at half-past ten. With well over four hundred patients in about twenty wards, it was a long task. The wards on the ground floor tended to be gloomy because of the colonnades, but the upper floors were brighter; they had all recently been refurnished with light iron bedsteads, much easier to keep clean than wooden ones. Some wards were specialised; patients who had undergone lithotomy,* a procedure pioneered by St Thomas's, were kept in a ward close to the operating theatre, where they were supervised

---

* removal of bladder stones

by Mrs Wilcox, a nursing sister experienced in such cases. There were four wards for 'foul' or 'unclean' (venereal) patients and St Thomas's was proud of being the first hospital in London to have such wards, with one for the 'immodest women' and another three for men.[19]

So attuned was St Thomas's to moral virtue and sexual segregation, there was even a separate operating theatre set aside for female patients – a unique feature among the London hospitals. It was believed that the extreme modesty of even working-class women made them appreciate being operated upon in a room that was never used by men (aside, of course, from the male surgeon, dressers, apprentices and pupils who attended the operations, whom the women were supposed not to notice).[20]

By the end of the ward round, James would have been keeping an anxious eye on the time; at one o'clock Mr Astley Cooper would begin his round at Guy's. A few minutes before the hour, James parted from the apothecary; passing out through the side gate into St Thomas's Street, he hurried along the narrow, twisting way to Guy's, where Mr Cooper held the post of senior surgeon. It was a rather grander edifice than St Thomas's; whereas the latter had grown over the centuries to fit its ground, Guy's had imposed itself on Southwark. A stately building surrounding a quadrangle fronted by high railings, it was modelled on the Palladian style.[21] James crossed the quadrangle to the main building, where a rapidly growing crowd of pupils stood on the steps.

The buzz of conversation, the air of expectation and excitement and the size of the assembly were all quite beyond anything at Edinburgh. By the time the hour chimed, about a hundred young men were gathered. As one they spotted the carriage turning in at the gate, and the atmosphere heightened – Mr Astley Cooper had arrived.

Although still some years away from his baronetcy, Astley Paston Cooper was already a colossus, renowned as much for his fabulous wealth (upwards of £15,000 a year) as for the professional brilliance and personal charisma that had earned it. He was a man of extraordinary gifts and amazing devotion to the minutiae of his science and craft.

Each morning Cooper would rise at six and spend an hour or two working in the dissecting room at the back of his house (his home being also his practice), incorporating a consulting room and bed chambers for a select few of his surgical patients. Having quenched his thirst for practical anatomy, he would deal briskly with some of the poor 'gratuitous' patients who flocked to his house seeking treatment. Only then would he allow himself a small breakfast before proceeding to the consulting room to attend to his private, paying patients. Eventually, before one o'clock, with the aid of his manservant, he would push through the crowds of importunate would-be patients (some having travelled from out of town in the hope of a consultation) to the door, mount his carriage, and travel from the City across the river to Guy's.[22]

One hundred pairs of eyes watched the carriage circle the quadrangle and halt before the steps; they observed the door swing open and the august gentleman descend. Forty-four years old and ageing gracefully, Astley Cooper cut a robust figure; heavily built (but stopping short of obesity), he had poise and dressed finely, wearing his white stock high under the chin and favouring dark coats and waistcoats, closely cut and with collars of velvet or fine black fur, giving him the air of a Romantic poet rather than a surgeon. His fair hair was receding, swept carelessly back and set off with sandy side-whiskers, his profile was stern, but his cheeks dimpled around the mouth, which tended naturally to smile, and he projected an air that inspired warmth and confidence among those who met him. His manner was cheerful and courteous, with a voice to match; the son of a Norfolk clergyman, he still spoke with the soft burring accent of his native county. Without exception, students admired and liked him: 'He was the idol of the Borough school,' one contemporary recalled.[23]

James Barry was susceptible to the charisma of great men – even more than young men generally are – and had a talent for attracting their attention and favour. James knew that from the moment of Cooper's arrival it was each man for himself in the contest to gain his notice, his favour, or even see anything at all. As perhaps the only MD present among the students, James had the advantage of medical as well as surgical knowledge. Cooper spoke first to his dressers* and the older, more knowledgeable students, who were asked for details of any particularly important or interesting cases; here James's qualifications and dedication would make him an outstanding informant. His reticence had been left behind in Edinburgh, the disguise having been thoroughly mastered.[24]

---

* experienced surgical apprentices or students employed to assist with preparing and applying dressings

Following Cooper on the wards was a very different experience from accompanying his counterpart, Mr Henry Cline, senior surgeon at St Thomas's. Cooper had been Cline's apprentice, and they were close friends, but as men they were different in almost every way. Cline was described by one surgical apprentice as 'a tall, sickly, and very plain man, marked with small-pox, and very shy; but when he spoke his smile was most pleasing and agreeable ... his hair was most oddly dressed, a sort of *toupet*, with longish hair combed down straight, and matted with pomatum and powder ... he looked as if he had put his head in the dripping-pan on one side, and the flour tub on the other.'[25] He was kind, but hadn't the charisma of Cooper, and his lectures, like those of Monro at Edinburgh, were monotonous and slow. Nonetheless, it was said that 'to have been a pupil of Cline, and to have carried a box* under his superintendence, always gave a man a character and lift in his after life'.[26]

As the crowd processed from ward to ward, interesting cases were discussed and commented upon by Mr Cooper – especially those needing or having received surgery. No operation was undertaken lightly, partly because of the risk, partly because of the distress to the patient. Any surgeon intending to operate was required to give notice to his colleagues, who often wished to be present.

So traumatic was it for the patient that they were given 4 shillings 'operation money' to buy extra comforts during their recovery. There was no notion of surgical hygiene; hands were washed *after* an operation to remove the detritus, never before; indeed, practitioners would frequently go straight from the dissecting room to the wards or theatre without washing their hands at all. Disease was believed to come from direct contact with a sick person or from foul miasmas in the air, and nobody suspected the existence of transferable microscopic agents of infection. The high mortality rates among women in childbirth, the sick and the recipients of surgery were attributed to constitutional weakness or bad environments. It would be another thirty years before it began to dawn on doctors that they were literally carrying the cause of the problem in their own hands.[27]

Once the ward round was complete, some students drifted away, while the rest of the procession hurried along the street to St Thomas's

---

* act as dresser

and piled into the anatomical theatre, where Mr Cooper would deliver today's lecture.[28] The Theatre for Anatomical and Chirurgical Lectures was notorious; cramped, poorly ventilated and stinking of putrefaction, it was so vile that many pupils avoided lectures, 'lest they should endanger their health, and perhaps their existence'.[29] James Barry braved it for the sake of the priceless knowledge on offer.

There were over forty lectures on Cooper's course, with subjects ranging from dislocation of the ankle to ulceration, gangrene, head injuries, suppuration, spinal injuries, urinary calculi and lithotomy, nasal polyps, hare lip, contusions, fractures and dislocations, hernias, and the most dramatic of all: amputation.[30] Of particular interest to James was a subject that came about three-quarters of the way through the course – femoral hernia, the subject of James's MD dissertation, which had cited Cooper's published notes as a source (observing with interest that his surgical method differed from that of other surgeons). Cooper had pioneered the anatomising of this condition, and now came the opportunity to hear it all from the man himself, who was as accomplished a lecturer as he was a surgeon:

> His clear silvery voice and cheery conversational manner soon exhausted the conventional hour … He had no pretensions to oratory, spoke with a rather broad Norfolk twang, often enlivened us with a short 'Ha, ha!' and when he said anything which he thought droll, would give a very peculiar short snort and rub his nose with the back of his hand.[31]

Watching Cooper operate was an inspiration. He was noted for his solicitude as well as his skill; he 'brought confidence and comfort; and … on an operating day, should anything occur of an untoward character in the theatre, the moment Astley Cooper entered, and the instrument was in his hand, every difficulty was overcome, and safety generally ensued.'[32] One former student recalled, 'I can never forget the enthusiasm with which he entered upon the performance of any duty calculated to abridge human suffering.'[33] When he carried out an operation at Guy's, the theatre would be crammed to the rafters with students and observers – 'packed like herrings in a barrel, but not so quiet'.[34]

> The elegance of his operation … all kindness to the patient, and equally solicitous that nothing should be hidden from the observation of the

pupils – rapid in execution – masterly in manner … The light and elegant manner in which Sir Astley employed his various instruments always astonished me.[35]

In an age when surgery was a pain-wracked, gasping horror, in which patients had to be held down while the surgeons cut and sawed, such reassurance was welcome. It was little wonder that his contemporaries' recollections of him strayed into the realm of hero-worship. Some of his pupils, as they grew older and took students of their own, wished that more would take Astley Cooper as a role model – not only for his skill but for his character, which provided a fine example for medical students, 'who sadly lack moral discipline'.[36]

The Borough High Street was still busy when James left the hospital a little after seven o'clock. The cold evening damp brought down the choking fog of coal-smoke into the streets, mingling with the thick odour of the huge brewery that sat on the far side of the Borough Market, its miasma of yeast and hops wrapping around the tower of St Saviour's Church and seeping through the windows of the lodging houses. James crossed the road and entered a narrow house, one of a row of near-identical old buildings in St Saviour's shadow, where he shared lodgings with his aunt. He had an hour to spare for a bite to eat before returning to St Thomas's for Mr Whitfield's evening round.

It was immediately obvious that something was wrong. Mrs Bulkley was ghostly white, and more agitated and upset than she had ever been before, her hands trembling violently. Lying open on the table beside her was a letter from their friend and benefactor – and James's tutor in Latin – Dr Robert Anderson. It was only too easy to guess what it was about.

Earlier that year, while James had been preparing for final examinations, he and Mrs Bulkley had been living on debts already totalling £80. Mrs Bulkley had again convinced herself that she could sell the *Pandora* for a good price, and had rushed to London.[37] While there she'd had to borrow more money, and at her request James had approached Dr Anderson for help. He kindly endorsed a bill of exchange for £70, made out to Mrs Bulkley, the sum to be repaid (without interest) in five months. Like many a generous person who'd backed bills for friends, Dr Anderson discovered the folly of kindness.

James looked despondently at the letter. Embarrassment and suppressed indignation were in every line:

> Yesterday, the bill bearing to have been accepted by you, was returned to me, protested in London for non-payment* when it became due; although Dr Barry received the money, not me, it became necessary for me, as the indorser, to pay the bill & expences.[38]

Eager to resolve 'this awkward business' in a way that would be least painful for Mrs Bulkley, Dr Anderson had had a new bill drawn up for the full amount. If Mrs Bulkley accepted and signed it, it would be due for payment in just ten days. It hurt Robert Anderson to have to take this step; he and his daughter had been very fond of James, and continued to wish him well.

The new bill was enclosed. This was excruciating and utterly impossible; they couldn't hope to raise over £70 in ten weeks, let alone ten days. The wretched *Pandora* still hadn't been sold, and they had nothing. Their only prospect was a remote one; a gentleman in Piccadilly had been encouraged by Lord Buchan to take an interest in the painting and it looked as if he might bite, but there was no certainty of it, and not the slightest chance of its occurring within ten days. Dr Fryer had tried to persuade James to become involved – not just for the sake of the sale but as a first step towards becoming a professional gentleman in London society; 'I wish after all that the Doctor would arrange the terms,' he'd written to Mrs Bulkley the previous week. 'It may make him known to people, who may be of use to him, and will initiate him in the business of negotiation – of treating in a matter of your interest and his.'[39] Margaret knew as well as Dr Fryer that if James Barry hoped to follow the lucrative path of the Anthony Carlisles and Astley Coopers of this world, such connections would be vital. But it was easier proposed than done; it would require Margaret to subject her disguise to an unprecedented degree of scrutiny where there were people who'd known Miss Bulkley before her transformation.

It was as if the Barry inheritance was cursed – Redmond had lost his portion and ended up in prison, while the anxiety of managing the estate had driven Mrs Bulkley to the brink of death. Margaret's share of the

---

* *protest*: a written statement of non-payment

fortune had been exchanged for an education that now looked endless, useless and laden with insoluble debt. Had she been born a man, with the patronage of the likes of Dr Fryer and the Earl of Buchan to call on, her future as a physician or a surgeon would be absolutely secure and literally golden.

For the time being, keeping James Barry alive was her only choice. A gulf had grown between James and the Margaret Bulkley who had first put on this disguise – a gulf of four years filled to the brim with knowledge, experience and new skills. It was Margaret who possessed all that, and the talents that had enabled it, and yet outwardly she had no existence. This struggle with identity was difficult, and must inevitably exact a price; a price in emotional stress that would grow with the passage of years.

Dr Barry left the house that evening with the dilemma unresolved, and returned to St Thomas's for the evening round. At about the same time, Astley Cooper, having dined, would be setting out in his carriage to pay calls on his richest patients – those who could afford his enormous visiting fees and who'd been known to tip him 1000 guineas for a single operation.[40] James could earn money by treating the working poor in this part of Southwark – a recourse often taken by impoverished medical students – without any risk of exposure, but the remuneration would be in shillings.

A week after receiving Dr Anderson's bill, they replied, stating that Mrs Bulkley would not sign it. Dr Anderson was saddened and wounded, and reminded them that the bill 'was judged to be the least expensive & most convenient way for you to repay the money I paid for you',[41] and that he had originally endorsed Dr Barry's bill out of concern for his welfare. 'In this case,' he wrote reluctantly, 'I have no alternative but to send the bill which you accepted to London to be put into the hands of a Solicitor.'

If the £70 was ever repaid, it left no trace in the historical record. Certainly neither Mrs Bulkley nor James Barry could raise such a sum without the sale of the *Pandora*, and that did not occur – their elusive buyer's interest fizzled out.[42] Possibly some compromise was reached, since James could not afford to alienate Dr Anderson and risk losing the support of his most influential patron, the Earl of Buchan.

James continued at the United Hospitals until April 1813. Finally, the decision about what to do with his future could no longer be postponed.

Private practice was as feasible as any other course; after all, there were cities other than London with wealthy inhabitants, where a medical man with powerful sponsors could do well and where Margaret Bulkley wasn't known. But something in her balked at this path. It would cost a lot of money to become established. Money could be borrowed, but Margaret had never known anything but trouble come from that. In the end, with money as the driving force, her adventurous spirit – the very same that had made her take on the guise of a man in the first place – probably guided the decision.

Some five years earlier Margaret had taunted her hapless brother about 'the wisdom or folly resulting from your substituting a musquet for a goosequill' and added with bravado, 'Was I not a girl I would be a Soldier!'[43] Now she had the opportunity to make that come true, exchanging James's tailcoat for a scarlet jacket.

Whether out of wisdom or folly, the decision was made. Dr James Barry would join the Army.

9

Qualified to Serve

Plymouth Hoe: Sunday 30 July 1815

The sun was going down over Plymouth Sound, illuminating the masts standing in thickets and copses here and there on the water, and picking out a great two-decked man-of-war anchored alone far off-shore, in the gap between Drake's Island and Mount Batten. Standing on the cliff at the point of the Hoe, a young officer with red-gold hair stood looking at the scene; the lowering sun saturated his scarlet coatee, glinted on its gold buttons and on the sword at his hip. He knew that ship's name – everyone in the Three Towns knew it; her arrival a few days earlier from Tor Bay had caused an epidemic of gossip and rumour in every parlour, tap-room and newspaper in the land about the infamous prisoner aboard her – the Thief of Europe, the monster, the usurper, the so-called 'Emperor', Napoleon Bonaparte. Just over a month had passed since his defeat at Waterloo, and he was now a captive. Taking advantage of a Sunday afternoon recess in the busy life of the Military Hospital, Acting Assistant Surgeon James Barry had walked down to the Hoe to see what all the fuss was about.

The ship was HMS *Bellerophon* – the very same seventy-four-gun ship of the line that had visited Cork in the winter of 1797, when a little girl named Margaret had seen her cutter sail up to the city. That little girl had not had the slightest expectation – although she'd had the fancy – that she would one day wear the King's uniform. Neither could she have imagined the journey that would take her from that day to this.

Margaret had been an infant when the French wars began, and war had been a constant background to her life. During the winter when James was at St Thomas's, there was conflict in the Americas, with forces from the United States attempting to wrest control of Canada from the British. At the same time, news came through of Napoleon's defeat in Russia. The retreat from Moscow had begun that October, and in early November there was news of a coup in Paris; by Christmas 1812 the last tattered remnant of the Grande Armée had left Russian territory. In Spain the British had been driven back to Portugal, but after Napoleon's defeat in Russia the French began to withdraw from Spain; Wellesley pursued and beat them decisively at Vitoria, advancing to the border of France.

At the same time, Margaret made her decision, and in June 1813, James Barry walked down Piccadilly, turned up Berkeley Street and ascended the steps of number 5 – the offices of the Army Medical Board. There he put his name on the list of applicants for the position of surgeon, giving his age as eighteen – a compromise between the truth of twenty-four and the appearance of about fourteen.[1] He was then directed to call at Horse Guards, the seat of the War Office.[2]

With the nation fighting on several fronts around the globe, Horse Guards was one of the busiest places in London. James waited for some hours in a corridor, watching the to-and-fro of officers of the staff in their bright, braided scarlet, with flashes of blue or green on a hussar. Eventually James was admitted to the office of Matthew Lewis, the Deputy Secretary at War, a dark-haired gentleman with fishy eyes and a perpetually flustered expression. He took James's details and provided him with a letter of introduction to the Royal College of Surgeons:

> Application having been made for Dr James Barry to be regimental assistant surgeon, I am directed by the secretary at war to desire that you will be pleased to examine the said James Barry and acquaint this office whether he is fitly qualified for the above station.[3]

James paid a fee of 5 shillings to Lewis's clerk and walked out into Whitehall with the letter securely tucked inside his coat. He'd completed his first step, and it was a momentous thing.

From Whitehall it was a brief walk to Lincoln's Inn Fields. There, facing authoritatively onto the greenery of the square was the brand-new pillared frontage of the Royal College of Surgeons of England (RCS), which was only that year being completed.[4] James presented his letter and had his name entered on the list of candidates, paying another 5-shilling fee to the College secretary, plus 2s 6d to the porter ('a lad must have his pocket regularly stripped by these associations, before he pretends to pass an examination,' the satirist George Cruikshank noted).[5]

As a symbol, the new building was not only a statement of authority, it was a bid for respectability. The Royal College had received its charter in 1800, and was still extricating itself from a centuries-old association with the trade of the barber-surgeon, setting itself on a footing with the more ancient Royal College of Physicians. It was a mighty task, and by 1813 had hardly begun. There was little in law to prevent any charlatan with a dubious diploma from calling himself a surgeon. Charles Dunne, a Royal Navy surgeon, complained:

> It is truly lamentable to see so many base quacks fostered in this country under the wing of our government, for the sake of the revenue produced by stamps … many empirics write over their door, '*Surgeon*,' without any legal qualification whatever, and that too in the very vicinity of the Royal College of Surgeons … Other worthless beings, who, by some stratagem, have obtained the college diploma, advertise to the manifest prejudice of the profession.[6]

The ability of 'worthless beings' to obtain diplomas from the RCS by 'stratagems' was indicative of a deeper problem, which the College had not even begun to address – the poorly regulated, easily subverted process by which its own examinations of prospective surgeons were conducted. Attempting to regulate the profession at large, it was scarcely conscious of the disorder and laxity in its own house. Likewise the medical departments of the Army and Navy were full of men who were 'preposterously ignorant of the profession of chirurgery, indeed of the rudiments of their own language'.[7] Dunne was far from alone in his views; another doctor wrote in 1810 that the 'enormous and complicated abuses' existing throughout the Army Medical Board were 'a grievance, not only involving the criminal expenditure of immense sums of the public money, but, in their consequence, affecting the health and life of the soldier, the rights and dignity of the Medical profession, and … the vital interests of the empire'.[8]

Besides harbouring poorly qualified men in surgical posts, the British Army appointed inexperienced men to the very highest positions, and it was rare to find a senior military surgeon who'd seen active service or been to the colonies. The system was riddled with favouritism, and despite official regulations, the promotion of unqualified and inexperienced men caused unnecessary suffering and death among British troops.[9]

That had begun to change. In 1808 the Parliamentary Commission of Military Enquiry had seized the Army Medical Board by its collective collar and shaken it until its teeth rattled;[10] the ensuing reforms were quick to initiate but slow to take root. Driven by the will of Lord Palmerston, in 1810 the Board was sacked, reorganised and regulations put in place for the proper qualification of medical appointments.[11] The Royal College of Surgeons of England, along with its Scottish and Irish counterparts, was the officially recognised authority on who was or was not qualified to practise surgery, its governors and examiners laying the rule against every candidate to determine whether he measured up. But in practice the College wasn't so reliable a regulator. An outward image of rigour was promoted by the College and its fellows – who had an interest in sustaining the mystique of their calling – but in fact the examination was childishly easy to pass.

On Friday 2 July, Dr James Barry returned to Lincoln's Inn Fields and entered the College;[12] he was directed to a hall at the foot of a grand flight of stairs, where he joined eight other apprehensive young men also waiting for their examination. (It was a quiet day; normally there would be up to thirty or forty candidates.) Most were apprentices from the provinces aiming for their diplomas, only two besides James seeking Army or Navy appointments. All were terrified by the coming ordeal, having been led by their mentors to believe that it would try them beyond their limits.

At the set hour, William Stone, the College beadle, clad splendidly in a long blue coat, tricorne hat, bright buckled shoes and an aura of enormous self-importance, strode out onto the half-landing above, struck the foot of his staff on the marble and called the names of the first batch of candidates.[13] The young men started, turned pale, and went hastily up the stairs, vanishing through the door into the examining room.

James, having registered late (something of a habit with him), was near the bottom of the list, and had to sit for an hour or more while the others paced up and down the hall or sat jiggling their feet or staring at the floor. At irregular intervals the beadle reappeared, the staff banged, and another batch of two or three would flinch and go to meet their doom. In each case, after a painful stretch of time, they would emerge again, either ashen or glowing, and resume their seats.

Eventually, 'James Barry MD!' came thundering down the stairs; he rose, and several pairs of eyes followed his diminutive figure up to the door.

James found himself in a large room in which the decorative theme was macabre grandeur.[14] A huge clock, ornately framed in gold, loudly marked the minutes, heavy, gold-fringed curtains flanked the windows, and paintings depicting anatomically curious subjects (including Saartjie Baartman, 'the Hottentot Venus') lined the walls. In a pair of niches in the wall behind the examiners stood the College's two notorious skeletons. One was of Elizabeth Brownrigg, hanged and publicly dissected in 1767 for the torture and murder of a female servant; her skeleton had been displayed in the old Surgeons' Hall next to Newgate Prison for years before the move to Lincoln's Inn Fields. It had lately been joined by the bones of Captain Joseph Wall, a colonial Governor and notorious drunkard who'd been convicted and hanged in 1802 for flogging several soldiers to death on the West African island of Gorée.

Beneath these exhibits stood the grand chair of the Master of the College, at the apex of the huge horseshoe table at which the examiners sat and scrutinised the unhappy candidates. On the floor in the centre of the horseshoe was a box of reference books, presided over by an assistant. The examiners – of whom there were eight in addition to the Master – were an assortment of elderly specimens, some well-dressed in the modern style, some clothed and wigged in the fashion of the previous century. They had an acute sense of their own eminence – many of them held appointments to the King, the Queen, the Prince of Wales or various high-ranking aristocrats and were immensely satisfied with themselves. There were fat faces and bony, harsh countenances and kind. While some of them studied James, others gave him barely a glance before resuming talking among themselves, consulting their papers, taking snuff, and in one case sleeping soundly, head back and snoring.[15]

Happily, there were at least two faces that were both friendly and familiar to James – Henry Cline, his former teacher from St Thomas's, and the elderly Mr George Chandler, also a long-serving surgeon at the hospital and the kindest of men. Patronage was still important, whether it involved money or simple favouritism based on professional connection (it had been known for certain examiners to vote to pass a candidate without questioning him, merely because he'd studied under one of that examiner's favoured former pupils).[16]

They conducted the examinations in pairs – one examiner quizzing the candidate on surgery, the other on anatomy – while the rest looked on, chipped in, or ignored the proceeding altogether. Some were fierce, others kind. George Chandler was said to have only ever failed one candidate, and felt so badly about it afterwards that he never did it again.[17] By contrast, Sir William Blizard, a formerly handsome man now aged and bony, was 'very stern' and 'delighted in terrorising the candidate';[18] he was also out of touch with modern anatomy, and sometimes confused candidates with his antique terminology.[19] The examination – which, unlike the MD, was conducted in English – consisted of a succession of deceptively simple, terse questions: 'Describe the organs of hearing, sir' … 'Where's the epigastric?' … 'How is bile secreted, sir?' … 'How would you treat a man who has ruptured some fibres of the gastrocnemius muscle?' Some of the elderly fellows were hard of hearing (at least two ear trumpets were on show), and any hesitant or soft-spoken candidate would be jolted by impatient barks of 'Speak up, sir!'

Some found the ordeal so distressing that their tongues locked up. 'It often happens,' wrote an examiner, 'that young men are exceedingly alarmed, and sometimes so much so, that they faint, or sit like statues, unable to answer a single question … We allow such candidates to retire for an hour or two, to recover their faculties, if they can.'[20]

But for a young man who was confident, who knew (or had skilfully crammed) his stuff or had the favour of an eminent member of the court, the ordeal was quite painless. So painless, in fact, that the young satirist George Cruikshank had posed as a candidate and passed, based solely on charisma, listening to the talk of the other candidates, and some slight experience of surgery. Despite the fearsome reputation of the Court of Examiners, the pass rate rarely fell below seventy-five per cent.[21] Contemptuous of the Royal College's pretensions, Cruikshank declared himself 'qualified to kill, hack and slay any or all of his majesty's subjects, without being indicted for murder'.[22] Other candidates, less cynical and insightful than Cruikshank, came down the stairs believing that their talent had seen them through – and thus the Court of Examiners continued to inspire fear or apprehension year after year, helped by the tales of candidates who'd been unlucky enough to be grilled by the few really harsh examiners.

James Barry was probably tested by Henry Cline, who, recognising his student, would have called him over, the other examiner being whichever fellow was next to him. James's experience of the much more demanding oral examinations at Edinburgh, together with the favour of Cline and the fact that he'd studied hard and was eminently prepared, must have made it a decidedly easy affair. He passed and was entered in the book as a prospective regimental assistant surgeon,[23] paid his 2 guineas fee (for civilians it was 22 guineas) and departed with his certificate:

Know all men by these presents, that we the Court of Examiners of the Royal College of Surgeons in London, have deliberately examined Dr James Barry, and find him fit and capable to exercise the Art and Science of Surgery; We therefore admit him as a Member of the College, and authorise him to practise the said Art and Science accordingly.[24]

At the same time, a letter was sent to the War Office:

To the Right Honourable the Secretary at War,
    … We have examined Dr James Barry, and find him qualified to serve as assistant surgeon to any regiment in his majesty's service. We are your most obedient servants, etc. etc.[25]

The final hurdle was another examination carried out by the Army Medical Board. Having passed the RCS on Friday, with barely a pause to catch his breath James was called to attend the Medical Board in Berkeley Street on Monday. This examination – also oral – explored the candidate's hospital experience, his mastery of anatomy, medicine, chemistry, *materia medica* (pharmacy) and botany.[26] The examiners were the three heads of the Medical Board, all still fairly new in their posts, having been appointed in the wake of the reforms of 1810. Unlike their predecessors they were all experienced military doctors with long service overseas.[27] They had reopened hospitals closed by their predecessors and improved the flow of surgeons and supplies to regiments serving abroad (though not nearly enough, as the aftermath of the Waterloo campaign would prove two years later).

    James passed, and his name was marked on the list as suitable to be a hospital assistant – the first rung on the ladder for a military doctor.[28] If he served satisfactorily, he would be promoted to assistant surgeon in due course.

Had Margaret been born sixty years later, her deception would have been impossible, due to a medical examination of an entirely different kind – a thorough head-to-toe physical inspection of the candidate, stripped to his skin. But in 1813, although recruits to the lowest ranks were stripped and scrutinised like cattle at an auction, the officer class was not subjected to such indignity; a gentleman's word was sufficient to certify him physically fit.[29]

When James Barry emerged from the office on Berkeley Street and walked down to Piccadilly on that summer day, he had crossed the Rubicon. As well as being a professional gentleman, he was now a soldier of the British Army, and getting out would be much more difficult than getting in. The only quick route back to civilian life would be through discovery, shame and ruin. Margaret was taking a terrible risk, without even the financial compensations that a society practice would have provided.

James's first posting was to the Military Hospital at Chelsea. Although it was only a few miles from London, this departure coincided with the fading away of the few ties Margaret still had in the metropolis, leaving a fog of uncertainty about what happened to her relationships with her mother, Dr Fryer and Daniel Reardon and his family, all of whom had been so vital in her career. Mrs Bulkley's letters to Mr Reardon in the spring of 1812 would be her last surviving correspondence, and the awkward business of Dr Anderson's bill of exchange was the last clear trace of her relationship with Margaret. James departed for Chelsea and didn't look back. It was as if, with the decision made and the die cast, Margaret was cutting off every link with the people who had known her before she became James Barry – just as she'd done to her father and brother, but this time the reason was unclear.[30] There was a new life ahead – yet it would continue to be haunted by the old, even decades later.

The York Hospital in the village of Chelsea was the great clearing-house for the sick and wounded from all the British Army's wars; they were sent here in their thousands and subjected to what Army regulations called 'a minute examination into their several conditions and capacity for further Service'.[31] Here it was determined whether they were fit, and if not, what manner of pension they would receive.

Most invalids – and most visitors – came to Chelsea by river. It was a pleasant journey upstream from the noisome press of London through the pastures and osier beds bordering the Thames up to Chelsea. They disembarked beside the main Chelsea Hospital, a handsome building set in formal grounds like a stately home, where only the most fortunate invalids would end up – those selected for a Chelsea pension (to 'get Chelsea' was a stock phrase in the Army, meaning an injury that was both severe and highly visible, such as a lost limb).[32] Newly arrived invalids were marched up through the village, past the Royal Military Asylum – another fine building, set aside for soldiers' children – and then into the warren of crowded, squalid streets surrounding Jews' Row, where York Hospital stood.

Overcrowded beyond bursting point, the York was set back from Five Fields Row, not far from Sloane Square, on the edge of the slum. A young Irish soldier, James Ewart, who'd lost an arm in the Peninsula and arrived at Chelsea in 1814, was shocked to find that 'the invalids, who by hundreds at a time were accustomed to congregate here, found it exceedingly difficult to procure a shelter, however humble, for their heads'. Failing to find accommodation anywhere, Ewart took refuge in the hospital chapel, which was already full of men and women who'd lit a fire in the middle of the floor and were 'smoking, drinking, and blaspheming to a degree which I had never witnessed even in Spain':

> The pictures which it recalls to my memory are loathsome in the extreme – for they represent the very squalor of poverty – with reckless and overmastering vice everywhere … and selfishness, the invariable attendant on these evils.[33]

By Ewart's reckoning, eleven thousand sick and wounded men were living rough in the area. When his case was eventually heard, like many others he received a crushing disappointment:

> I had flattered myself, and others also assured me, that my pension could not fall short of a shilling a day,– but we were in error. Their Lordships told me that I was young, and had served but a short time, and sent me about my business with the pittance of sixpence daily.[34]

It was in this environment that James Barry had his first experience of service with the Army Medical Department, as a hospital assistant on

6s 6d a day.[35] Since 1810 it had become standard practice for all new entrants to serve a short period at the York in order to give them a severe blooding before sending them out on active service. Most would be going to regiments in the Peninsula or the colonies, and they needed to be toughened up; in this respect, the York was the nearest thing the Army Medical Department had to a medical school.[36]

James Barry left no record of the four months he spent there. A fellow novice, William Gibney, who'd been a year below James at Edinburgh and joined the Army shortly after him, looked back on his time at the York with loathing:

I found myself something like a fish out of water among the comical set of fellows I met with at the York Hospital. Physicians, staff surgeons, hospital assistants, apothecaries, and the queer lot generally, composing the staff ... The principal medical officer was a stout, jolly looking Irishman, who somehow had obtained his position without having previously occupied any of the inferior grades.[37]

The hospital assistants worked under the direction of the surgeons, each taking it in turns to be officer of the day and deal with the overwhelming influx of wounded and ill. 'This duty came round disagreeably often,' wrote Gibney.[38] Conditions for the junior staff weren't much better than for the inmates; 'it was the bad commons and disgusting bedding which tried one most'. The officers' mess, known as 'the Ordinary', was 'very bad':

Our pound of beef was anything in the shape of meat, and as tough as shoe leather; the potatoes bad and badly boiled; one pound of bread of the brickbat nature; and a pint of porter sufficiently sour to necessitate our practising on ourselves the cure for diarrhoea; as for the bedding it was damp and dirty, with sheets so coarse as to act like nutmeg graters.[39]

For this miserable posting, James Barry had declined the lucrative prospect of setting up in private practice. But at least here, as one of the 'queer lot', and surrounded by misery, there was little chance of anyone noticing anything unduly remarkable about James's voice, physique and beardless face, other than his unusual youthfulness.

Wretched as it was, the York served its purpose in introducing new doctors to the character of British troops and their various wounds, illnesses and foibles:

> Some of them were really good, brave, and heroic fellows, who submitted to every kind of treatment and operation with undaunted courage; but others were most obstinate and discontented, using every kind of dodge to impose upon us young doctors, and to avoid being sent back to duty. To this end, some even of the younger soldiers, benefiting by the instruction given to them by old malingerers, caused sores and slight wounds ... to become inflamed and daily worse ... Fits were common and constantly enacted in the barrack yard, lameness was a general complaint, and not a few declared themselves to be hopelessly paralysed.[40]

Some of these 'malingerers' must have been suffering from traumatic stress, but in 1813 that condition had not even begun to be recognised by doctors.

Gibney endured the York for just six weeks before being gazetted in the 15th Hussars and heading off to war. But James Barry had to suffer the place for much longer; although his work was good, and he was appointed acting assistant surgeon after three months, his age had come into question again. He'd declared himself eighteen, but people wouldn't believe it, and the authorities would not send him to a regiment or overseas posting, nor confirm his assistant surgeon's rank.

Once again, the Earl of Buchan came to the rescue. Despite the painfully awkward episode with Dr Anderson and the bill of exchange, James's standing with Buchan had not been damaged, and although he had few Army connections, His Lordship lent his weight to the cause. A posting was found for James at the military general hospital at Stoke Damerel, Plymouth.[41] This wasn't quite the adventure the teenage Margaret had had in mind when she dreamed of a sword and colours, but it was progress. With autumn setting in, James packed up his kit and left Chelsea for Devon.

Plymouth was one of the engines of Great Britain's maritime power. The mouths of the rivers Tamar and Plym formed the huge natural anchorage of Plymouth Sound, with ready access to both the Channel and the

Atlantic. To landward stood the Three Towns – Plymouth itself, with its
harbour and fortified citadel, then the smaller settlement of Stonehouse
half a mile to the west, and finally the great military enclosure known as
Dock,* a vast fortified base and dockyard belonging to the Royal Navy,
where a large part of the fleet was built, berthed and serviced. Out on
the Hamoaze,† warships of every description, from trim little sloops to
mighty three-decked men-of-war, rode at anchor, with swarms of cutters,
tenders and bumboats darting among them.

Just inland from Dock, on the steep slope above Stonehouse Creek, in
the parish of Stoke Damerel, stood the Military Hospital, a chain of four
grey stone pavilion blocks three storeys high, fronted by a colonnaded
ambulatory running the full length of the building.[42]

Upon arrival, James reported to the Principal Medical Officer, Dr
Joseph Skey. In his late thirties and in the prime of his career, Dr Skey was,
in order, an Englishman, an Edinburgh graduate, a physician, an amateur
geologist and a veteran of service in the West Indies.[43] He was also deeply
shocked by the appearance of Acting Assistant Surgeon Dr James Barry.
As an Edinburgh man, Skey was acquainted with His Lordship the Earl
of Buchan (and presumably also with his eccentricities), and had taken
Barry upon his recommendation; but the person who presented himself
was a mere boy. This would not do at all.

Skey wrote immediately to Lord Buchan to protest, and was astonished – and not a little put out – to be told imperiously that it was 'not
desirable to agitate the question' of Dr Barry's age or suitability.[44] Taken
aback, Dr Skey reluctantly accepted Dr Barry onto his staff and set him
to work. Happily, within a few weeks James had proven his worth and
skill, and Skey wrote again to Lord Buchan, this time in a much more
positive mood. Buchan reported this outcome to Dr Anderson:

> Inclosed I send you a letter relating to poor James Barry which came
> to my hand a few days ago from Dr Skey ... to whom I had recom-
> mended him. Dr Skey's hand writing is almost illegible but I made it
> out after a good deal of decyphering and find that he has found favour
> with his principal whom I intend to thank for his attentions & request
> the continuance of them.[45]

---

* now Devonport
† Tamar estuary

Since James was clearly not going to escape this reputation for juvenility, he began to admit to it. Despite having given his age as eighteen when he enlisted, he eventually confessed that he had been born 'about 1799'.[46] As a result, he was denied the possibility of active or colonial postings for another three years. Inside the disguise, Margaret was now twenty-four years old, and yearning to escape. The fortunes of war in Europe were turning against Bonaparte, and it might not last; for Margaret it seemed that the opportunity for adventure and glory would elude her.

While Dr Barry eked out his service at Stoke Damerel, the wars on the Continent and in North America entered their final acts. In Europe, Bonaparte, in his ever-shrinking empire, fought a series of losing battles against the overwhelming forces of the Sixth Coalition. In March 1814 the allies entered Paris, and in April, Napoleon abdicated and was sent into exile on Elba.

The European war was over. The news, slow to reach the far southwest of England, burst dramatically – the *Royal Cornwall Gazette* announced the return of 'the good old times' and an 'honourable peace'. 'The glorious Era has at length arrived. Europe is Free!! – The reign of Tyranny and of Desolation is at an end; and the resplendent beams of Universal Peace and Happiness once more shine in dazzling radiancy!'[47] Ambitious officers subsided in disappointment or seethed with frustration. But within the year it would be realised that these declarations were premature; in February 1815 Bonaparte escaped from Elba and began his stunning return to power. The British government hastily got up off its rump, straightened its hat and got back on a war footing.

Having been wrong-footed once, the nation was rigid with tension through that unseasonably autumnal June when Napoleon set out from Paris with his reinvigorated army, heading for Brussels. The border was defended by the scattered, ill-prepared forces of the Seventh Coalition under the Duke of Wellington. The clash came at the end of the third week of June – a ferocious, pitiless campaign that was as brief as it was bloody, culminating on Sunday 18 June in a decisive battle in the farmland between the villages of Mont St Jean and Plancenoit, just south of Wellington's headquarters at the obscure village of Waterloo.

Away from the battlefield, conflicting reports were heard: Napoleon had been defeated; no, on the contrary, he had routed his enemies, taken

Brussels and was advancing on Antwerp; nonsense, the allies were in Paris ... Hope and panic bubbled up erratically everywhere. At last, on the following Thursday, four days after the battle, Wellington's official report was announced by the government. It was victory.

From London the news spread, carried along the highways and turn-pikes by mail coaches decked in laurels and emblazoned with triumphant posters, the coach guards blowing extravagant fanfares on their horns as they clattered into each town. It took a long while for the London coaches to arrive at the furthest parts of the nation, and it was on Saturday morning that the West Country mails reached Plymouth. From the coffee rooms of the coaching inns the news spread through the town – the battle had been a 'most sanguinary' one, in which whole regiments had been cut to pieces, but had culminated in final victory.[48] There were spontaneous celebrations – houses were illuminated, bonfires lit, there was gaiety and drinking in the streets.

Reports from Belgium indicated a battle so violent and costly that it had shocked even the most hardened veterans. There had been a dire shortage of surgeons and hospital assistants. Each regiment had one surgeon and two assistant surgeons, in addition to the staff complement at the main hospitals. So many amputations were performed that the surgeons' knives were blunted by use. Charles Bell, a private practitioner who went to Belgium to observe and assist, was exhausted by the demand, operating from six in the morning until seven in the evening: 'All the decencies of performing surgical operations were soon neglected. While I amputated one man's thigh, there lay at one time thirteen, all beseech-ing to be taken next.' His clothes, saturated with blood, turned stiff as it congealed, and his arms were 'powerless with the exertion of using the knife'.[49] Piles of severed limbs grew outside the houses and barns used as makeshift hospitals. Some witnesses suspected that 'many a poor fellow had a limb cut off when it was not necessary, just that the young doctors might try their skill.'[50]

A good surgeon could perform a simple amputation in a few minutes; in both military and civilian life it was one of the commonest operations, carried out for compound fractures, gangrene and any untreatable injury or infection of the limb, and every surgeon's instrument case contained an amputation kit – long knives, a saw and tourniquets. There were two main methods. The commonest, used if the limb was to be removed above the knee or elbow, although classed as a 'capital' (major and potentially dangerous) operation, was relatively straightforward, and all surgeons were well practised in it.

First a tourniquet – in the form of a buckled canvas strap – was bound about the limb above the intended incision and pulled extremely tight. Then, using his largest knife (which often had a curved blade like a sickle to maximise reach), the surgeon reached around and under the limb, and, with a bold, sweeping cut around the circumference, incised through the skin and flesh down to the muscle. Most surgeons took two cuts to complete the incision, but a really skilled one could do it in a single stroke. An assistant would then roll back the skin and flesh from the upper edge of the incision, and the surgeon, using a similar stroke close to the folded edge, would cut through the muscle down to the bone. Then a cloth or a purpose-made metal plate was used to pull the mass of muscle and flesh upwards to expose a length of bone. The surgeon took his saw and cut through the bone, again working close to the pulled-back soft tissue. If he was an expert, a mere two minutes might have elapsed since the tightening of the tourniquet.

Now came the slower part of the operation – tying off the arteries with fine thread. Once that was done, the tourniquet was loosened, the retracted muscle released and the skin unrolled, providing a neat covering for the exposed end. The standard method was to fold it over like the end of a parcel, which in a well-provisioned hospital would be held in place by straps coated with a special oily adhesive plaster.[51] The whole procedure was quick; but where the limb had to be removed at the shoulder or hip, the operation was far more complicated, dangerous and time-consuming.[52]

Recipients of battlefield amputations were noted for their calm during the procedure, probably because their injuries were so painful that the surgeon's knife was barely noticeable. Survival rates were not good, especially in overcrowded, unsanitary military hospitals; after Waterloo, as many as nine out of ten amputees died. One eminent military surgeon reflected sadly on 'the poor sallow dejected beings that have pined in the hospitals' and recalling 'the flabby non-adhering inanimate stumps, lined with a discoloured half-digested sanies,* which have disappointed my most sanguine hopes – I shudder.'[53]

James Barry's experience thus far was confined to home service, but he knew all this intimately: the horrors of the operating theatre and the

---

* mixture of pus and blood serum

death-haunted surgical wards, the well-used knives and saw in his own surgical kit — and like other surgeons he had become inured to them, focused on the scientific fascination of the case. He would learn in due course how these miseries could be redoubled in the disease-ridden conditions of colonial outposts and on active service.

In the mass euphoria triggered by the news of Waterloo, while most were eager to celebrate, some people's thoughts were spared for the dead and wounded. During the first week of July the wretched aftermath appeared in England with the arrival of the first transports of wounded. The British went to the York in Chelsea (whose overcrowding must have become truly horrific) and the Isle of Wight, while thousands of French prisoners — wounded and unwounded — came to Plymouth.

On 7 July the first transports docked at Stonehouse Point. Two hundred Frenchmen — the first of an expected eight thousand — were marched through the town under a guard of Royal Marines. They wore ragged, filthy remnants of uniform, and many were bootless (they'd been thoroughly plundered by Prussians during the rout following the battle). The wounded were distributed among the Army and Navy hospitals while the walkers were marched off to the prison depot on Dartmoor. Many were veterans who had been prisoners in the last war, and were heard to remark 'that they knew the road to Dartmoor better than the Marines did'[54] (indeed, some of them had helped build it). The less fortunate were taken to the hulks anchored in the Hamoaze. Over the coming weeks, the prisons and hospitals filled with Frenchmen. Most were simply glad that the war was over; they exhibited 'the same frivolity and thoughtlessness which has always characterised the French nation', and 'not a single cry of "Vive l'Empereur" was heard among them'.[55] This was perhaps fitting, because that gentleman would soon be joining them as a prisoner himself.

From the cliff on the rim of Plymouth Hoe, James gazed at the ships anchored in the Sound. He cut a small but proud figure; having left behind the habit of shy withdrawal that had marked him in the early days of the disguise, he stood as tall as his five feet permitted, resplendent in a red coatee and Hessian boots, his small hand resting self-consciously on the hilt of his sword (surgeons, as members of the officer class, were expected to wear one, and James was uncommonly proud of his).[56]

Out on the Sound, HMS *Bellerophon* stood out amidst the flocks of small boats already beginning to surround her as sightseers came to gawp at the infamous visitor. Although Plymouth had been among the last places in England to hear of Bonaparte's defeat, it was one of the first to learn of his fate. In the weeks after Waterloo, contradictory rumours had come from France – that he'd been captured, or assassinated, or had escaped. In fact, he had made for the coast at Rochefort, hoping to flee to the United States, but had found the port blockaded by the Royal Navy. After prolonged negotiations, the fallen Emperor finally surrendered to Captain Maitland of HMS *Bellerophon* (known as 'Billy Ruffian' to her crew). Maitland set sail for English waters and dropped anchor in Tor Bay; the news was sent to London, and the government wondered frantically what to do with their captive. *The Times* called pugnaciously for 'that bloody miscreant who has so long tortured Europe' to be severely punished. 'The cruelty of this person is written in characters of blood in almost every country ... and if he be not now placed beyond the possibility of again outraging the peace of Europe, England will certainly never again deserve to have heroes such as those who have fought and bled at Waterloo.'[57]

While Whitehall havered, *Bellerophon* was ordered to move from Tor Bay to the more sheltered waters of Plymouth Sound. The news ran like a wind through the Three Towns, and soon every man, woman and child was heading for the water's edge to behold the ship. The cliffside roads became clogged with carriages, while legions of ladies and gentlemen, soldiers, sailors and idlers went out in boats to try to catch a glimpse of the bloody tyrant himself. Being vanity personified, Napoleon obliged, showing himself at the stern windows and strolling on the quarterdeck – a portly, green-coated figure accompanied by his military aides and his ladies. When several transports filled with French wounded sailed in, Napoleon 'earnestly looked at them from the stern gallery' as they passed.[58]

All the while the crowds of sightseers increased. Two frigates and a flotilla of guard-boats were stationed around the ship to keep them at bay. By Sunday, people had started arriving in Plymouth from all over the kingdom and hiring every boat and barge for miles around. Captain Maitland observed that 'the crowd of boats was greater than I ever remember to have seen at one time', estimating that 'upwards of a thousand were collected round the ship':

The crush was so great, as to render it quite impossible for the guard-boats to keep them off; though a boat belonging to one of the frigates made use of very violent means to effect it, frequently running against small boats, containing women, with such force as nearly to upset them, and alarming the ladies extremely. The French officers were very indignant at such rude proceedings, saying, 'Is this your English liberty? Were such a thing to happen in France, the men would rise with one accord and throw that officer and his crew overboard.'[59]

On several occasions, 'Billy Ruffian's' marines and crew were obliged to fire muskets and cannon to discourage the crowds.

The spectacle went on for more than a week, while the government's plans for Bonaparte were finalised. He was to be sent into exile on the remote island of St Helena, with a British regiment to guard him; Napoleon 'expressed the most violent determination'[60] not to suffer this fate, but he had no choice. On Friday 4 August *Bellerophon* weighed anchor and, towed by rowing boats in the slack breeze, departed from Plymouth Sound. A few boats followed as far as the open sea – one entirely occupied by ladies 'frequently standing on the thwarts of the boat, and waving their handkerchiefs' as Napoleon made a last appearance at his cabin window. At last the show was over, and the occasion memorialised in a popular song of the time:

> Boney went a-cruisin'
> Aboard the Billy Ruffian.
> Boney went to Saint Helen',
> An' he never came back agen.[61]

For one slight, red-coated, strangely youthful member of the Plymouth garrison, this would not be his last connection with the former Emperor or his fate.

After more than two years of home service, James's career began moving forward at last. On 7 December 1815, being now deemed about sixteen years old and with a reputation as a child prodigy, he was gazetted to the rank in which he'd been serving in an acting capacity since October 1813:

In the Name and on the Behalf of His Majesty

GEORGE the Third, by the Grace of God of the United Kingdom of Great Britain and Ireland, King, Defender of the Faith, &c. To our Trusty and Welbeloved James Barry, M.D. Greetings: We do by these Presents Constitute and Appoint you to be Assistant Surgeon to the Forces.

You are therefore carefully, diligently to discharge the Duty of Assistant Surgeon ... And you are to observe and follow such Orders and Directions from Time to Time as you shall receive ... according to the Rules and Discipline of War. Given at Our Court at Carlton House the Seventh day of December 1815 in the Fifty Sixth Year of Our Reign.

By Command of His Royal Highness the Prince Regent in the Name and on Behalf of His Majesty.[62]

It was probably to mark this occasion that James commissioned a mini-ature portrait of himself. It was common for young officers to commem-orate their commission in this way, and for James Barry this miniature would be the only image of him in youth that would ever be made (or at least survive). The tiny portrait – small enough to fit easily into his little palm – was made in bright oils on a wafer of ivory, and depicted a confident-looking youth in uniform, with red-gold curls cut in Roman fashion, a large nose and wide, blue-green eyes.[63]

In August the following year, Dr Barry at last left English shores for his first overseas posting – the Cape of Good Hope, in one of the furthest reaches of the Empire. Finally Margaret's foreign adventure, postponed four years earlier by the arrest of General Miranda, was beginning. As she sailed south, through the Bay of Biscay, past Portugal and Cádiz, she came close to the place where, just a month earlier, on 14 July 1816, Francisco de Miranda had died in his Spanish prison, aged sixty-six and utterly broken. He was buried in a mass grave.

Part II

More Than a Father
1816–1831

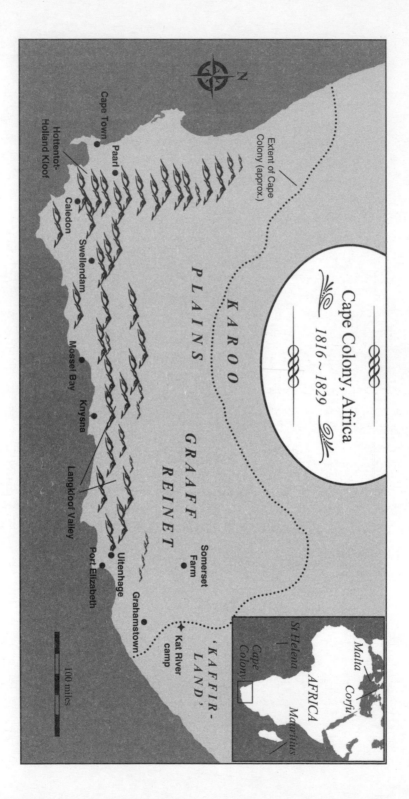

Cape Colony, Africa
1816 ~ 1829

N

Cape Town
Hottentot-
Holland Kloof
Paarl
Caledon
Swellendam
Mossel Bay
Knysna
Langkloof Valley
Port Elizabeth
Uitenhage
Grahamstown

Extent of Cape
Colony (approx.)

KAROO

PLAINS

GRAAFF
REINET

Somerset
Farm

'KAFFIR-
LAND'

Kat River
camp

100 miles

Malta
Corfu
St Helena
AFRICA
Mauritius
Cape
Colony

The Cape of Good Hope

The Atlantic Ocean: September 1816

Broad-beamed, tall as trees, the East Indiaman *Lord Cathcart* pushed hard through the swells, her yards set with canvas pot-bellied with the northeasterly wind, heeling to starboard with spray bursting over her rail.

Bound for the Cape! Margaret had grown up with the sea, but her sailing had been limited to the little workaday vessels plying around the British Isles. She'd seen many Indiamen and countless other merchantmen and warships come and go at Cork, with their salted sails furled and their timbers impregnated with the farthest seas – now at last her own feet were on the tilting deck, flying out across the ocean, outward bound. Or rather, James's feet were. Margaret – at least the idea of Margaret, the spinster, the governess, the would-be wife – was fading into the distance until she was hardly visible. Physically, of course, she was still with James – an irremovable stowaway.

It was a good time to be leaving England, a place beset by the gloom of a post-war recession. To crown it all, that year the whole of Europe fell under a dust cloud carried by air currents from the eruption of Mount Tambora in the Dutch East Indies. It suppressed temperatures and led to the 'Summer that Never Was', in which crops withered and people starved. The far south of Africa – where the sun still shone – was the place to go.

Yet the voyage was daunting even for the adventurous. It took the better part of three months – or even longer if one encountered any of the notorious Atlantic storms – and was arduous even for the wealthiest, most luxuriously accommodated passengers.

James Barry had concerns that his fellow passengers were not subject to – for three months he would have to live, eat and sleep alongside a fixed set of people in greater confinement than ever before, in or out of the

Army. Cabin space was at a premium; Indiamen were not purpose-built
as passenger ships – they were armed merchant vessels equipped to defend
themselves in time of war and against pirates. They sailed in convoys of a
dozen or more, sometimes with a Royal Navy escort, and larger Indiamen
were built with a gun deck, like a frigate, and carried upwards of eighteen cannon. *Lord Cathcart* was small for an Indiaman, but was otherwise
standard,[1] and on this voyage she was full to bursting with a company of
soldiers, part of a battalion bound for the garrison of the Cape Colony.[*]
The troops were accommodated in the dark, dank steerage and the orlop
deck, while the better-off paying passengers took accommodation in
cabins made up of collapsible wooden or canvas partitions, either on the
gun deck aft, in the roundhouse[†] or the great cabin,[‡] which enjoyed the
advantage of the stern windows. A cubicle here, with one window and
barely enough room to set up one's cot, cost at least £200.[2] The roundhouse was the most expensive – £1000 bought a few feet of space, with
the noise from the poop deck above as sailors worked the mizzen sails
and spanker boom and the poultry squawked in their coops.

At least there was light, privacy and fresh air; the less well-off passengers – probably including James Barry – had to make do with a cabin on
the gun deck. One person who experienced such accommodation recalled
the 'variety of inconveniences, the grand one that of being completely
debarred of all daylight in tempestuous weather' when the gun ports
were closed; yet the sea still found a way in, 'for I was often set afloat in
my cabin by heavy seas breaking against those dead lights'; sometimes
'it poured in in torrents, beating even over my bed'.[3]

For a young man in England facing his first oceanic adventure, there
was plenty of information available, and the wiser travellers – of whom
James was one – read all they could in order to prepare themselves. James
knew he would have to live in such conditions, closely confined with men
who hadn't any occupation to distract them from scrutiny of their fellow
passengers. At least he'd have privacy in attending calls of nature – passengers were entitled to use the enclosed privies in the ship's quarter-galleries,
while the soldiers and ordinary sailors had to use the open-air heads at
the bow or the communal pissdales[§] built into the ship's waist.

---

[*] officially named the Cape of Good Hope, often referred to as the Cape Colony
[†] enclosed area below the poop deck
[‡] area below the aft end of the quarterdeck
[§] urinals

Passengers, whatever their station in life, had to get used to the strict, even draconian, discipline on board ship – all men, civilian and military, ascending from the gun deck to the quarterdeck had to touch their hats to the captain, and 'a breach of this rule would be considered grossly insulting, and might induce to a rebuke, by no means pleasant to the feelings ... of a gentleman.'[4]

As the convoy approached the Equator, a more exacting ritual loomed – one that would be particularly unpleasant, even dangerous, for James.

Every guide and memoir described the customary ritual of 'crossing the Line', when neophyte passengers and crewmen who'd never before crossed the Equator were ritually 'shaved' and ducked by the crew, under the direction of the god Neptune – a veteran seaman adorned in a makeshift costume and riding on a car made from a gun carriage. Women were exempt from this treatment, but the custom made no allowance for rank or class – gentlemen were treated the same as common men, and it was a vigorous, hearty and sometimes violent business. A huge butt was filled with water and a plank laid across it. The initiates were brought up one at a time, blindfolded, from below decks and seated on the plank. The victim's chin was 'lathered' with a mixture of tar and grease, then 'shaved' with a piece of rusty barrel-hoop that was notched like a saw on one side; those who resisted were given the notched side. When the shaving was done – to uproarious hilarity from the spectators – the plank was suddenly pulled away and the victim tipped backwards into the butt of increasingly tarry, oily water.

The ritual served in part as a safety-valve; for a few hours, the hard-worked crew ruled the ship and had the opportunity to mistreat their betters. If the initiates were reluctant, their treatment could turn violent. On one voyage, a passenger who resisted 'was roughly handled, and had not the captain interfered, would have suffered much more'.[5] On another vessel, 'Two or three of the passengers, who had given offence to the sailors, had all their faces covered with tar, and the brush rammed into their mouths, and were then ducked two or three times in the dirty water. Six gentlemen defended themselves in their cabins with pistols and small swords.'[6] Published accounts abounded in the period before James Barry took ship for the Cape, and one popular book, published in 1813, added a blood-chilling detail to the scene, describing the plank 'whereupon the victim is seated in a state of nudity'.[7]

For those who took the trouble to inform themselves beforehand, there was a way out. Neptune and his fellows could be bribed — the usual fee being a gallon of rum and a pound or two of sugar.[8] Given the thoroughness of study and precaution taken by James in his professional life, he would have followed this advice — carefully giving his bribe well ahead of the event — and been able to observe the crossing of the Line as a spectator.

As the weeks passed and the temperatures grew more sultry, life for passengers was a constant dream-like limbo, in which boredom was staved off by smoking (if it was allowed), playing cards and chess, talking, and walking on the little deck when it wasn't busy with hands at work; those who were daring and nimble might be allowed to climb aloft. The sights ranged from nocturnal trails of phosphorescence to vast daylight shoals of flying fish breaking the waves, and occasional landfalls at Madeira, the Canaries and the Americas.[9] Having crossed the Equator well off the coast of Brazil, the ship continued following the coastline southeast and southwards, holding the northeasterly trade winds, before eventually turning southeast and catching the westerlies for the long, difficult crossing to the Cape of Good Hope, in which ships could be hit by storms or becalmed.[10] For James Barry it was a blessedly easy and brief passage, and at last, on a day in late October — the mild early summer of the southern hemisphere — *Lord Cathcart* dropped anchor in Table Bay.[11]

*   *   *

From the ship's rail, James looked for the first time at the land that would be his home for the next ... well, there was no telling how long he would be here — months, years — or whether the future awaiting him on that shore would involve prosperity, drudgery or ruin.

Whatever it held in store, it was a wonderful sight — as stark and green as the Scottish Highlands, with every detail lit by a sun more potent than James had ever known, and domed by a subtropical sky the colour of copper sulphate. The Cape Peninsula* was an astounding, jagged-toothed jawbone of land and mountain; it was as if a divine hand had taken a

---

* The Cape of Good Hope is a southern headland of the peninsula, and the name was used as a synecdoche for the whole region, and for the British colony.

piece of Africa's mountainous coast and dragged it several miles seaward, stretching behind it a broad isthmus of flat land edged north and south by sandy bays. On the northern bay, in the lee of three massive peaks that stood behind it like a theatre backdrop – the conical Lion's Head, the fang of Devil's Peak and the vast, flat-topped Table Mountain – lay the thriving little white-stucco settlement of Cape Town.

Although smaller than either Cork or Plymouth, it was the principal watering place for ships travelling to and from India and the Far East; yet it contributed little trade of its own to the flow. The huge Cape Colony, stretching away inland beyond the mountains, had only received limited development, its boundaries still dominated by hostile tribes. East Indiamen and warships stopped here, took on food and water, and departed again; for this reason, Cape Town had no harbour, no quays; ships anchored in Table Bay and boats plied to and from the single jetty.

A flotilla of rowing boats and single-masted shallops came out to *Lord Cathcart*. The soldiers filed up from below, toting their heavy packs, rubbing their eyes in the blazing sunlight and staring in stupefaction at the scenery. While their officers began the slow process of loading them into boats, the paying passengers were already on their way to shore. ·

James's boat pulled in at the jetty beneath the promontory of the 'Castle', a squat, star-shaped fort, much like Plymouth's citadel, which dominated the bay and the western fringe of the town. His trunks, besides holding his worldly goods, his books and his precious surgical kit, also contained a letter of introduction to the Governor of the Cape of Good Hope provided by Lord Buchan. Officially Dr Barry was a mere assistant surgeon, here to take up a post at the Military Hospital (a nondescript building on the edge of the beach close by the Castle), but after four years of grinding away, honing his skills in similar establishments in England, he had more elevated hopes.

The figure walking up from the jetty into the town, followed by the porter trundling the handcart, looked subtly different from the officer who had gazed out at Plymouth Sound. He still wore the same uniform, the spurred boots and the shining sword, with a black bicorne hat covering his golden curls, but he was a little taller and appeared a shade broader in the body. Anyone who looked closely would notice that the boots had two-inch heels, while the lining of his coat had been stuffed with kapok.[12]

Cape Town was still decidedly Dutch in character; established by the Dutch East India Company a century and a half earlier, in recent decades it had changed hands several times. The British had seized it by force in 1795 in order to keep it out of French hands, then gave it back to the Dutch in 1802 at the Peace of Amiens, only to capture it again in 1806. Britain eventually acquired possession permanently as part of the fiendishly complicated exchange of rights and territories following the first defeat of Napoleon in 1814. Although it had a British administration and garrison, the Union flag flying over the Castle and a budding British population, most of the people were Dutch-speaking, the streets had Dutch names and the architecture was distinctly Netherlandish.

Having reported to the Principal Medical Officer at the Military Hospital, James sought lodgings for himself (it was customary for officers to arrange their own accommodation). He found a very satisfactory set of rooms in a 'lodging house of high repute' at 12 Heerengracht, run by the Widow Sandenberg.[13] Heerengracht ('gentlemen's walk')* was a broad, tree-lined avenue that at one end overlooked the open space of the Grand Parade and at the other abutted the Company's Garden, the long, verdant botanic park that was Cape Town's centrepiece.

Once he'd settled in, James lost no time in venturing out into Cape society. He put on his best uniform, retrieved Lord Buchan's letter from his trunk, and set out for Government House, the residence of the Governor of the Cape of Good Hope, Lieutenant General Lord Charles Henry Somerset.[14] It was a large but understated building: low, exquisitely refined in white stucco with a simple pillared carriage porch facing the town and a more ornate frontage with a veranda facing the Company's Garden. Having delivered his letter, James retired and waited to see whether an invitation would come. The eccentric Lord Buchan could be relied on to give James a good recommendation, and he and Lord Charles were not unknown to each other; Buchan's younger brother, Lord Thomas Erskine, had been part of the Prince Regent's social circle in his Brighton days, as had Lord Charles,[15] and the two had been privy councillors together. Yet James was not guaranteed a welcome; the Governor had reason to be wary of doctors.

Lord Charles Somerset, younger brother of the 6th Duke of Beaufort, had been Governor at the Cape since its formal acquisition in 1814. Prior to that, after a career in the Army he had resided in England, living the

---

* now Adderley Street

life of an aristocrat: socialising, riding to hounds, gambling, holding a seat in Parliament and taking a good living from a sinecure as a Paymaster of the Forces. Wrangling between Whig Members of Parliament and Lord Liverpool's Tory government had caused trouble for him, with the result that he was sent into a kind of exile; by arrangement between his brother the Duke, Lord Liverpool, and Earl Bathurst, the Secretary of State for War and the Colonies, he was appointed to the governorship of the Cape.

For a man who'd been largely devoted to leisure, Somerset took his position very seriously, throwing himself wholeheartedly into governing the Colony, extending its bounds, encouraging its growth and acting like a viceroy more than an administrator, caring for the Colony as if it were his own personal estate.

But there was a pall of sadness behind Lord Charles Somerset's public life – Elizabeth, his beloved wife of twenty-seven years, had died little more than a year after arriving at the Cape. They'd had an appalling voyage – long, uncomfortable and racked by storms – and Elizabeth had spent much of it in a state of terror and dreadful seasickness.[16] She was never really well afterwards, and lived on for just over a year. On 11 September 1815 she died. Lord Charles was almost prostrated with grief. They had met and fallen in love in 1788, when Lord Charles was a twenty-year-old infantry captain; Elizabeth Courtenay had been three years older and noted for her looks and charm. Charles's father, the 5th Duke, disapproved of the match, not for social reasons – Elizabeth, as daughter of Viscount Courtenay, was as high-born as the Somersets – but because as a second son, Lord Charles would not inherit and was expected to hunt down a rich heiress. But there was no stopping the impetuous, love-smitten Charles. He and Elizabeth eloped and were married at Gretna Green. Besides her looks and pleasant company, Elizabeth was a loving and faithful wife and mother, always putting her own needs second to those of her husband and children – even when she was ill she played her public role as a governor's wife. By the values of the time, she was the perfect woman, and Lord Charles loved her. Without her he was not the same man. A few days after her death, he wrote to his brother, the 6th Duke:

> You will I am sure hear with great concern that it has pleased God to visit me with the severest Affliction in depriving me of the best, the most attached and the most affectionate of wives, and my Children of

the Tenderest and Best Mother ... I have felt this severe blow perhaps
the more forcibly by being entirely unprepared for such a Visitation of
Providence ... My mind is as yet scarcely composed enough to view
the Magnitude of the Calamity that has befallen me – the more I think
the more weighty it appears, and if I look back to the Happiness which
her attachment and affection for me have afforded me I am in a state
almost of Destruction and Despair.[17]

Bewildered by grief, and perhaps haunted by the memory of his father's
disapproval of his marriage, he signed this letter to his brother 'your most
dutiful and affectionate son'.

Through negligence or ignorance, all three doctors who had attended
her had completely misjudged the case, and had misled Lord Charles about
the patient's condition. He'd been deeply concerned about her, but they
had assured him, right up to a few hours before her death, 'that there
was not the slightest cause for apprehension; indeed they went further
and quite derided my fears.'[18]

When Dr James Barry arrived with his letter of introduction, Lord
Charles had been a widower for two years, and had an understandable
distrust of medical men. But when James set himself to charm, he could
overcome most men's resistance; bright, pleasant and well-informed,
he possessed great force of character. Almost immediately he had the
opportunity to prove himself and enhance his standing; Miss Georgiana,
Lord Charles's elder daughter, was ill – by all accounts dangerously so.

Since their mother's death, the twenty-three-year-old Georgiana and
her younger sister Charlotte, who was seventeen, had had to take over the
role of hostess in their father's household. They were as grief-stricken as
he was, and Georgiana seemed especially prone to melancholy and sickness. Whatever was ailing her now, the doctors had not been able to cure
it, and in the wake of his wife's death Lord Charles feared for Georgiana's
life. Dr Barry's arrival could not have been more fortuitous; a dazzling
reputation had accompanied him from England, where he was said to
be renowned as a prodigy who had earned his MD when still a child;
moreover, he was already an experienced doctor despite still looking like
a half-grown youth. He was quickly appointed to Miss Somerset's case,
in the hope that he would succeed where the older doctors had failed.

James threw himself into the care of his patient in a manner that would
prove to be his hallmark. When Dr Barry took over a case, he did so

absolutely – all previous treatments and medications were dismissed and discarded with a contemptuous flourish, as if they were the concoctions of quacks; he insisted upon his patients following his instructions to the letter, and could become furious if they disobeyed.[19] (Such is the nature of people that this tyrannical, charismatic force added to his reputation as a doctor.) His handling of this case was by all accounts exemplary, and despite the failures of the other medical men and the fears of Lord Charles, James restored Georgiana to health.

Lord Charles's admiration and gratitude were immense. From being an unknown outsider, newly arrived and only one step from the bottom of the Army's professional ladder, James was welcomed into the bosom of the Somerset family. He became a close friend of both Georgiana and Charlotte, and a favourite of their father. Having only just set foot on Cape soil, his reputation and social standing here were sealed.

In truth, his spectacular 'cure' of Miss Somerset may have been as much a product of his bedside manner as his *materia medica*. She was homesick, grieving for her mother, and had a tendency to emotionally induced illness. Her life as a young lady, with no occupation but to entertain visitors, attend galas and hope for romance and a husband, was wearisome and dull, and perhaps little was needed other than some stimulation of the mind and soothing of the emotions to effect a cure. Perhaps James – or rather Margaret – recognised Georgiana's affliction from personal experience, and acted with a natural empathy.[20]

Table Bay: Friday 17 January 1817

The neat little Royal Navy brig HMS *Griffon* rode at anchor in Table Bay, timbers baking under a high summer sun. Her captain had gone ashore some hours ago to call on His Excellency the Governor. *Griffon*, which had just arrived from St Helena, was carrying an important passenger, and the captain, who had orders to deliver him to the Cape of Good Hope, needed directions on what to do with him.

On board, *Griffon*'s passenger bided his time, strolling on the deck and enjoying the beautiful view of the mountains. Although only in his early fifties, his receding hair was grey and his thin face aged with stress and ill health. Emmanuel, Comte de Las Cases was a small man, slightly built, dressed in a tailcoat and black stock, looking more like a scholar than a diplomat, while his assured manner was more that of a distinguished visitor than a prisoner; until now he had been confidant and aide to the exiled Napoleon Bonaparte. In the wake of Waterloo, Las Cases had ridden out of Paris in the imperial coach with the abdicated Emperor (acting at one point as a decoy to fool the teeming mobs, who might have raised their old leader on high or torn him limb from limb with equal passion); it was Las Cases who had negotiated Napoleon's surrender, sailed with him on *Bellerophon*, and accompanied him into his final exile on St Helena.[21]

Trouble had begun with the arrival on that island of General Sir Hudson Lowe, the new Governor, who'd been sent out to St Helena to act as Napoleon's 'custodian' but saw himself more as a gaoler. He and the former Emperor had got on badly – following the government line of refusing him his titles and calling him 'General Bonaparte' didn't help. They quarrelled, and Lowe imposed severe restrictions on Napoleon's life and movements. Napoleon's retinue regarded Lowe as a martinet – a view shared by some of the British community and a few prominent voices at home, including the Duke of Wellington.[22]

Las Cases began working to open a secret line of communication between Napoleon and his contacts in Europe, but the plot unravelled when an agent was caught trying to leave St Helena with a letter stitched inside his waistcoat. Lowe, identifying Las Cases as the instigator, first removed him to a different part of the island, then decided that he should be sent beyond reach of anyone connected with Napoleon. He selected the Cape of Good Hope, and packed Las Cases aboard ship, along with his fourteen-year-old son, Emanuel. The captain was provided with a letter to Lord Charles Somerset explaining the situation and specifying that Las Cases was a prisoner and was to be treated as such.[23]

When *Griffon*'s captain returned from delivering the letter to Lord Charles, Las Cases thought he seemed 'no longer the same man; his behaviour was cold and embarrassed.'[24] Lord Charles's order was that the prisoner be kept aboard for two days while suitable accommodation was prepared. When Las Cases and his son were eventually rowed ashore, they were taken to the Castle, where they were confined in three rooms that were little more than a dungeon – dusty, wretchedly furnished and, as it turned out in the coming days, exposed to sweltering day-long sun through shutterless windows. 'This circumstance,' Las Cases wrote, 'did not afford me a very high notion of the regularity, precision, or promptitude of the new authority under which I was now placed ... I was informed that I must not communicate with any one. I now found myself literally a prisoner.'[25] A fine way to treat the man who had ensured Bonaparte's surrender, even if he was suspected of trying to arrange his escape.

The next day, he was visited by a British officer who had been at St Helena. Knowing that the Count's son was ill, the officer brought a young doctor with him from the Military Hospital. The introduction caused a moment of embarrassing misunderstanding: 'I mistook the Captain's medical friend for his son or nephew,' Las Cases recalled. 'The grave Doctor, who was presented to me, was a boy of eighteen, with the form, the manners, and the voice of a woman.'[26]

Such a near guess, and yet the Count little realised how close he was. So complicated and subtle were the nuances of posture, gesture and demeanour in an age when gender differences were at their utmost peak, that there were plentiful signs detectable by an acute observer, and Margaret had never yet succeeded in acting the man authentically in voice or manner. Other people who met James noticed his effeminacy and his struggle to overcome it.[27]

Dr Barry was described to Las Cases as 'an absolute phenomenon' who 'had performed extraordinary cures at the Cape, and had saved the life of one of the Governor's daughters, after she had been given up, which rendered him a sort of favourite in the family'.[28]

Las Cases, who had spent ten years in England during the Revolutionary Wars and spoke good English,[29] engaged James in conversation. It may have crossed James's mind that the last time he'd been in proximity to this man had been at Plymouth, with the waters of the Sound and a vast swarm of sightseers between them. Las Cases and Dr Barry became good friends; James returned regularly to the Castle to treat young Emanuel, and grew fond of him. He talked at length with Las Cases, who profited by gleaning information about Lord Charles Somerset with which to guide his diplomacy.

Over the next few days, Las Cases made several fruitless attempts to improve his situation; he wrote to Lord Charles pleading his case, asking that he be allowed to write to the British government and to the Prince Regent; that he be sent to live in England; that he be given better quarters. Lord Charles rebuffed them all, declaring flatly that on the word of Sir Hudson Lowe 'he considered me as a prisoner ... and condemned me to remain at the Cape, until instructions arrived from England'.[30]

Lord Charles did grant permission for young Emanuel to go to Europe alone; but the loyal son refused to abandon his father in a foreign land, regardless of his own health, and wrote to the Governor telling him so – 'I prefer dying by his side to living at a distance from him.'[31] The letter impressed Lord Charles, who passed it on to his two daughters. They in turn told James, who was deeply moved.

The feelings awoken in Margaret must have been intense; perhaps memories of a little girl left behind in Ireland, a mother left in London, or a hopeless, negligent father who'd helped ruin his own daughter's prospects, meagre as they were. Margaret constantly longed for a father figure – a role that had been filled in succession by Miranda and Buchan. The next day, Georgiana and Charlotte took James in their carriage to the Castle. Leaving the women in the vehicle, James hurried indoors. On seeing him, the Count began trying to persuade him to use his influence as a doctor to induce Emanuel to leave, but James didn't even listen; instead, brushing past Las Cases, 'he hastened to Emanuel's chamber, and embracing him, expressed his approval of his conduct, observing that he should not have respected him had he acted otherwise.'[32] He led the young man to the window, threw it open, and introduced him to the two young ladies.

After this, apparently on the recommendation of Dr Barry, who warned that Emanuel's health was clearly being harmed by confinement and lack of exercise, permission was given for him to go out whenever he liked (under guard) for walks in the town.

As the days of the Count's confinement dragged by, the only person he saw was Dr Barry, who'd become a frequent visitor (all others were kept away by the officer in charge). 'I found his company very agreeable,' Las Cases recalled. 'He constantly recommended me to take care of my health.' Intuiting that the Count's own health problems were psycho-somatic and rooted in depression, James explained that:

He could guess the seat of my disorder, and regretted that it was out of his power to prescribe any remedy for me. I assured him that the greatest favour he could confer on me would be to procure a person who could read to me and write to my dictation. This I had been vainly soliciting since my arrival, for the state of my eyes precluded all occupation, and my son was strictly desired to abstain from all sedentary employment. I therefore laboured under an intolerable depression of spirits, in being thus wholly abandoned to my melancholy thoughts.[33]

James informed him that as Lord Charles was about to depart on a three-month tour of the Colony, he was unlikely to take time to make new arrangements for the prisoner. Alarmed, Las Cases wrote immediately to the Governor, describing at length the wretched, sweltering conditions of their prison. With all the pitiable dignity he could muster, he asked for a house in the town, to be run at his own expense, with whatever guard his excellency thought fit to provide. It was a cleverly composed letter, 'calculated to lead to a decisive result',[34] and as a diplomat and politician who had ranked high with Napoleon Bonaparte, the Comte de Las Cases was well qualified. The effect – probably vouched for by James's personal recommendation – was extraordinary. Lord Charles reversed his attitude; he gave immediate orders for the improvement of the Count's quarters, and for new accommodation to be found for him. Meanwhile, he permitted the Count and his son the use of Newlands House, his country residence in the hills about five miles from Cape Town, during his absence. Accordingly, on 29 January the Governor's aide-de-camp brought a carriage to drive Las Cases and Emanuel to their luxurious new accommodation (well-guarded by soldiers), where they would spend the rest of the summer – 'removed from a prison to a Paradise'.[35]

Meanwhile, Dr Barry, as an ever more favoured member of Lord Charles's family circle, prepared to accompany the Governor on his grand tour of the Cape Colony. For the first time he was going to see the untamed interior of Africa.

'Savage Neighbours'

This Colony, which is distant a voyage of just three months from the port of London, comprehends all the southernmost points of Africa, and lies in a temperate healthy and delightful climate ... The healthiness of the air in every district, is known to all who have breathed it ... nor are there any prevailing fevers, nor what may be called seasoning disorders ... That it is congenial to human life, is indisputably proved by the vigorous appearance of its present inhabitants.[1]

So said a book published in London with the purpose of encouraging British farming folk to emigrate to the Cape and bring its hundreds of miles of wild veldt under civilised cultivation. Lord Charles Somerset was an instigator of this drive to expand, improve and civilise. His tour from January to April 1817 was conceived with the purpose of surveying the land and its scattered settlements, and also of gauging (and hopefully pacifying) the native peoples.

The tour contradicted the guidebook's rosy view from the outset. It was high summer in the southern hemisphere, and conditions were intense; 'from the great heat of the weather,' wrote Lord Charles, 'I must necessarily be exposed to much inconvenience, and from the nature of the country to the greatest privations.'[2]

His travelling party was a small one. Aside from Lord Charles himself, there were Georgiana and Charlotte, and Lieutenant Colonel Christopher Bird, the Deputy Colonial Secretary, who'd lived at the Cape for thirteen years, knew its land and people, and was a fluent Dutch speaker.[3] Also in the party was Captain Thomas Sheridan, Colonial Treasurer and son of the playwright Richard Brinsley Sheridan. 'Captain Tom' was a one-time soldier, theatrical manager, dramatist and failed politician. His energy was fast running out; suffering from tuberculosis, he'd come to the Cape for the healthy air, and would be dead before the year was out. Completing the small party was Dr James Barry, just three months into his posting at the Cape and rising with amazing rapidity.

Although the party was modest in size, the convoy that would carry them the hundreds of miles across the Colony was not. There were horses for the travellers, as well as wagons for baggage and personal transport (carriages wouldn't have survived the punishing road ahead, so sturdy wagons would have to do); there were grooms, valets, maids and cooks, all of whom required conveyances; on top of personal baggage there were tents, camp furniture, equipment and supplies, and a convoy of heavy wagons to carry it all, each pulled by a team of up to sixteen oxen.

On 27 January, a bright Monday morning, the whips cracked, the drivers roared, the wheels creaked, and the great convoy, full of gear and purpose, moved off along the eastward road out of Cape Town. That morning's journey brought them some twenty miles to a green land dotted with sheep farms. Beyond loomed the forbidding wall of the Hottentots Holland mountains, which cut off the Cape isthmus from the rest of the Colony. Travelling southeast until the glittering sweep of False Bay came into sight, the convoy made for the only viable pass – the notorious Hottentots Holland Kloof.[4]

Everyone who'd made the journey regarded it with apprehension, and to those like James Barry who had no experience of mountains, it seemed impassable. Before even reaching the pass, the horses and oxen had to heave the grumbling vehicles up a rising road into the Roode Hoogte, the hills of hard red earth that formed the feet of the mountains; then the steeper slopes of the mountains began; yellowing vegetation clung in banks and patches between the jutting red rocks that stood up in startling combs and fringes from the ridges of folded bedrock – as if giant tormented creatures had been crushed into the landscape, leaving vast heaps of twisted bones, spines and scales.

Up and up the crude, narrow road went. Those who could left the confinement of the wagons and took to horseback – even James Barry, who was far from an experienced rider.[5] Straddling his mount alongside Lord Charles and the other travellers, he urged it up the perilously steep track. It was scarcely believable that wagons could be brought this way, but they were – not only the touring party's but locals transporting produce from the interior to Cape Town – so many that the passage of their wheels had worn grooves in the rock. The ordeal for the draught animals was dreadful; the pass echoed with the cracking of the drivers' whips and the thwacks of the vicious *sjamboks*.* The cruelty was unavoidable, not only to drive the beasts up the tortuous slopes, but to ensure their total obedience; it was a narrow, lethally dangerous road, twisting alongside sheer drops, and if the oxen deviated in the slightest, or became restive, the whole vehicle – animals, wagon, driver and load – could slip over the edge, and frequently did. This was another good reason to take to horseback.

At the summit of the pass, the party paused for a rest. Looking back the way they had come, they had an awe-inspiring view across the whole isthmus, from False Bay to the Cape of Good Hope, Table Bay and the tiny dot of Cape Town in the shadow of Table Mountain under its 'tablecloth' of cloud.

James, having studied botany and natural *materia medica*, took an interest in the plants that grew in abundance by the roadside. Among the scrubby grasses were splashes of bright pink *Erica taxifolia* and *E. fascicularis*, and large bushes of *Protea speciosa*, which the locals called *suikerbos* – sugarbush. James was intrigued by the medicinal potential of plant species, and the possibility of new discoveries excited him.[6]

With the eastern descent, the first great ordeal of the tour was over, and the convoy passed into the gently rolling green downland around Swellendam. It was alive with wildlife – especially the elegant bontebok, a chocolate-coloured species of antelope about a yard high with a broad white blaze and a pair of lyre-shaped horns. Local people had hunted them almost to extinction, a fact that concerned Lord Charles Somerset – probably with prompting from James, who was fond of animals and detested destruction. The following year, a proclamation would appear in the *Cape Gazette* that bontebok were not to be hunted, 'as these animals are so scarce that His Excellency forbids them being destroyed'.[7] A few years later he extended this protection to the eland and hippopotamus.[8]

At the Gourits River they had to descend a two-hundred-foot gorge with no bridge. The rear wheels of the wagons were locked to prevent them running away. Once across the water, the ascent provided (according to one British traveller) 'one of the most animating and picturesque

---

* heavy crop or whip made from hippopotamus or rhino hide

scenes imaginable'; the wagons were hauled 'up a broken road which in other countries would be deemed impracticable, with a long line of, in some instances, thirty six oxen … the shouting of the drivers, the echoes occasioned by the cracking of their huge whips, and the passengers in every direction climbing amongst the rocks in pursuit of the nearest way to the summit of the ridge.'[9]

Life on the great east–west route through the Colony's interior followed a pattern into which all travellers fell; as soon as a grazing place was reached, the oxen were unyoked. The saddle horses could be let loose, as they would stay close to their riders, while oxen could roam free – 'In these wild parts of the Colony there is little fear of the cattle straying, for they are too much in fear of wild beasts to wander far from protection'; fires were lit, food cooked, and the wagon teamsters made their camps under their wagons. At dawn the signal would be given, the teams yoked, the whips cracked and the convoy moved on again. 'Such is the history of every day, and of the whole journey.'[10] For James Barry, it was an entirely new world – the land, the life, the people, as unlike anything in his or Margaret's experience as an adventure in a book.

Sometimes the wild penetrated even the security of the camp. One night shortly after crossing the Gourits, the Somerset party camped on the flat plain near Mossel Bay. As they slept, a lion slunk into the camp. Normally lions would stay away from large groups of people, but it wasn't unknown for individuals, hungry from scarcity of prey, age or injury, to turn man-eater. Such beasts became the stuff of folklore, entering human settlements at night in search of easy meat. If there were camp guards posted, this cat crept by them. A young Khoikhoi boy, one of the wagon teamsters, asleep in the open rather than under the wagons with his fellows, was seized and carried off. His screams shook the whole camp awake. Some men who'd been sitting up gave chase; their noise and fury startled the lion and it dropped the boy and ran off. He was carried back, and Dr Barry examined him; the lad had been amazingly lucky, his injuries limited to minor bite marks and scratches from being dragged.[11]

Towards the coastal region of Knysna, the plains gave way to a region bordered by high mountains, 'clothed along their skirts with majestic forests … irregular, dark, hoary with moss, and ancient-looking almost as the rocks'.[12] Beyond, lay Kaaimans Gat,* an even more formidable

---

* Crocodile Gorge

barrier than the Gourits – a huge wooded gorge named after the massive
crocodile-like iguanas inhabiting it. Tales were told of wagons breaking
and oxen falling to their deaths on the descent to the beer-brown waters
roaring through it:

> The traveller must pass over rocks, in steps of from one to two feet ...
> the waggons bouncing down, reeling from side to side, and but for the
> management of Hottentots accustomed to such service, in continual
> danger of oversetting. They support the waggon, by thongs fastened
> to each side, pulling with all their might, either to the right or left, as
> otherwise, in several places, the waggons with all their contents, and
> the poor beasts staggering before them, would be precipitated into the
> abyss beneath.[13]

Besides the iguanas, there were monkeys and flamboyantly plumed birds
thronging the trees, and each evening meal was haunted by the nearby
howling of jackals.[14] Yet strange as it all was, for James Barry the chief
danger still lay ahead, and came from his own species.

At Knysna, the party rested at the famously hospitable farmstead
of George Rex, an Englishman with a vast estate of twenty-five thousand acres. He was said to be the natural son of King George III; this
was universally believed on account of his name, his wealth and his
resemblance to the King. The tale was that he'd been granted riches
and sent into exile. However, the truth – which he must have actively
suppressed – was that he was the son of a London distiller called John
Rex;[15] having risen through the ranks of the civil service and made
money in commerce, George had come to the Cape as an administrator
in 1796. He'd since retired from the service and gone into the timber
business; he was in his early fifties, 'of a strong robust appearance, and
the exact resemblance in features to George III'.[16] And so the royal
legend flourished.

But George Rex's equally legendary hospitality was no myth: travellers were welcomed warmly and encouraged to linger and be entertained.
His home – named Melkhout Kraal after the squat milkwood trees growing thereabouts – stood on a rise above a marshy lagoon through which
the Knysna River flowed into the Indian Ocean. For the Somerset party,
Rex laid on river excursions, fishing and shooting parties, and social
gatherings in the evenings.

It was noticed that Dr Barry took a keen interest in George Rex's large brood of children. Most were the offspring of his relationship with Johanna Rosina van der Caap, who had once been one of his dozens of slaves. Strictly, Rex's relationship with Johanna Rosina was illegal under colonial racial law, but he disregarded it openly and with impunity.

It wasn't in James Barry's nature to approve of slavery, and perhaps this influenced his fondness for the Rex children, whose lives intertwined with those of their father's slaves. James gave them lessons; it was as if Margaret was reverting to a life before medicine, before the existence of James, and she allowed them a degree of intimacy that James had never given to any other person. The children got sufficiently close to detect the kapok stuffing in the lining of the doctor's clothing, and they sensed something else about him as well; lacking the discretion of the English, they nicknamed Dr Barry the *Kapok Nooientjie* – little kapok maiden.

The phrase took root among the Melkhout slaves, but apparently didn't affect the integrity of his disguise. Yet it did seem to make James much more sensitive to breaches, and more inclined to fear them – a sensitivity that would grow sharper as he grew older. (George Rex himself believed that Dr Barry was a woman in disguise, but treated the matter with discretion – one of the English traits he retained.)[17]

On 27 March, a full two months after setting out from Cape Town, the Governor's party reached Somerset Farm, an experimental project established by Lord Charles in 1815 to supply frontier troops with provisions.[18]

Although satisfied by the growing prosperity of the Colony, he had remained dismayed by the 'aggravating conduct' of its 'savage neighbours'.[19] The frontier districts had seen violent turmoil between European settlers and the so-called 'Kaffirs' – the restless, displaced Xhosa tribes who had been raiding and despoiling the settler farms.* Eastward expansion of the Cape Colony had slowed due to the presence of the Xhosa, who had been displaced as European settlement expanded, condensing their populations, exacerbating existing inter-tribal tensions and leading to Xhosa incursions into Cape Colony territory.

---

* *Kaffir*: umbrella term (now extremely pejorative) for various peoples, including Zulu and Xhosa; other groups such as San ('Bushmen') and Khoikhoi ('Hottentots') were regarded as distinct from 'Kaffirs'.

In December 1811 there had been a crisis when Xhosa groups under their leader, Chief Ndlambe, invaded the Colony. The *landdrost** of Graaff Reinet had been set upon and speared to death, along with eight farmers and Khoikhoi workers, and others wounded.[20] In a bid to stamp out such depredations once and for all, Governor Sir John Cradock (Lord Charles's immediate predecessor) ordered the destruction of all 'Kaffir Kraals' within Cape Colony territory, 'laying waste their gardens and fields, and in fact totally removing every object that could hold out to their chiefs an inducement to revisit the regained territory'.[21] Ndlambe and his people were driven back across the Fish River (another formidable watercourse, forming the eastern boundary of the Colony). This retreat heightened inter-clan tensions and ratcheted up the pressure across the eastern Cape.[22] Xhosa raids continued, and a drought in 1817 had made the situation still worse.[23]

Lord Charles was determined to work out 'some system for preventing those repeated irruptions of the Savages' that were gradually driving out the settlers.[24] He was concerned also about the settlers' reprisals:

> I have hitherto endeavoured to impress upon those in authority in these remote districts the policy of treating the Caffres with mildness and kindness, of rewarding every instance of fair dealing, and while Caffre marauders in our territory should be followed and punished ... as their crimes deserve, I have strictly prohibited all instances of retaliation ... It has been my anxious hope that a perseverance in this system of mildness ... would gradually bring about a sense of the benefit of friendly intercourse in the breasts of the Caffre Chiefs themselves.[25]

Thus far he'd been disappointed; even stationing troops at Uitenhage had been ineffective. The problem was aggravated by roaming bands of 'Bastaards'[†] – men born to mixed white, Khoikhoi or slave parents – who lived as bandits, trading with the white settlers and raiding and plundering in 'Kaffirland'.[26] Lord Charles intended to offer diplomacy with a sharp edge; he'd invited Chief Ngqika to conference 'to demand his aid in repressing the outrages' and 'to notify to him the vigorous measures

---

* regional administrator
† hybrids (Dutch)

His Lordship was determined to adopt in future, and the retribution he should henceforth require'.[27]

At the Fish River, a large military escort was gathered, and in splendid array the Somerset party crossed into native territory, heading for the Kat River, where the conference was to take place. The main pillars of Britain's imperial forces were present: the 21st Light Dragoons, dashing in blue jackets and shakos with red and white plumes; a small detachment of the Royal Artillery; the 83rd (County of Dublin) Regiment of Foot; the 72nd Foot, marching along in their tartan trews; and several companies of the Cape Regiment, white officers in command of mainly Khoikhoi troops in green and brown uniforms, their cavalry armed with sabres and double-barrelled carbines carried brigand-style in their boots.[28] At the head of the column, alongside General Lord Charles Henry Somerset, rode the slight figure of Assistant Staff Surgeon Dr James Barry, in cocked hat and scarlet coatee, booted and spurred, with his long sword jingling at his hip. If the little girl Margaret had been granted a glimpse of her future self, she could hardly have wished for better.

This force came down to the Kat – a small river winding through a broad green valley fringed to the east with table-top hills. A camp was made on the west bank, and Major Fraser of the Cape Regiment was despatched to deliver Lord Charles's invitation to Chief Ngqika. He found the Chief nervous and reluctant to meet the Governor;[29] his uncle, the raider Ndlambe, and some of the other chiefs argued that the British had come to avenge the murder of the landdrost. Lord Charles's predecessor, at the close of that war, had declared himself happy that his troops had spilled sufficient Xhosa blood 'to impress on the minds of these savages a proper degree of terror and respect',[30] and five years later the fear was still there. It didn't help that the tribesman who was said to have thrown the first spear at the landdrost was present now. Eventually Ngqika was persuaded that Lord Charles's intentions were diplomatic, and he agreed to come to the conference. He set out with his retinue of subordinate chiefs and followers, together with a bodyguard of three hundred armed warriors.

They reached the Kat in the late morning of 2 April, and paused, surveying the sight before them. On the opposite bank, the scarlet, blue and green-clad British troops were formed up in long lines, motionless, sweating under a sun ascending towards noon; its light glinted on bayonets, sabres and cannon barrels, and on regimental colours twitching in the breeze. On the east bank, about half the British numbers but equally formidable, stood the ranks of Xhosa warriors, their naked skin the colour of polished rosewood, decorated with beadwork, plumes and fringes, carrying long hide shields and deadly-looking assegais.*

In the conflict-ridden fringes of the British Empire, it wasn't at all unknown for such parleys to turn into bloodbaths, and there was never any way of telling which side would have the upper hand. In the centre of the British lines a marquee had been set up as a meeting place, its sides let down so that the meeting would be visible to all. To Ngqika and many of his people it looked like a trap. His warriors instantly formed a defensive square around their chief, while some of the lesser chiefs' followers fled for the hills. Major Fraser assured Ngqika that it was safe. To prove that they weren't about to be gunned down, he and some of the frontier landdrosts linked arms with Ngqika and Ndlambe to walk across the river, while the warrior guard formed a line again.[31]

James Barry, in one guise or another, had been on the fringe of affairs of state several times, but he'd never seen anything like this: the pale, slender Lord Charles Henry Somerset, in a general's uniform, flanked by his troops, greeting the Xhosa Chief and his retinue of ferocious-looking warriors. Ngqika was middle-aged, but had the face of a boy, which sat oddly on his bulky, heavily built body; his breast was hung with beaded necklaces, and he was draped in a long leopard-skin cloak, decorated with buttons. The two men sat down to negotiate. It was a complicated business; Lord Charles spoke in English, which was translated into Dutch by one of the landdrosts and then into Xhosa by a Khoikhoi interpreter, with some Xhosa-speaking colonists certifying his translation. The Governor offered the Chief concessions: the freedom to enter the Colony for trading purposes, and British government recognition of Ngqika as the chief of all native chiefs. This was a clever step, and a common instrument in Britain's colonial diplomacy; it would consolidate Ngqika's status among his subsidiary and rival chiefs (which had been declining lately), and bring with it special bargaining rights. But he would also be personally responsible for his people's crimes against the Colony. Ngqika understood, and promised to 'punish with death all such as steal from the Colonists, telling them they make him appear as deceiving the Governor'.[32]

---

* long, leaf-bladed throwing spear (different from the Zulu assegai, a stabbing spear)

The conference concluded with the presentation of gifts to the native chiefs, including a very fine grey horse for Ngqika and a sack of parcelled presents that had been chosen for their 'civilising' influence – shoes, handkerchiefs, shawls and buttons. Ngqika was very taken with the looking-glasses, knives and tinder-boxes he was given, and later asked for more. A Christian missionary, one Mr Williams, who'd been foisted upon the Xhosa by Lord Charles as part of the agreement, observed that the Chief seemed eager to depart once the negotiations were complete, and was reluctant to linger for the opening and explanation of individual presents. Williams interpreted this as a greedy impatience to be away with his booty: 'When he had done receiving,' Williams wrote, 'he fled instantly, like a thief, to the other side of the river' where his warriors awaited him.[33] This prejudice can't have boded well for Williams's future relationship with him.

Diplomacy served, the two forces withdrew from the banks of the Kat – the British marching west and the Xhosa melting into the green hills.

Lord Charles was well satisfied.[34] But the meeting did not see the end of the conflict – on the contrary, it very nearly led to catastrophe for the British eastern Cape two years later, when Ndlambe, responding to a punitive raid by the British, led a force of ten thousand Xhosa warriors against Grahamstown, defended by a garrison of only 333 mixed British, Dutch and Khoikhoi troops – the opening of what became known as the Fifth Frontier War. Steady nerves and disciplined firepower repulsed the attack, but Lord Charles was badly shaken by the outbreak.[35] Relations with the natives of 'Kaffirland' were what they were, and nothing would fundamentally change.

12

A Prodigy in a Physician

The touring party returned from the eastern territories by a much quicker route through the Karoo plains, an arid, semi-desert region, reaching Cape Town less than three weeks after the meeting with Chief Ngqika. Winter was coming: chilly after the roasting summer but not nearly as cold as the English freezes to which James was accustomed.

He settled back into his duties at the Military Hospital, but at the same time began acquiring other patients through his social connections. He renewed his acquaintance with the Comte de Las Cases, who was neither a happy nor a healthy man. His stay at Newlands House, the Governor's country residence, had got off to a shaky start when he had discovered a portrait of Napoleon – a 'wretched sketch' by one of the young Somerset ladies in imitation of a well-known depiction of him, sullen and flabby aboard HMS *Northumberland*. The Comte's son, Emanuel, penned a verse on the paper in reproof:

> Sous vos doigts élégans tout devrait s'embellir;
> C'est aux belles surtout à peindre le courage:
> Du héros des héros, du Mars de l'avenir,
> Comment avez-vous pu défigurer l'image?[1]

> (In your elegant hands all should be embellished;
> It is above all for the beautiful to depict courage:
> Of the hero of heroes, of the Mars of the future,
> How have you managed to disfigure the image so?)

Las Cases placed this in a box, along with a medallion bearing 'a more faithful representation of Napoleon', hoping that Miss Somerset would find it.

He and his son had spent three months at Newlands, socialising with visitors under the eye of General Hall, the Deputy Governor. But when Cape Town was visited by Lord Amherst, former Ambassador to China, stopping en route to Britain and allotted Newlands for his use, Las Cases and his son were moved to Tygerberg, a newly settled farming area fifteen miles from Cape Town. The accommodation chosen was, according to Lord Charles, 'Apartments in the best house ... with every convenience which this Country affords and beyond what is usually met with, by every room in the house being provided with a fire place'.[2] But after Newlands, Las Cases thought Tygerberg a sparsely populated 'desert'.[3]

While there, he received secret visits from French sympathisers and an American sea captain who offered to smuggle him away from the Cape. Las Cases declined; he hoped to achieve freedom by negotiation with the British government.[4] That hope was gradually failing; he fell into a depression and felt more and more unwell. His illness 'attacked all parts of my head, under various symptoms and with various degrees of pain, without leaving me even a single day's respite'. Beside the pain he had 'an intolerable ringing in my ears. I was seized with deafness.' He also claimed to suffer swellings that hampered speech, and outbreaks of pimples on his scalp.[5] He remonstrated with Lord Charles, pleading to be allowed to move back to Cape Town; but the Governor had resumed his cold-shouldering of the Frenchman, regarding his grievances as 'in every point exaggerated'.[6] Anxious to give the Comte the very best medical assistance, however, in June he sent Dr Barry (now acting unofficially as physician to the Somerset family) to see him.

James's report came back promptly; he'd found Las Cases 'apparently feeble & anxious', complaining of 'occasional affections of his bowels' that the patient believed came from his damp bedchamber, as well as 'great agitation of his mind'. Las Cases feared that if he or his son fell seriously ill, medical help could not reach them in time. James examined both of them, and found nothing physically wrong with either. 'It is my opinion,' James wrote, 'that the Count cannot be benefited at this moment by medicine, and except the languor, debility and irritability which his body labours under, from a mind ill at ease, and a sedentary habit, he has no actual malady.'[7] (He could have added that the case was not unlike that of Miss Georgiana Somerset.) James sympathised with the Count – he concurred that the bedchamber was damp, the locale 'very dreary' and a long way from medical help, and recommended that Las Cases be allowed to return to town.

He visited once a week and prescribed treatments (tonics, cordials, exercise, fresh air), while Las Cases bombarded Lord Charles and the Colonial Secretary with letters, asking that he be moved to live close to Dr Barry. Despite the doctor's charitable suggestions, Lord Charles declined to act. And indeed James's original diagnosis of depression brought on by confinement was proved right – when Las Cases was finally given leave to sail for England, he seemed to shake off his illness with astonishing alacrity, rushing about making arrangements and social-ising.[8] In August he and Emanuel departed; barred from ships that might touch at St Helena, they were sent aboard 'an extremely small brig, an absolute cock-boat';* but 'I would have jumped into the sea rather than have delayed another moment.'[9]

Meanwhile, James Barry went on consolidating his standing in Cape society. His association with Lord Charles brought him wealthy and devoted patients. Most, unlike Las Cases or Georgiana Somerset, had very real afflictions, and some were beyond the skill of any doctor.

Lady Isabella Brenton, wife of Vice Admiral Sir Jahleel Brenton, the Cape Naval Commissioner, had been ill for years, and by early 1817 her husband was beginning to despair – he wrote heart-rending letters to their children describing his beloved's deteriorating state. They had retreated to the peaceful environment of Wynberg, not far from Newlands, but Lady Brenton got weaker by the day. Eventually Sir Jahleel sent for Dr Barry.

Like everyone else, Sir Jahleel had heard about the doctor's amazing precocity, of his having qualified at fourteen, and like most people he believed it entirely, knowing that James had 'practised with the most extraordinary success' at the Cape. He was impressed by the young doctor's manner and thorough assessment of the case – almost to the extent of allaying his sense of doom: 'Had not a firm conviction taken place in my mind, that the nature of my beloved Isabella's disorder was beyond the reach of human skill, I should have derived the most sanguine hopes from his advice'; however, 'I knew that Omnipotence alone could restore her.'[10] From the description of her symptoms, Lady Brenton was

* small rowing boat

probably suffering from tuberculosis. Dr Barry 'pronounced the case to be very alarming, and declared strong measures to be necessary'. This would have included bleeding, fresh air, possibly a milk diet, and in the last extremity laudanum to relieve the suffering. The treatment went on for some time, but 'Her state was soon pronounced hopeless.'[11] She clung on for several more weeks before dying on 29 July. The bottom fell out of Sir Jahleel's world. Yet he was grateful for the work that Dr Barry had done in easing his wife's last weeks, and they remained friends for years to come.

Other cases were more successful. Captain William Dillon, commander of the frigate HMS *Horatio*, was taken ill within a short while of dropping anchor at Simon's Bay: 'I was attacked by a violent inflammation in both eyes, the result of a cold caught in the late gales.'[12] The ship's surgeon 'inflicted upon me some painful trials', bleeding him from the temple and scarifying both his lower eyelids as a means of counter-irritation, 'which only produced temporary relief'. Dillon was desperate. Inevitably he heard the remarkable reports of the Governor's physician, who 'was in the Army and considered extremely clever'. Dillon heard gossip: 'Many surmises were in circulation relating to him; from the awkwardness of his gait and the shape of his person, it was the prevailing opinion that he was a female.' (In fact it wasn't the prevailing opinion at all, other than among those who most relished scandal; most people simply wouldn't credit that a woman could do such a thing.) Despite Dr Barry's oddity, Dillon was impressed: 'He was extremely assiduous, but did not approve the remedies resorted to, plainly telling me that a milder treatment would have sufficed.'[13] James waived the customary fee, asking only for his travelling expenses from Cape Town.

His situation with regard to fees was a delicate one; as an Army surgeon he wasn't a free agent. Despite practising semi-permanently for the Governor, he severely disapproved of military doctors taking payment for private work. There was only one possible solution to his situation – to make it official. This was done on 7 December 1817, and the following week the proclamation was issued:

His Excellency the Governor has been pleased to appoint Dr James Barry, M. D. to be Physician to His Excellency's Household, and Vaccinating Physician to the Vaccine Institution at the Cape.[14]

The position carried an annual salary of 600 rixdollars* (about £45),[15] a very modest sum for a physician's services, and likely just a retainer, with fees and expenses paid on a case-by-case basis. James also received a grace-and-favour residence in the grounds of Government House, which saved him a good deal of expenditure and put him close to the flow of the Governor's friends and visitors.

James's second appointment bolstered the official nature of the arrangement. The Vaccine Institution had been founded in 1807 by one of Lord Charles's predecessors for the purpose of inoculating the population against smallpox. The disease wasn't endemic in the Colony, but there had been outbreaks brought in by ships – the last one in Cape Town itself in 1812, when hundreds had been afflicted, necessitating the establishment of a quarantine colony at Paarden Eiland; dozens had died.[16] 'Variolation' (named after *variola minor* and *major*, the medical name for smallpox) – a method that applied infections prepared from the scabs of smallpox sufferers through abrasions in the skin – had been developed during the eighteenth century and introduced into the Cape by the Dutch. However, in 1796 Dr Edward Jenner had developed a much safer method using a cowpox-based preparation; this was named 'vaccination' (after *vaccinia virus*, the scientific name for cowpox).[†]

The Vaccine Institution was small, housed in civil offices in Church Square, Cape Town, and had just three officials: the Senior Member, a Mr William Henry Lys (an Army surgeon), a secretary, and now Dr James Barry as Second Member. All vaccination in the Cape Colony was under their control.[17] It wasn't an easy task; because the authorities were concerned about 'improper assemblage' of common folk and natives, so Mr Lys and Dr Barry were obliged to conduct their vaccination programme laboriously house-to-house, one town at a time.[18]

James's salary for this part-time appointment was 1200 rixdollars (about £90).[19] On top of his Army pay of 7s 6d a day,[20] and salary from Lord Charles, this brought his annual income to a little over £270;[‡] not at all bad for a young fellow who (according to popular belief) was not

---

* *rixdollar*: international European currency used in some British colonies; 1 rixdollar = about 1s 6d.

† *virus*: poison (Latin). Viruses were not identified, let alone understood, until the late 19th century.

‡ over £200,000 in terms of average 2016 incomes, but much less in actual purchasing power

quite out of his teens, and a fitting close to a year in which James Barry's life and fortunes had been transformed. Just over twelve months earlier he'd been an obscure assistant staff surgeon, a stranger newly arrived at the Cape, his only claim to friendship a well-travelled letter from the Earl of Buchan (which admittedly was rather more than most young surgeons could boast). In that busy year, he'd acquired a reputation and position, if not at the peak of Cape society then in its shade.

For his private cases, James took only expenses or sometimes a payment in kind. On one extraordinary occasion he was called out to Great Westerford, near Newlands House, to attend one of the Governor's neighbours, a Mrs Cloete. She was suffering from pneumonia, and believed to be dying; her family had consulted Lord Charles, who immediately recommended Dr Barry.[21] As soon as he received the call, James got in his buggy and drove out to Great Westerford.

With pneumonia there wasn't a moment to lose, and this sounded like an advanced case. As one lung specialist noted, 'A fatal termination is frequently a speedy consequence of neglected pneumonia.'[22] Venesection – bleeding – was the first resort, according to the established principle that it reduced inflammation (or 'excitement') by lowering blood pressure; 'By producing copious evacuations of blood,' wrote the same specialist, 'the violence of excitement is diminished with great celerity.'[23] However, it was thought unsafe (indeed sometimes fatal) to bleed a patient more than three or four days into the illness; in that case a variety of external treatments, including blistering (a stimulant) and cupping (using a vacuum glass on the skin to draw out toxic substances), could be used. An alternative to bleeding, only recently introduced, was a medicine made from *Digitalis purpurea*,* which lowered blood pressure and inflammation by reducing the action of the heart; but again this was only appropriate in the early stages.[24] Mild (*not* strong) purgatives might also be required to clear the bowels, and steams of *Althaea officinalis*,† camomile flowers and vinegar were to be inhaled regularly.[25] However, the sense of foreboding attached to Mrs Cloete's case, and its advanced state, suggested that the inevitable outcome would be death, or at best development of irreversible phthisis.‡

---

* foxglove
† marshmallow
‡ tuberculosis, believed at the time to sometimes follow pneumonia

James was met by a servant who conducted him with great solemnity to the sickroom. The bedroom door opened, releasing a fug of hot, stale air like the blast from an oven. Inside the darkened, stifling room there was a veritable crowd of anxious, depressed family members and servants; the windows were firmly shut, and the patient lay in a four-poster bed with its thick curtains drawn, struggling to breathe. It was the worst conceivable state for anyone with a lung disease. James's temper snapped. He stamped his foot in anger, hurried to the window and heaved up the sash, letting in a rush of air; then he strode to the bed and furiously tore aside the curtains, revealing the distressed Mrs Cloete.

While fresh air flowed around the bedroom, Dr Barry 'proceeded to give the bewildered Mrs Cloete and her mournful attendants such a scolding as they had never had before'.[26] He examined the patient, pressing an ear to her chest to listen to her breathing (the stethoscope – a peculiar new instrument resembling an ear trumpet – had been invented two years earlier in France, but had not yet reached the colonies) and percussing the chest with his fingers to hear its resonance (another relatively new technique, developed late in the previous century). With some relief, he found her to be past the crisis point of the disease; there was little to be done. And with that – without explanation, with no further treatment or prescription, nor any instruction other than to keep the room properly ventilated – he turned on his heel, left the house, mounted his buggy and returned to Cape Town.

To the patient and her friends, the outcome was amazing. Mrs Cloete – her life having been all but given up – rallied with astonishing speed, and within a few weeks she had entirely recovered her health. Her illness was probably lobar pneumonia – quite different from bronchopneumonia and relatively rare in the modern world – which produces a 'crisis' moment, at which point the sufferer's system overcomes the infection and the lungs are cleared. The recovery is so rapid as to appear miraculous.

Mrs Cloete was profoundly grateful, but James declined to take any fee. So instead she selected two very fine black horses from her stable and sent them to Cape Town for the doctor to keep and use; she also arranged for regular wagons of fodder to be delivered for their maintenance. James was delighted; he adored the horses and rode them often, immensely proud of their beauty. Years later, when he eventually left the Cape, he returned them to Mrs Cloete, 'who for many years would never tire of telling how she had been saved from death by the doctor who went into a frenzy of rage over her'.[27]

James became known as an enthusiastic rider and huntsman – during a stay in the country with Lord Charles, one female patient among the party recalled him coming to her bedroom 'booted and spurred, ready for the hunt'.[28] Very fond of Dr Barry, she didn't experience his temper, and found he had 'impeccable bedroom manners', with a kind voice and soft touch; when he left, the patient said to her maid: 'It might have been a woman touching my head: the doctor's hands are so light'; indeed, James Barry's 'beautiful small white hands were the envy of many a lady'.

A little under a year after being appointed Governor's Physician, a much more testing case came James's way and gave him occasion to truly earn his retainer – Lord Charles himself fell seriously, mortally ill.

Newlands: Saturday 17 October 1818

The neat little buggy clipped briskly along the road from Cape Town, the equally neat little figure of Dr James Barry at the reins. Of all the roads in the Cape of Good Hope, this was one of the most pleasant; now in the rising spring it was positively idyllic. From Cape Town the road took a great sweep around the foot of Devil's Peak – the massive outthrust spur of rock that formed the end of the Cape Peninsula's spine – before curving south into the rolling wooded country nestling beneath the vast bulk of Table Mountain. It was in this region that the upper classes of the western Cape's society had made their country retreats – including the Governor. Newlands House was a large, exceptionally fine residence, noted for its elegant garden wing built in an unusual shape with semi-circular ends (anticipating Art Deco by more than a century) topped by a dainty cupola. The estate stood on steep green hills with the spectacular mountain cliff-face towering over it.

But for all the pleasant scenery, Lord Charles's life was hanging in the balance. It had begun exactly four weeks earlier, on a Saturday afternoon in Cape Town.[29] His Excellency had complained of feeling ill; his symptoms weren't recorded in detail at the time, but based on the eventual outcome the pattern would be all too certain. First came a feeling of malaise, of being strangely out of sorts; there was a headache, and a slightly flushed sensation.[30] Nothing to be unduly concerned about in his own opinion, and that evening he felt fit enough to attend the theatre, despite Dr Barry's contrary advice. There were no immediate ill effects, but he obediently stayed indoors for the next two days. However, by Tuesday his restless spirit, which hated confinement, induced him to call for his carriage. In the doctor's view this was a grave error – and he was right, for after driving around the town for a short while, Lord Charles returned to Government House 'in a state of great debility', in the words of Colonel Bird, 'and has not been up since'.[31]

A week passed, and Lord Charles's condition grew alarmingly worse – a high fever, extreme fatigue, bradycardia* and mild delirium. To Dr Barry's eye, this was the *typhus mitior*, the nervous fever that gave typhus its name.[32] But there was more – pain and distension in the abdomen and diarrhoea; according to contemporary medical science, this could be one of two things. One was *typhus gravior* – also known as putrid and malignant fever – but Lord Charles did not have the black tongue, the acrid odour or the rapid, fierce onset of symptoms. The other was typhus with dysentery, which was seen as a common pairing. Dr Barry was almost constantly at the Governor's bedside – ear pressed to his fevered chest, listening to the slow heartbeat and (as the illness progressed) the labouring of the congested lungs, watching the eyes flutter and stare in delirium, studying with marvellous detachment the efflux of the loose bowels (the consistency of pea soup) – and settled inevitably upon this diagnosis: typhus with dysentery.[33]

And what a depressing diagnosis it was; James felt that Lord Charles's habits of temperance should help him withstand the illness (at fifty-one he led a rather healthier life than in his prime when he'd been one of the Prince of Wales's Brighton bucks), but, as Colonel Bird wrote to Lord Bathurst, 'Dr Barry nevertheless expresses so much apprehension that I cannot delay making your Lordship acquainted with the state in which he now is.'[34] Orders had been given that the colonial schooner, *Mary*, be prepared to carry the sad news to London 'should an unfavourable turn take place'.

For James Barry it was a personal and professional challenge of huge proportions. Where would he be without his patron? He had acquired status and influence in the Cape of Good Hope, but his position was hardly settled; the whispers behind his back about his peculiar effeminacy

---

* slow heartbeat

were a real danger. Without Lord Charles, the world of new friendships, of socialising and hunting and lively, educated conversation, which had taken such a surprisingly short time to build, must surely collapse. He would have to revert to being a mere assistant staff surgeon, toiling away in the Military Hospital, where the gossip about him was especially marked. And that was far from all: Lord Charles Henry Somerset was not only his patron and protector; he was becoming the centre of James Barry's world, a close friend, successor to Francisco de Miranda's role of beloved father figure, and possibly more than that.

Treatment was a matter for much consideration. It was conventional to bleed a patient with dysentery, but if there was fever and the pulse was weak, that was ruled out.[35] A mild emetic in the evening and an occasional saline purgative in the morning to clear the stomach and bowel were recommended, and perhaps a diaphoretic.* As a fall-back one might try *vitrum antimonii*† coated with wax. If the sufferer was already retching or vomiting, then these treatments were ruled out – instead, draughts of camomile tea were recommended, to evacuate the stomach. Hip baths and abdominal massage might also be tried. The list of possible treatments varied according to the precise symptoms and the preferences (and inward desperation) of the physician.

Those were just the dysenteric symptoms; then there was the typhus. This was thought to be fearfully contagious, and the patient had to be isolated from all persons other than their medical attendants, due to the miasma – the contagious vapour – that was thought to emanate from the sufferer. Anything the patient had contact with – garments, linen, utensils – had to be cleansed before leaving the room. The room must also be thoroughly aired to dilute and dissipate the miasma. Treatment could include a mild emetic; a laxative might also be given, to 'dislodge, and bring off whatever feculent matter may be contained in the bowels, which by retention might be likely to prove highly offensive, as well as irritating'.[36] Sponging with cold water was highly recommended, but only in the late evening, when the fever tended to be at its height. In the early stages of the disease, it was suggested that the patient be doused with cold water from a pail or a garden watering can. Purification of the skin with soap and water was also desirable.

---

* a drug inducing perspiration
† glass of antimony, an emetic

Because of the patient's strict confinement, all these treatments would have to be applied by Dr Barry, or in his absence by a nurse; given his notorious intolerance of meddling and insistence on precise obedience to instructions, not to mention his fond devotion to his benefactor and the paramount importance of the case, James almost certainly did everything himself. From collecting Lord Charles's stools for inspection to listening to the heart, bathing him and sponging his perspiring, shivering body – all would have been taken care of by those small, white hands, fighting tenaciously to pull him back from the brink of death.

The *Mary* did not sail with her dreadful news. Instead, on the thirteenth day of His Excellency's sickness, Colonel Bird was able to write to Lord Bathurst that 'Lord Charles Somerset has rallied a little and was last night without fever. He is certainly in a state of great debility, but considerable hopes are now entertained that he will do well.'[37]

In a little over a week, he was well enough to be moved to the fresher air of Newlands, where Dr Barry continued to visit him.

Bringing his buggy to a halt on the drive and hurrying into the house, James found Lord Charles in his usual state: attending to business and fretting over government policy. Britain had threatened to impose duty on wine imported from the Cape, which vexed him greatly; he was dictating a furious letter to Lord Bathurst, Secretary of State for War and the Colonies.

'I am really hurt and alarmed at the thought,' he declared, as his daughter struggled to keep up. 'As it is, the price which Cape wines fetch in the London market does not pay the exporter of them.'[38] He was considerably paler than normal, and much thinner too; the ordeal had tested him to the limit of his constitution, and had also been exceedingly trying for Dr Barry. He wasn't well enough yet to write letters for himself, and there was no secretary present, so he railed on while Georgiana followed: 'so much capital has now been embarked as well in addition to plantations of vine (not yet come to bearing) as in the building of capacious cellaring and storehouses and in the fustage* necessary for a permanent export trade ... that nothing short of absolute ruin to all concerned can be anticipated from a change of policy in our regard.' He concluded: 'Just convalescent from a severe illness I avail myself of an amanuensis in addressing your Lordship, because I would not delay an instant endeavouring to interest

---

* vats, tubs and utensils using in wine-making

you in a case of such vital importance to us. I remain etcetera etcetera ...'
There was nothing, apparently, that could divert this man from his duty.

Their enforced closeness – and its outcome – had cemented their friendship and increased James's influence on Lord Charles; it was during these weeks of convalescence that he issued the decree banning the hunting of bontebok. By the beginning of November his recovery was sufficiently assured for him to publish a statement in the *Cape Gazette*: 'His Excellency begs to offer his most sincere and grateful thanks to all those who have with the kindest solicitude made such constant and anxious enquiries for him during his late illness.'[39]

His Excellency's opinion of James Barry – which had always been high – now knew no bounds. A few months later, Sir Hudson Lowe, Governor of St Helena, wrote to Lord Charles and happened to mention that Lady Lowe was unwell. Lord Charles suggested that she be brought to the Cape of Good Hope, where the climate was so much more healthful; moreover, 'I have, however, beside here quite a prodigy in a physician [in] Dr Barry whose skill has effected wonders since he has been here, indeed it would be worth while for an invalid to come here solely for the purpose of obtaining his advice.'[40]

James's position at the Cape was more elevated and secure than ever. And yet there was a danger that beneath the disguise Margaret might grow complacent, overplay the part. Moreover, the stress of sustaining the charade so publicly was beginning to take a toll.

13

The Most Wayward of Mortals

A garden in Constantia: dawn

The pistol felt surprisingly heavy in James's hand; so much weight and purpose in so small a thing. A work of death; and yet also a work of strange beauty: the dull steel of the barrel merging with the polished wooden stock and in one elegant sweep turning into the grip, the bulbous butt-cap giving the whole an outline not unlike a femur, with vein-like chasing on the silverwork glinting softly in the dawn light. Beauty, weight and purpose. As the seconds moved apart and the brass-bound pistol box snapped shut, from the corner of his eye James watched his opponent – the handsome, golden-haired cavalry captain – cock his piece. James imitated the action, using his left hand to draw back the lock with an oily click.

The two combatants walked to the marks from which, on the signal, they would level and fire. Two officers of the British Army, one a man of healing, each endeavouring in earnest to kill or maim one another. How had it come to this?

Within James Barry's skin, Margaret was growing ill at ease. It was ten years since she'd packed away her dresses and bonnets, ten years in which to forget what it was like to be a woman and acquire the ways of a man; but it was an imposture that was ultimately impossible to perfect. And James's professional and social success at the Cape of Good Hope, glorious as it was, brought danger with it; he was far more prominent, more exposed to attention than he had ever been in Edinburgh or London, or even in the hospitals at Chelsea and Plymouth. And attention from the multitude must inevitably bring suspicious scrutiny; there had been rumours whispered behind his back, and each new telling, each new acquaintance, must increase the precariousness of the situation.

On at least one occasion it came to a crisis. There was an English nurse who had a high reputation and was often employed on cases he attended, and one night both she and James were staying in the house of a female patient. The nurse found the patient in need of immediate attention, so she sent for Dr Barry, and waited. He seemed to be taking a long time, so she ran to his room and – as was customary with nurses fetching doctors to an emergency – burst in without knocking. Precisely what he was doing was never recorded, but the nurse saw enough to know that Dr Barry was a woman. From that day onward, their working relationship was finished; Dr Barry 'displayed the most implacable dislike to her' (wrote a friend to whom she told the story years later), and refused to attend any patient who employed her. As long as James lived at the Cape the nurse was absolutely silent about what she had seen, but the risk and the fear were always there, and in the end Dr Barry's enmity was sufficient to drive her out of the Cape for good.[1]

James had pursued his male persona to the extent that he'd become known as a ladies' man – a 'perfect dancer who won his way to many a heart', one woman noted, as if he were a latter-day Orpheus, beardless and effeminate but enchanting: 'In fact he was a flirt … He had a winning way with women.'[2] If this was a deliberate act to deflect suspicion, it must have been hard to sustain. The effect of relentless stress was there for anyone to see, and he was becoming known for his irascibility, abrasiveness and outbursts of rage. James's contemporaries would expect him, as a redheaded Irishman, to be hot-blooded and choleric (if not actually insane), and he acquired an extraordinary reputation for ill temper. Yet his genius usually preserved him from censure.

Dr Barry had never been tolerant of other doctors' contrary opinions or their (in his view) ineffectual treatments; now he became fierce and his patients sometimes experienced the brunt. Certain incidents became legendary, passed down with the folklore of the Cape for generations afterwards. 'Fine and delicate as a dragonfly', one chronicler recorded, Dr Barry 'could be as angry and reckless as a ruffian'.[3] So long as his patients, their nurses and servants complied perfectly with his instructions he would be the embodiment of gentleness; but if any stepped out of line – omitted a medicine, failed to follow an instruction, burned a broth – his inner ruffian came shrieking out. It wasn't unknown for him to storm out of an uncooperative patient's sickroom, 'slamming the door behind him with such violence that the whole house echoed with the noise',[4] not caring whether he upset the patient. When one patient's room had not been ventilated according to his order, he flung open the sashes with so much force that the glass smashed. Nurses and maids were regularly given shrill scoldings, accompanied by the violent stamping of the doctor's tiny foot, and on occasion bottles of medicine that had been neglected by the patient would be flung at the walls.

And yet, according to the same chronicler, 'despite all of this, his patients remained loyal to this little tyrant':

> He had the eye of a hawk, from which no detail escaped, summing up a situation at a glance. And following this assessment, the patient and his relatives were able to witness how the sickness would resolve. His practice was extraordinarily successful, and he combined his clarity of vision with firmness of hand and strength of will.[5]

Sometimes James took out his anger by more measured means. When a clergyman sent a polite note asking him to remove a tooth, Dr Barry exclaimed, 'Does this stupid parson suppose that I'm a vulgar tooth-drawer?' He called on his local farrier, who had experience with horses' teeth, and told him to go to the clergyman's house, where a 'donkey with toothache' needed his attention; the innocent farrier went, equipped with a hand-vice, pincers and a couple of brawny assistants, and asked the clergyman to show him the donkey with tooth trouble. The cleric complained to the Governor, only to be advised that Dr Barry's antics were to be tolerated, and that the reverend gentleman had better just 'join in the laughter against you'.[6]

Even Lord Charles Somerset himself was not exempt from the Barry temper. In the period following his convalescence, the Governor failed in some way to comply with his treatments, with the result that James told him he could prescribe for himself if he thought he knew better, and abandoned him.[7] Lord Charles, who doted on James, soon submitted to his medical authority, and confided his feelings about Dr Barry to George Keppel, a young infantry lieutenant (and earl's son) who visited the Cape in 1819. He told Keppel that Dr Barry was 'the most skilful of physicians, and the most wayward of mortals'.[8] Keppel 'heard so much of this capricious, yet privileged gentleman, that I had a great curiosity to see him'. He soon had the opportunity, when they sat together at a regimental mess dinner:

> I beheld a beardless lad, apparently of my own age, with an unmistaka-
> bly Scotch type of countenance – reddish hair, high cheek bones. There
> was a certain effeminacy in his manner, which he seemed to be always
> striving to overcome. His style of conversation was greatly superior
> to that one usually heard at a mess-table.[9]

Margaret never could succeed in imitating the male persona entirely – it was apparently not in her.[10] Another problem, which would only get worse with the passing years, was that although James appeared in most people's eyes to be a youthful twenty, beneath it Margaret was a decade older; soon the first signs of ageing would become visible (if they were not already – the Cape sunlight must have been harsh on her pale com-plexion). The skin would start to slacken and the crow's-feet begin to grow, yet James would continue to be beardless and delicately featured long after the excuse of juvenility had expired.

The stresses would never go away, and James's notorious temper would continue. Keppel, who was so intrigued by Dr Barry that he fol-lowed his later career, recorded that he 'was considered to be of a most quarrelsome disposition. He was frequently guilty of flagrant breaches of discipline ... but somehow or other his offences were always condoned' by the powers above.[11]

That gift of acquiring patrons and protectors was an indispensable barrier against the worst consequences of that explosive, uncontainable temper. Lord Charles Somerset was quickly proving the most benefi-cent of all his protectors, often tested far beyond what most men in his position would consider the limit. One day James was out riding with a group of fellow officers when one of them – an ill-bred, ill-mannered fellow – drew his mount up close beside James's and drawled, 'By the Powers, you look more like a woman than a man!'[12] It was like prodding a cobra – James instantly lashed out with his horsewhip, laying a dreadful cut across the officer's cheek. By the custom of the day the officer was entitled to demand satisfaction by means of a duel; but surprisingly there was no meeting, no challenge; instead he sought redress by appealing to his superiors. Like the clergyman with toothache, he took his complaint all the way to Government House, and instead of provoking disciplinary

action against Dr Barry, the officer was astonished to find himself removed
from the Cape garrison and posted to a remote island station. As one
chronicler noted, 'Powerful influence was ever at Barry's back.'[13]

The relationship between James and Lord Charles was a peculiarly
complex one: the bond between physician and patient mingled with
that of father and son. In the sickroom James was the paternal one, but
elsewhere the roles were the other way round. And there must have been
another dimension; James had spent hours, day and night, nursing Lord
Charles during his illness, in intimate physical contact. At some point,
Lord Charles – who was far from inexperienced with women – must
have sensed that James was female. It may have been this shared secret
that increased Lord Charles's protective instinct; Margaret grew to love
him, and the feeling appeared to be reciprocated. What manner of love
it was, from either side, would be impossible to identify with certainty
in those early days, but there were signs that James was jealous of his
patron's affections, and the jealousy had a discernible sexual colour to
it. It seems that James Barry was in love with Lord Charles Somerset. If
so, it must have added still more depth to James's stress, frustration and
outbursts of rage. In different ways during the coming years, it would
eventually lead both of them to the edge of ruin.

That year, 1819, it threatened to extinguish James altogether, when
jealousy happened to coincide with a gross miscalculation in Margaret's
understanding of masculine values. One spring morning, James found
himself at Government House, kicking his heels in the Governor's outer
office, and fell into conversation with one of his aides-de-camp, Captain
Josias Cloete of the 21st Light Dragoons, who had recently returned
from war in India.

This good-looking young man was the sprig of a very well-to-do local
family with an estate not far from Newlands (relations of Mrs Cloete,
the pneumonic patient who had given James those fine horses). He was a
striking sight beside Dr Barry; they resembled each other astonishingly.
Cloete had blond hair (a shade brighter than James's red-blond), coiffed
in the Caesar style, and his face was almost feminine: the very same soft,
pink complexion, large, wide-set eyes (watery blue, while James's were
blue-green), a similarly long, curved nose, full lips with a Cupid's bow,
and a narrow button chin. But with the exception of his nose, which
was finer than James's Ciceronian prow, Cloete's features were broader,
heavier, more distinctly on the masculine side of androgyny.[14]

Cloete had position and influence too. The third son of vineyard owner Pieter Lourens Cloete, Josias had been fourteen years old when the British captured the Cape in 1806.[15] His father, adapting quickly to the new regime, sent him to the Royal Military Academy at Great Marlow (a few years prior to its move to Sandhurst), and he was commissioned as a cornet in the elite 15th (the King's) Hussars in 1809. By 1813 he had returned to the land of his birth.

Cloete's career at the Cape had also mirrored James Barry's: he was aide-de-camp to Lord Charles, who considered him a 'young officer of considerable talent and acquirements' and 'in every respect trustworthy'; considering it politically desirable to place Dutch colonial officers in British regiments, in 1816 Lord Charles made him commandant of the small military force sent to seize Tristan da Cunha – the most remote inhabited island in the world – to prevent its being used as a base for attempts to rescue Napoleon.[16] After that, Cloete's regiment had been despatched to India to take part in the Third Anglo-Maratha War, and it was only recently – September 1819 – that he'd returned to the Cape,[17] where he found that the Governor had a new favourite in this odd little doctor.

Cloete was a seasoned war veteran, and exactly the kind of *beau sabreur* that little Margaret Bulkley had once dreamed of being. Although Captain Cloete had the greatest respect for Dr Barry's medical skill, which he said 'combined in an extraordinary degree, the rarest qualities of Esculapian* Talent', he was jealous, and regarded him as a usurper and a schemer, with 'the most mischievous propensities of a Monkey, and all the subtle wiles of the Serpent', who had worked his way into Lord Charles's affections while Cloete had been away on active duty.[18]

This mutual suspicion and jealousy apparently led James to his first great blunder. While he and Cloete chatted in the office, a buxom, attractive and wealthy woman entered and was quickly shown through to Lord Charles's inner sanctum, on 'business of a private nature'.[19] Who this lady might be, and the nature of the 'business', was not recorded, but she was shut in with the Governor for a very long time.[20]

James, deeply uncomfortable, tried to relieve his feelings through a little masculine banter with his companion. 'I say, Cloete,' he said with a sneer, 'that's a nice Dutch filly the Governor's got hold of.'[21]

---

* or Aesculapian, after Asclepius, Greek god of medicine

It was a stunning *faux pas*, doubly surprising in someone who had
studied so hard to play the man. It simply wasn't done for an officer
to speak in this disrespectful manner to another officer about a lady –
even mentioning a lady's name in the officers' mess was prohibited by
custom – and James had compounded the outrage with his imputation
about the Dutch.

'Retract your vile expression, you infernal little cad,' said Cloete.

Taken aback, James obstinately refused to retract or apologise. Cloete,
despite his anger, refrained from striking the fragile little doctor; instead
he delivered the conventional alternative to a blow: he stepped up, seized
James's 'long ugly nose' and pulled.

It would have been comical if the implication hadn't been so serious.
The affront was impossible to ignore, and James's temper impossible
to contain. Other than an unseemly brawl, there was only one possible
response for an Irishman (the Irish code of honour being exceptionally
harsh); summoning as much dignity as he could muster in the circumstances, James challenged Captain Cloete to a duel.[22] One or other of
them would gain satisfaction by combat. Declaring that his second would
call upon Captain Cloete's, James left, seething.

He had possibly made out his own death warrant; Josias Cloete was a
real martial soldier, while James Barry, for all his sword, spurs and gold
buttons, was not. What chance would he stand in a duel? Influence with
Lord Charles would not help him out of this; Cloete stood high both in
the Cape service and in society. There was no choice but to meet.

How different the beautiful southern road seemed in the cold hour before
dawn, with death waiting at the end of it. The coach rattled along with
James inside, accompanied by his second, a fellow Army surgeon,[23] past
Newlands and on through the gloom. At last they reached the Cloete
family estate, Alphen, and drew up in front of the house, a large building in white stucco, square and blockish, with minimal ornament: neither wholly Dutch nor especially English. In daylight it was elegantly
restrained and quite pleasant, but in the cold dawn light it looked grey and
grim, the Cape Dutch windows, chequered with tiny panes, resembling
the gratings of a madhouse.

This was the appointed place, chosen by Captain Cloete's second
(whose right it was to determine the scene of action).[24] Behind the
house the ground sloped away through lawns and shrubberies, and in

the distance – just growing visible in the eastern light – it swooped up to the vineyards on the foothills of Table Mountain, whose summit was already bathed in light. The meeting place was on a lawn a short distance from the house. Like James, Captain Cloete was in uniform – in his case, the full dress rig of a light dragoon: dark blue jacket with pink collar and cuffs, braided and buttoned with gold, Hessian boots, and a peaked shako topped with a feathered plume. The notion of duellists facing one another in shirt-sleeves was a romantic invention; gentlemen wore their best, including hats and coats if the weather required it. This carried an inherent risk, and James would be acutely aware of the danger of cloth being carried by a bullet into a wound, where it would fester.

A gentleman was present to act as loader, as well as the customary surgeon. The seconds met and spoke, inquiring whether either gentleman wished to issue an apology or retraction. Neither did. There followed a pause while the seconds paced out the ground and placed marker stones twenty paces apart. (The practice of combatants starting back-to-back, pacing out their own distance, was also a theatrical invention.)[25]

The loader came forward, producing a flat, brass-bound box from beneath his cloak: rather like a surgeon's instrument case, and with contents equally terrifying to the uninitiated. He primed the pieces, inserting new flints, ramming home the loads. Honour stipulated no double shotting, no rough balls that could cause severe wounding, and minimal, lightweight wadding, to reduce the risk of gangrene (like clothing, it tended to get stuck in wounds).[26] The seconds chose a pistol each – half-cocked – and walked back to the principals, still standing aloof from one another (communication between them at this stage was forbidden). James took his piece, a thing of beauty and violence. He was quite accustomed to handling complex devices designed to puncture human flesh, but none that was designed expressly to maim or kill.

He walked to his marker stone and placed the toe of his right boot against it, then turned side-on towards Cloete, with the pistol cocked and lowered; Cloete did the same. The sky was brightening now, the light clear, every detail of the scene standing out in crisp detail. There was no turning back; even the humane option of deloping* was closed to James, since the Irish code forbade it.[27] Both the English and Irish rules insisted that combat, once begun, must continue, shot after shot, until one man

---

* firing deliberately into the ground to terminate a duel without bloodshed

was wounded or dead. Any wound 'sufficient to agitate the nerves, and necessarily make the hand shake' was regarded as decisive.[28] One way or another, someone would be leaving his blood on the grass.

The seconds retired to a safe distance. From the corner of his eye, James could see that the surgeon had his instrument case open and his medicine bottles laid out. The signal came suddenly – the quick flutter of a white handkerchief; James's arm shot up, rigid, the pistol poised, his opponent's face a pale smudge above the barrel. Both fired simultaneously; James's flint struck the frizzen, the pan erupting in a cloud of sparks and smoke; there was an instant's silence, then the loud double crack sent birds fluttering from the trees.[29]

James's aim was the better – his bullet struck Captain Cloete square in the middle of the forehead. It was deflected by the peak of his shako, which broke off and went spinning away. As Cloete staggered and regained his poise, James noticed a dull throb coming from his thigh; there was a rent in his breeches near the groin, and blood was beginning to seep.[30]

The surgeon hurried to him, whipping out a pair of scissors. James knew exactly what he intended to do; the wound was high up on the thigh, necessitating the cutting away of his breeches. He ordered everyone to stand back and insisted on binding it hastily himself, then got to his feet and went to exchange formalities with Captain Cloete. They declared honour satisfied, and shook hands.

Back in the cottage in the grounds of Government House after a long and anxious drive from Alphen, Margaret locked herself in, pulled off breeches and drawers and examined the wound. Despite the blood, it was a flesh wound, and easily dressed. An inch or so further in, it would have hit the femoral artery and the bleeding might have proven fatal before it could be staunched. Or had it dug a little deeper into the flesh, it would have been beyond self-treatment, and Margaret's exposure would have been certain.

A chilling realisation. She must have foreseen this complication, yet it hadn't discouraged the challenge. And it wouldn't inhibit James in the future – incredibly, Dr Barry's temperament was unaltered.

James's standing with Lord Charles wasn't materially harmed by the duel. However, Captain Cloete didn't remain an aide-de camp to the Governor; he was appointed acting deputy quartermaster general, a promotion of sorts, but also a post that would require his removal to Algoa Bay, where a new settlement was taking root.[31] His career was becoming distinctly more prosaic, having been placed on half-pay in January 1820 pending the disbandment of the 21st Light Dragoons.[32]

For Dr James Barry, nothing immediately changed – other than walking with a limp for a week or two and adding to his reputation for volatility. So perhaps his influence with the Governor – or at least his manifest value – was greater than Cloete's after all. Perhaps most surprisingly, despite having gone as far as to fire pistols at one another, James Barry and Josias Cloete ended on good terms and remained so for decades, keeping in touch as they rose through the ranks.

14

A Change of Circumstances

James Barry didn't confine his attentions to the ruling classes of the Cape; he also worked among the poor. Aside from his work for the Vaccine Institution, he took a sympathetic interest in the plight of the Colony's black population – particularly the slaves. There were tens of thousands of them, and no sign of emancipation in sight, despite the abolition movement in Britain. The indigenous Cape peoples – mostly San and Khoikhoi – were protected by law from enslavement, but were sometimes little better off than slaves. There was a constant state of insecurity and suspicion among the whites towards the black people of the Colony, which had been heightened in early 1819 by Ndlambe's assault on Grahamstown.

Occupying an uneasy middle ground between slavery and freedom were the 'Bastaards' and the so-called 'Prize Negroes', people who'd been abducted by Portuguese slavers from Mozambique and Madagascar then captured by Royal Navy patrols. Rather than being liberated, these slaves were taken as 'prizes' – part of the perquisites of victorious naval commanders.[1] Since they couldn't be traded, they were 'apprenticed' in the Cape Colony, where they lived in a state that was scarcely distinguishable from slavery. The apprenticeship was fixed at fourteen years – a period judged to be 'most likely to fix them in habits of industry' and prevent them lapsing into delinquency and 'retiring in idleness to the interior'.[2] Some of them were drafted into the Cape's garrison as reserve manpower.[3]

Life was bitterly tough for the Africans in southern Africa. Some local natives ended up in apprenticeships as repressive as those of the 'prizes'. One in particular, in whom James Barry took a keen interest, was a young San boy known to the whites as Hermes. He was kept by a Dutch woman who treated him abominably and was threatening to have him thrown in gaol over some trivial act of theft. James, taking pity on the boy, bought the woman's contract rights over him. He placed Hermes in the care of Sir Jahleel Brenton, who'd been in low spirits since his wife's death, and welcomed him into his family.

Hermes's character was not unlike James's, which might explain his particular interest; according to Brenton he 'gave remarkable evidences of intelligence and quickness' but could be 'irritable and revengeful when wronged', yet was 'in no ordinary degree attached and grateful when treated kindly'; it was hoped that 'this child of the wilderness' might eventually be sent back to his homeland 'as a messenger of peace, and a herald of mercy to his persecuted and benighted countrymen'.[4]

When Brenton gave up his post and sailed for England in late 1821, he took Hermes with him. But despite the family's fondness for him, the boy was a mere object of fascination in English society – little more than a freak. He couldn't adapt to his situation, and his health suffered in the climate; 'the irritability of his temper and restlessness rendered it inconvenient to retain him in the family'. He was sent back to the Cape, with the intention that he be placed in a suitable occupation. There, his 'original nature' resumed; he vanished from the Colony and went to live in the bush, where he became 'the wild timid wanderer that he had been'.[5]

Everything changed for James in January 1820, when Lord Charles Somerset left the Cape for England. Within a few weeks James would also depart, in the opposite direction.

Still concerned about Georgiana's health, Lord Charles believed – apparently on James's counsel – that the voyage might do her good.[6] (James knew well that there was nothing physically wrong with Miss Somerset, and might have guessed – correctly as it turned out – that she needed jolting out of her lassitude.)[7] Lord Charles's friend the Prince Regent had granted him a period of leave, and so he and his daughters sailed for home.

Management of the Cape Colony was handed to Acting Governor-General Sir Rufane Shawe Donkin. Lord Charles had appointed him without knowing him well, and could scarcely have made a worse choice. Donkin was a Whig, and hostile to Lord Charles's Tory politics. His ideas about running the Colony were quite different; whereas Lord Charles's approach had been nurturing, based on economic development,

conciliation and bargaining, Sir Rufane Donkin was abrasive and dictatorial, disdainful of committees and strong on personal power.[8]

His first challenge came within days of the Somersets' departure. In late
January the Royal Navy brig *Hardy* arrived from Mauritius with alarming
news: there was cholera on the island, a disease that had always before
been confined to India. Thousands were reported dead.[9] Donkin immediately proclaimed strict measures for the Cape's protection: 'undoubted
information has been communicated to me,' he announced publicly,
'of a malignant Disorder having broken out in the Island of Mauritius,
which is said already to have carried off (after a few hours illness only)
vast numbers of the unfortunate Inhabitants.' All vessels arriving from
Mauritius or Madagascar were subject to quarantine, and anyone breach-
ing it would be 'liable to the punishment of Death, without any form
of Trial'.[10] The British government endorsed Donkin's measures (while
hoping that the threat of death was just a deterrent, and not intended to
be carried out).[11] Donkin's second action was to despatch the brilliant Dr
James Barry to Mauritius.[12]

It was a two-week voyage – around the tip of Africa, bearing northeast
past Madagascar and across the sweltering Tropic of Capricorn. Mauritius
had been a French possession for nearly a century before its capture by
British forces in 1810. It resembled the Cape Peninsula – jagged mountains rearing up hard behind the coast, a tiny scatter of buildings that
made up the capital – yet it was lusher, more verdant, the sands whiter
and the sea an even crisper blue-green. Port Louis was much smaller than
Cape Town, but equally orderly and provided with an excellent enclosed
anchorage. From a distance it appeared a paradise.

For James this was his first experience of a disease that would be
one of the great challenges of his career. The cholera epidemic was
fascinating, complex, devastating; the disease was known in India, but
was now beginning to appear for the first time outside the Indian subcontinent. It was believed to have arrived at Mauritius with the Royal
Navy frigate *Topaze*, out of Ceylon, which had anchored at Port Louis
on 29 October 1819. Dozens of her Indian passengers were sick with
a gastric disease believed initially to be dysentery, and they were taken
ashore to be cared for. Three weeks later, on 18 November, the first
cases diagnosed as cholera morbus* occurred in the town, and on the

---

* then a blanket term for gastroenteritis, including cholera

29th it appeared among the soldiers of the 56th Regiment, spread to the island outposts, and appeared 130 nautical miles away on the Île de Bourbon,* in spite of 'a most rigorous quarantine' at Mauritius.[13] It was almost always fatal.

In the first quarter of the nineteenth century there was a scientific debate over whether cholera was contagious or environmental – the ferocity of epidemics seemed to argue transmissibility, but their tendency not to spread far beyond the point of outbreak (or at least to spread slowly and sporadically) argued that it was something in the environment.[14] It would be decades more before the cause (contamination of water or food by *Vibrio cholerae* bacteria) was identified. In 1820 it was seen as a contagion spread by foul airborne miasmas emanating from the sick. Yet no seamen aboard *Topaze* developed the disease after her arrival, despite constant traffic between ship and shore – it was confined to the thirty people who had arrived with it.[15]

James learned that the epidemic, which had peaked in December, had subsided in January and was now almost over. The 56th Foot had suffered dreadfully. The regimental hospital had only one surgeon and a young hospital assistant, Dr John Kinnis,[16] to handle dozens upon dozens of dying patients. Kinnis had studied the disease closely, and later produced a detailed report. There had been 138 cases in the regiment alone, and uncounted numbers among the civil population – a frightening epidemic in such a tiny place.[17]

Symptoms were typical of Asiatic cholera – the victims began with headaches, vertigo, lassitude and acute abdominal pain, with diarrhoea developing later; this was described by Dr Kinnis as 'a clear colourless fluid, thinly interspersed with white flakes, and strongly resembling pus diffused through water'.[18] There followed a period of vomiting and ferocious thirst, in which drinking merely triggered more vomiting. Soon after, 'the muscles of the extremities were attacked with spasms; their bellies swelled up into hard knots ... and became the seat of insupportable pain.'[19] At that point, death was not far away. There was little the doctors could do, and their treatment consisted mostly of relieving the suffering with warm baths (to ease the muscle cramps) and laudanum.

For a keen professional like James Barry, it was a simultaneously tragic and enthralling epidemic. He was witnessing a local outbreak of a much

* now Réunion

larger pandemic – indeed, the world's first known cholera pandemic. It had originated in Calcutta in 1817 and during the next seven years would spread to the East Indies, Arabia, Persia and eastern Africa (most likely carried in ships' water supplies).[20] The total number of fatalities on Mauritius was never recorded, but the 56th Foot had been literally decimated.

Although James's visit to Mauritius provided him with valuable first-hand experience, there was little left for him to do, and he soon returned to Cape Town bearing the good news of the epidemic's abatement.

He found the Colony in crisis. A large and growing influx of would-be settlers had been coming from Britain, attracted by glowing reports of a land of plenty. Nobody had imagined that the response would be so huge, and the facilities and available land grants were hopelessly insufficient; emergency measures were being put in place to succour the starving people and settle them throughout the Colony, but they were inadequate.[21] The situation didn't reflect well on either Lord Charles, who had encouraged the influx, or Sir Rufane Donkin, who had failed to manage it.

Throughout the rest of that year and the next, James carried on with his work, with two unhappy and trying circumstances; one was the continuing absence of Lord Charles and the presence of the abrasive General Donkin, and the other was that from 21 May 1821 the Army put him on half-pay.[22] In a fit of post-war cost-cutting, Horse Guards was deactivating and disbanding regiments all over the globe, and placing hundreds of semi-redundant officers on the half-pay list, as Cloete had been for over a year. James was now more dependent than ever on his colonial appointments.

Table Bay: Tuesday 30 November 1821

Dr James Barry and Brevet* Major Josias Cloete, in full dress uniform, were face to face once more. This time they sat in the bows of the largest and finest launch that Cape Town possessed, heading for the frigate HMS *Hyperion*, which lay at anchor a few hundred yards out. The ship had just

---

* courtesy commission conferring rank in the Army but not in a regiment, often a preliminary to substantive promotion

arrived from England with Lord Charles Somerset aboard, returning after nearly two years' absence.

Major Cloete and Dr Barry were piped aboard *Hyperion*; her officers were lined up, brilliant in their blue and gold, in honour of His Excellency the Governor. Lord Charles was in the after-cabin with the captain, where the two young men presented their warm greetings before conveying some grim news: the Colony was in a 'very precarious situation'.[23] Aside from the settler crisis, the frontier was shaky, Donkin having utterly neglected Lord Charles's programme of defensive forts and troop deployments, with the result that Xhosa bands had been coming across the Fish River at will to raid and steal cattle. It would take months of arduous work to put everything right in the Colony (a bitter feud would later erupt between Somerset and Donkin, played out in a blizzard of letters between each of them and Lord Bathurst).

Then came Lord Charles's news. There was a young woman present in the cabin – an attractive, cheerful and finely dressed young lady aged about thirty. Lord Charles beamed at her – could this be another of his many children, perhaps?

He introduced her proudly to James and Cloete – Lady Charles Somerset, his new wife.

15

Heaven and Earth

Lord Charles had married Lady Mary Poulett, sister of the 5th Earl Poulett, on 9 August 1821, shortly before embarking for the Cape, while *Hyperion* waited for him at Plymouth. The ship had lain for months while Lord Charles dallied in England, claiming that he had horses and belongings to organise, but in fact courting this young woman. He was nearly fifty-five, Lady Mary just thirty-three, a bare year older than Margaret. It was a warm, enthusiastic marriage – despite the modest size of *Hyperion*, husband and wife had enjoyed a connubial voyage, and Lady Mary was pregnant by the time they landed at Cape Town.[1]

If Margaret's private feelings about Lord Charles were as they seemed to be, this marriage must have caused her immense pain, and he might well have known it. But she couldn't be a woman again for him or anyone, whether he wished it or not. However prodigious her talents, the idea of there ever being a Dr Margaret Bulkley, MD, Member of the Royal College of Surgeons, was as remote and absurd as ever.

Outwardly, James Barry continued to thrive; his career was still advancing. During the Governor's absence, Sir Rufane Donkin had reorganised the administrative structure of medicine in the Colony, abolishing the moribund Supreme Medical Committee; when its last remaining member died that year, Donkin, with an authoritarianism that sat rather strangely in a Whig, replaced it with a single new office – Colonial Medical Inspector. The post was combined with that of Director of the Vaccine Institution, which gave the appointee effective authority over all of the Cape Colony's public health, medical practice and practitioners.[2] The man appointed was Dr John Robb, a senior Army surgeon with more than two decades' experience.[3]

When Lord Charles Somerset took back the reins in late 1821, he decided not to overturn Donkin's reorganisation, which was apparently more efficient and slightly cheaper than the old system. But in early 1822, when Dr Robb resigned (having inherited a fortune), Lord Charles had the replacement already lined up. On 18 March, a rather terse letter was received by James:

> Sir,—Dr Robb who is on the eve of returning to England having resigned the Situation of Colonial Medical Inspector, I am directed by His Excellency the Governor to acquaint you that he has been pleased to appoint you to succeed thereto.[4]

The appointment was publicly announced four days later.[5] It was scarcely decent – in fact, by all the lights of civil and military protocol it was wholly improper to appoint a youth with little experience and scarcely any rank to such an elevated post. It was a role for a man of high standing – Robb had been a senior officer of command rank: a brevet inspector of hospitals, equivalent to a general, yet here was Dr Barry, a mere assistant staff surgeon, equivalent to a lieutenant – and on half-pay, to boot – being handed this exalted position on a plate by his acknowledged patron. It was favouritism of the most blatant sort. To sidestep this awkward fact, Lord Charles suggested that James resign from the Army altogether. James considered the idea, but declined.[6]

And yet the British Army ran on patronage and privilege. Wealthy men frequently leapfrogged their peers by purchasing commissions – the Duke of Wellington himself had purchased his way to lieutenant colonel. There might be resentment from those who lacked funds or friends, but the system ticked on in the same old style, fuelled by nepotism and hard cash. Even so, an instantaneous leap of such magnitude, without an accompanying promotion in Army rank, was decidedly unusual. (Possibly Lord Charles was aware of his marriage having hurt James and was trying to make amends; equally possibly it was a simple expression of his faith in James's talents.)

The office of Colonial Medical Inspector – as formalised by a government proclamation in September 1823[7] – gave James Barry huge powers. He had responsibility for prisons, civilian hospitals, regulating the treatment of lepers, the insane and the impoverished sick, together with provision of medico-legal opinions to the colonial government.

Then there was the control of drugs and patent medicines – particularly in respect of their quality. The Colonial Medical Inspector was responsible too for marine quarantine regulations, and certifying the qualifications of apothecaries, midwives and accoucheurs,* as well as surgeons. The credentials of every doctor arriving at the Cape from overseas – of which there was a steady stream – had to be inspected and verified. And the Colonial Medical Inspector also had to undertake the professional examination of any locally trained candidate who wished to be licensed. (This would later prove an awkward sticking point for James, who didn't rate local qualifications highly.) Additionally, Dr Barry helped to codify the conditions of service and the duties of district surgeons, and to regulate their fees. Prevention of 'public nuisance', from pollution near the towns' slaughterhouses to the inspection of sewerage and fresh water pipes, also featured among his responsibilities.

In short, James had authority over every medical practitioner in the Cape. In truth, it was too much responsibility for any one person to handle effectively, especially if that person was at all conscientious, as James was to an extraordinary degree. It was physically demanding too; the only way to travel around most of his area – the core of which stretched from Cape Town south to Simon's Town, and east to towns on the far side of the mountains – was on horseback. His salary for all this was a mere 2400 rixdollars, plus 1200 rixdollars as Vaccinating Physician and 600 as Governor's Physician,[8] giving him a total official income that was still only a little over £380 (less than the average vicar, and much less than a good private doctor might command).

James threw himself into his work. He was described variously as 'imperious and dictatorial', 'skilful and sympathetic'.[9] Whatever James Barry believed to be right, he promoted and defended to the utmost – fearlessly and recklessly – and attacked whatever was wrong. His terse descriptions and observations – often laced with waspish turns of phrase, sarcastic asides and unflinching finger-pointing – went down badly with the officials involved. Dr Barry seemed less concerned with the lower echelons of staff supervising the prisoners, paupers and insane; rather, he targeted those in charge – the men in positions of authority who had it within their power to bring about improvements yet did nothing.

---

* male midwives

From the outset, the poor conditions and dreadful practices James uncovered in the Colony's institutions fixated him. His predecessors – first the derelict Supreme Medical Committee and subsequently the short-lived Dr Robb – had failed to tackle or even acknowledge the problems. The new Colonial Medical Inspector undertook a task that had simply never been done before. As there existed no proper records (he began in the job without even the most basic documentation of surgeons' drug stocks)[10] he had to create his own modus operandi from scratch, taking on the issue of public health decades before that term was invented. What he considered to be abuses of any description, he exposed, no matter who had to be brought to account. It was courageous, for there could be no surer path to ruin.

He brought the renamed Vaccine Office under the same roof as the Colonial Medical Inspector – the roof in question being that of his own little cottage by Government House (it was an indication of how the role had been allowed to lapse that there was no office provided). He obtained himself a writing desk and a 'case for papers',[11] and got on with the business of inspecting.

One of his first tasks was a deeply upsetting one; he was asked to provide an expert opinion on the case of a slave who had allegedly been beaten to death by his master. The slave, named Joris, was owned by the Reverend Gebhard, minister of the Dutch Reformed Church at Paarl, a settlement about thirty miles from Cape Town, who also owned a vineyard at nearby Klapmuts.[12] The unfortunate Joris's transgression was habitual slowness in his work. The minister's twenty-two-year-old son, William Gebhard, had administered the punishment himself. The official indictment stated:

> That you [William Gebhard] ... went to said Joris ... and admonished him to be quicker in his work, which said Joris, on account of his weak corporal constitution ... could not perform according to your approbation; when you, on that account, caused him to be laid down on the ground, and taken hold of by four other slaves who were on the spot, and punished him with your own hand, with some bundles of branches of quince trees ...
>
> That ... you directed him to be dragged to the Wine Store ...
>
> That then and there, and by candle-light, you caused him to be laid down on the ground, and having been held fast by four Slaves, you

directed him to be punished by the Slave November, with a piece of Bullock Harness, long about four feet, and about one inch thick, in a cruel manner, by applying on his bare body many stripes.

That as you could not satisfy your cruelty on said Slave, you had given directions to fetch bundles of branches of quince trees ... [and] said Slave Joris was punished therewith, on his bare body, and in an excessive manner, by said November ... during which punishment, you threatened said November to punish him, should he not flog said Joris with force;– during which punishment, and by your order, salt and vinegar were brought to the spot, which you caused to be applied to the bleeding and chastised parts of the body of said Slave, by large quantities, on which parts you caused him to be flogged with the quince branches repeatedly, so that said Slave remained senseless on the ground, when you poured vinegar in his mouth; and he was, at last, in a state of senselessness ... The consequence of which cruel ill-treatment was, that the said Slave, Joris, of Mozambique, died the next morning, at about eight o'clock.[13]

A fellow slave, seeing that nothing would be done, took it upon himself to walk the ten miles to Stellenbosch, where he reported the matter to the local landdrost. The landdrost brought in the district surgeon, Dr Robert Shand, who conducted an autopsy.

Shand found no internal injuries or signs of disease, but externally 'the loins were one complete mass off extravasated blood, coagulated lymph, and bruised muscular substance.'[14] The muscles of the back were so damaged 'that their fibres could not, in many parts, be distinctly traced'; the loins were a 'heterogeneous mass of coagulated blood, effused lymph, and bruised muscular substance'. Shand concluded that death was caused by the external injuries, 'producing so much constitutional weakness, exhaustion and pain, as gradually to paralyze the action of the heart'. Gebhard was arrested and charged with wilful murder.

The Gebhard family fought back – they commissioned their own autopsy, which flatly contradicted Dr Shand's. It was conducted nine days after death by a Dr Tardieu, a Frenchman with a practice at Paarl. Tardieu claimed to find 'no signs of swelling ... and only one open wound on the buttocks'.[15] He continued that 'one could here and there, perceive the marks of the twigs with which he had been punished'. (This was only to be expected – after more than a week of springtime weather, the putrefaction of the corpse must have been extensive.) Tardieu then reached his astonishing assessment of the situation:

> The said slave was a great eater in his lifetime, a disorder known by professional men under the name of Bulimia, and which occasions to those afflicted with it, faintness, meagrin [migraine] and oppression ... The undersigned asserts that a cold in bed by night, the lock jaw [tetanus] and fainting oppression and want of prompt assistance or medicine might have been the cause of his death.

Lord Charles himself read this report, and was 'reluctantly led to attribute the giving of such a certificate to the worst motives',[16] but he was obliged to weigh it in the balance. He called in the Colonial Medical Inspector for his opinion.

James gave it with typical forthrightness – Tardieu's report was 'the most incorrect and unprofessional production that I have ever read or even heard of ... Tardieu seemed to think that bruises could not cause death, only cuts'.[17] James condemned this as ignorant or mischievous in the extreme, 'as it is a well-known fact that contusions or bruises occasion death very frequently indeed, and that a clean cut ... is not near so dangerous, unless a vessel of importance is opened'. He made an analogy: 'This is easily exemplified by rolling an orange on a table. If the skin or peel be not broken, the whole of the internal substance is destroyed, but if the peel is broken, a little only of the juice escapes and the inner structure remains intact.' In Dr Barry's opinion there could be 'no doubt that the slave died in consequence of the flogging'. He recommended that Shand's original findings be accepted and Tardieu's dismissed as 'ignorant and contemptible'. Tardieu's report was not admitted in evidence at the trial. After a fairly short hearing, William Gebhard was found guilty of wilful murder and sentenced to hang. Dr Tardieu, having proven himself either incompetent or corrupt (or both), was struck off the medical register.

Dr Barry had always been known for his intolerance of incompetent practitioners. Now he had the power to bring the Colony's quacks to account. Another was a Mr L. J. Bianchi, a shopkeeper whose premises were inspected and found to be stocked with medicines that Bianchi was selling without licence. James reported that 'upon more than one Occasion it has fallen under my notice that he practises Medicine in this

Colony to the destruction of the Patients – in one instance I witnessed the death of a poor man unskilfully treated by this Person.'[18]

Bianchi was far from unique, and the local apothecaries and druggists had been fighting a losing battle to prevent his kind from practising. They appealed to Dr Barry, and he took the complaint to the government, stating that 'Medicines are sold by almost every description of Shopkeeper without either Professional Knowledge or Licence.'[19] He added that it was 'also a well known fact that the most deleterious Drugs are vended and dispensed ... under the denomination of Patient Medicines ... to the personal risk of the Purchasers', and 'fatal consequences have ensued' from the administering of these substances 'by ignorant and mercenary persons'. The products often contained dangerous quantities of ingredients like arsenic, lead, mercury and opium (all of which were used in orthodox medicines too, along with other toxic substances such as antimony).

This trade was illegal,[20] but had been allowed to run out of control. James reined it in, and in September 1823 the Governor issued a proclamation providing additional regulations barring apothecaries from practising medicine, surgery or midwifery, and physicians and surgeons from preparing and dispensing their own medicines. It also empowered the Colonial Medical Inspector to make quarterly inspections of drug stocks and to 'condemn, and order to be destroyed, such as may appear to him improper, or unfit for use', as well as to take licences away from repeat offenders and punish them.[21]

This may have seemed like a radical start, but there was much more to come; the medical life of the Cape Colony was about to be turned upside down and shaken until all its concealed abuses fell out into the light.

Hottentots Holland Kloof: Friday 25 October 1822

Dr Barry's horse breasted the final rise of the mountain pass; ahead lay the rolling lands of the eastern Colony. More than five years had passed since he'd first come this way with the Governor's cavalcade; this morning he was alone, apart from his single manservant, Danzer.

Danzer was a boy of Khoikhoi or San origin from Graaff Reinet, about twelve years old. He was formally indentured to James, with the intention that he be trained as a groom and coachman. He was about five feet tall and lightly built. He dressed dandily in a glazed hat with a cockade, a blue jacket, striped waistcoat and light pantaloons. A restless spirit who was happy in James's service but uneasy so far from his homeland, in June of that year he'd run away in an attempt to return to his family, passing over the mountains with a wagon train.[22] Eventually he'd returned to James's service – whether by choice or laid by the heels was never recorded.

The previous day's ride had brought them to the foot of the mountains, and now it took another half a day to reach their destination in the valley between the town of Caledon and the sea. A contemporary visitor described this area as 'one of the most fertile and beautiful spots in the Colony; well-supplied with water … the air exceedingly pure'.[23] The deep valley was surrounded by rocky mountains, rich in flowers and shrubs, with scarcely any human habitation – just two buildings, one a modest house; the other, set some distance apart, an incongruous prison-like structure with high windows, surrounded by a scatter of little huts known locally as *ponthokkies*. As James rode between the huts, curious dark faces peered at him from the shadows, a few bolder ones coming out to watch the fine horse and the beautifully dressed gentleman ride by, with his rather splendid servant in train. Many of the faces – most of them Khoikhoi – were disfigured by tumours, and the figures moving about did so in a halting manner, some of them missing the extremities of their limbs. This place, the prison-like building, the spread of poor huts and the land all around, was called *Hemel en Aarde* – Heaven and Earth – and an aura of dread, palpable for miles around, hung over it, for it was where the Cape Colony housed its lepers.

James had been partly responsible for the Leper Institution. During the tour of 1817, Lord Charles Somerset had been struck by the plight of lepers, and with encouragement from Dr Barry he had taken action immediately, issuing a public proclamation:

Whereas it has been represented to me … that, that melancholy and distressing disorder, The Leprosy, has of late years considerably encreased within this Settlement … so that as an impression obtains (which the most learned of the Medical Profession hold to be erroneous) that the disorder is contagious, the distressed sufferers are frequently left in a state of abandonment, which is shocking to humanity to reflect upon.

And whereas it appears expedient to allot to Hottentots, Bastaards, Freeblacks, and Slaves labouring under this evil, a healthy and airy spot, where they may retire to, and where they shall receive such aid as necessary to their future subsistence and comfort, but to which place the safety of the Public requires they should be confined.[24]

A somewhat self-contradictory proclamation, this, pandering to public fears while nodding to medical wisdom. (In fact, the medical profession was wrong about the non-contagiousness of leprosy, but correct about it not being as contagious as was popularly believed.)[25] The farm at Hemel en Aarde was purchased for the purpose, and a new building completed in 1820.

A few months into his tenure as Colonial Medical Inspector, James had asked Lord Charles to add the inspectorate of the Leper Institution to his duties. He was concerned; passing through Caledon some months earlier (probably on his vaccinating business) he'd heard rumours that lepers had escaped from the institution in a bid to complain to the authorities, claiming that they were in an 'actual state of Starvation'.[26] Now he had come to see for himself.

Accompanying him was the Reverend Dr Thom, minister of the Dutch Reformed Church at Caledon, who was responsible for the spiritual care of the inmates. James had also asked for Dr O'Flinn, the Surgeon Superintendent of the Institution, to be present, but he was away on a call – perhaps fortunately for him, given Dr Barry's temper and what he found within the walls.

It fulfilled the worst of the rumours. James reported that the medical treatment of the lepers 'is so entirely neglected that as far as I can learn, no attempts to care for the patients have been made'.[27] Dr O'Flinn, who lived at Stellenbosch on the other side of the mountains, visited only once a fortnight, and then only if the weather was fine. There were currently 150 residents; the hospital was crowded and dirty with insufficient bedding, and the lepers were clothed in unclean garments with a rough texture that aggravated the diseased skin.

James asked the Reverend Thom to introduce him to the inmates and explain that he represented the Governor, who wished to do all he could to help them and make life better for them; therefore, if there were any complaints, now was the time to speak up. Those who were able stood up and told of their hunger, lack of personal comforts and inhumane treatment by their keepers, that they were forced to labour in the garden, and were punished if they were unable to do so, either by reduction in diet or confinement indoors – there were even complaints of flogging. One remarked that it was 'surely better to die of Disease rather than Cruelty and Hunger'.[28] Their food was poor, scarcely fit to sustain life, and utterly inadequate as a diet for the sick. This was the institution that James, full of good intentions, had helped bring into existence.

The patients didn't even get the benefit of the pleasant setting; 'These miserable people,' James reported, 'were confined to a small space of the Valley' in which most of the 'beautiful and ample portion of Lands allotted to them and intended by His Excellency to be appropriated for their use & Comfort' they were forbidden to use.[29]

There was a steward called Parker, who had neglected the general care of the lepers, while Dr O'Flinn – whom Dr Barry finally tracked down and interviewed – 'seemed to take not the slightest Interest in the poor People entrusted to his care'. Subjected to James's furious interrogation, 'The Doctor, the Religious Instructor & the Steward were completely at variance among themselves – one accusing the other.'[30] James ordered increased rations and measures to improve the lives of the lepers, and shortly after his visit all three men were dismissed from their posts.

Over the following months James ordered a thorough reorganisation of Hemel en Aarde and issued his own instructions for the lepers' care, lodging and diet. He made the punishing 150-mile round trip many times to check on progress, and by March 'found the whole Establishment much improved – the people looking better, and cleaner, not having the least disposition to mutiny nor to escape'; they were also satisfied with Mr Leitner, a Moravian missionary who had taken the place of Reverend Thom, living on-site and running the institution day-to-day with his wife's help. James himself replaced O'Flinn as medical officer.[31]

Harmony didn't last long. Mr Leitner felt that Dr Barry overreached himself, exerting authority in non-medical areas that Mr Leitner believed were his own sole responsibility.[32] He complained, asking that Dr Barry act as a consultant, not a manager, which enraged James, who was insulted by the suggestion that Leitner be allowed to call on him 'as upon his Apothecary for a dose of Physic ... when it shall please him to think such assistance necessary ... any thing so absurd and offensive needs no Comment.'[33] In truth, James couldn't bring himself to entrust another person with a matter this dear to his heart. He even attempted to bring the Leper Institution directly under his eye by proposing that it be transferred to Simon's Town, twenty miles from Cape Town.[34] The friction was only eased by the intervention of Lord Charles, who ordered Leitner to follow Dr Barry's medical instructions. After that, the Leper Institution continued on a more or less even keel, its dark days behind it.

Hemel en Aarde was just the beginning. There were other institutions mired in the Slough of Despond, some within Cape Town itself. On 4 March 1824, on the Governor's orders, Dr Barry inspected the Somerset Hospital, a small establishment on the edge of Cape Town. It had been founded in 1816 by an English naval surgeon called Bailey, with a blessing and a land grant (but no cash) from the Governor. Within five years Bailey had run his hospital into severe debt, and it had been taken over by the Burgher Senate.* Now, three years on, it was giving cause for concern, particularly in the care of the mentally afflicted.

'I visited the Lunatics at the Somerset Hospital last Thursday in company with Mr McCarthy, the Colonial Paymaster,' Dr Barry reported. 'We found 15 individuals (13 men and 2 women) denominated insane. The whole Establishment appears void of Cleanliness, Order or Professional care.'[35] In James's opinion, five of the fifteen were either not insane at all or were suffering physical complaints – including a man with a head injury who had been 'totally neglected' and needed proper hospital treatment to save his life, and a centenarian woman 'in her second childhood' who was provided with neither a bed nor a blanket. The Governor, dismayed (particularly as this hospital bore his name), ordered James to make regular inspections and instructed the Burgher Senate to allow him 'every facility' for the purpose.[36] Change was slow to come; when James visited in November, he reported that 'its general state is by no means improved; the wards are as dirty as the Patients themselves.' He went on:

> The Lunatics are in the most squalid & wretched condition that can be imagined; Medical Treatment certainly never has been resorted to – some of these poor wretches are totally destitute of Clothes or Beds. The Keepers say 'They might tear them' & that 'they never leave their Cells for any purpose lest they should do mischief.' It would be endless (and I am fearful useless) were I to enter into any further detail. I shall therefore conclude by saying, a general reform of some kind becomes necessary in this Establishment which certainly does not deserve to be dignified with the title of Hospital.[37]

---

* town council responsible for public services and regulating traders

Lord Charles agreed, and a three-man commission headed by James was formed. Its report was equally damning. Many of the hospital's rooms were either empty or being used as quarters for servants of the Burgher Senate, and as general offices – 'contrary to the principles in which hospitals for the sick are usually instituted'.[38] There was no resident doctor, the dispensary was disused, and hygiene and nursing were virtually non-existent. They found 'a dying man in agony with the only attendant, a fellow patient, flapping away the flies from his face', while 'Lunatics were kept in filthy cells better calculated for the confinement of brute animals than for the accommodation of beings visited with suffering, the most calamitous that the dispensation of Providence has hitherto inflicted on humanity.'[39]

The report ran to fifty densely written pages, virtually all of it by Dr Barry. He designed reforms, from staffing to facilities, medical care and daily management; he recommended that a scheme be introduced for giving free care to paupers, while treatment for slaves should be provided by an owners' subscription; the medical and psychiatric sides should be separated and sufficient nursing provided. Some of these recommendations were carried out – a resident surgeon appointed, the dispensary re-established, and the hospital generally improved. The logical step of removing administration from the Burgher Senate wasn't adopted – the colonial government wouldn't take on the expense. The Somerset Hospital was now on a sounder footing, and would eventually go on to serve as Cape Town's main public hospital for more than a century.

Like most reforming practitioners Dr Barry saw corruption and incompetence everywhere, and sooner or later his zeal to eradicate them would get him into trouble. James Barry had an ungovernable impulse to speak truth to power; but power did not like the sound, and stopped its ears. So James spoke louder, shriller, and in his passion he blurred the distinction between truth and fancy, fact and prejudice, and in so doing he gave power the weapons it needed to silence him.

16

'If Rumour Speaks Truth'

Cape Town: Tuesday 6 April 1824

Early in the evening, Dr Barry set out from his residence, walked through the Company's Garden and along Heerengracht, towards Strandstraat. In his new role he'd taken to wearing civilian clothes, and had a penchant for satin waistcoats and an ultra-fashionable coat in a style made absolutely the thing by the English dandy Joseph 'Pea-Green' Hayne, who'd acquired much of London's limelight since George 'Beau' Brummell's enforced exile to Calais.[1] The coat was double-breasted with broad lapels and a full knee-length skirt, quite unlike the cutaways that had been standard in Brummell's day. If worn fully à la Hayne, it should be accompanied by a chequered cravat and a tall hat.

Despite this modishness Cape Town had not caught up with England, where trousers were now the fashion, and James still wore stockings and the tight breeches known as 'inexpressibles' (a euphemism coined by ladies and later adopted ironically by the dandies). In England, inexpressibles had now become thoroughly unfashionable (it was said that the middle-aged Prime Minister Lord Liverpool lost his position as adviser to George IV because he 'refused to compromise his inexpressibles', for which the fashion-conscious King had developed a 'most unqualified dislike').[2] This change in style had yet to catch on in the Cape.

Dr Barry was an extremely busy official. Besides his government responsibilities, he continued as family physician to the Somersets, where James's unusual skill in midwifery had been in demand: since reaching the Cape in 1821, Lady Mary had produced a son and daughter (bringing Lord Charles's surviving brood to eight) and was very near her term with a third pregnancy. Any feelings Margaret had about Lord Charles's apparently happy marriage and Lady Mary's infants, she kept buried.

Nonetheless, James had drawn closer to Lord Charles than ever, in a manner that was beginning to excite surreptitious, scurrilous comments in Cape Town.

James paused at the junction with Strandstraat. Opposite, between the Custom House and the corner of a narrow lane, stood the edifice known locally as the 'Tronk' – Cape Town's prison.* A two-storey block of white stucco with plain mouldings, it wasn't particularly unfriend-ly-looking. Its outward atmosphere was certainly less unpleasant than the town shambles – the meat market and abattoir – which stood on the other side of the Post Office, filling Strandstraat with charnel-house odours whenever the breeze was off the sea. But despite its appearance the Tronk had a sinister reputation in the town.

Waiting for him was Judge George Kekewich of the Cape's Vice Admiralty Court,† a pleasant fellow described by Lord Charles as 'very mild, sensible, gentlemanlike',[3] who was to be James's colleague for the visit. They rapped on the door of the Tronk and announced that they had come on the instructions of His Excellency the Governor to make an inspection.

The great door creaked inwards and the gaol smell – composed of slops, gruel and uncleanliness – poured out, along with the deep, distant rumble of a treadmill. James had never, strictly speaking, set foot in a prison before; but Margaret had, sixteen years earlier when she visited her uncle Redmond at the King's Bench. The Tronk was a fraction of the size of the King's Bench, but just about its equal in misery.

James and his companion, conducted by the prison keeper, were shown cells that in James's eyes resembled medieval dungeons more than the accommodations of a modern gaol – no beds, no buckets, no furnishings at all.[4] One was opened by the turnkey to reveal a wretched-looking man, naked, unwashed and stinking, lying on a filthy stretcher. James could see he was injured, and on examining him found that he had a fractured femur. In excruciating pain, the man gave his name as Jacob Elliot, and claimed (in the presence of the prison keeper, who didn't contradict him) that he had received no medical attention at all; just once in twenty-four hours he'd been given a bucket of water and the meagre prison ration of

---

* *tronk*: prison, gaol (colloquial Cape Dutch). Possibly a loan word from Malay *trungku*: to imprison, or Portuguese *tronco*: trunk, box.

† British colonial court with jurisdiction over maritime legal matters

food; he'd been placed on this stretcher just before Dr Barry's visit – prior
to that he'd been lying on the bare floor. 'I do here, my Lord, declare
that I never witnessed any scene more truly appalling than this,'[5] James
reported. Judge Kekewich, lacking Dr Barry's strong stomach, had to
withdraw from the cell in disgust.

James asked the keeper sardonically whether there were any more
broken bones in the prison; he was taken to another cell and shown a
prisoner whose condition was identical to Elliot's: 'This poor wretch
had one of his legs fractured and the other carefully surrounded with
a heavy chain.'[6] James couldn't bring himself to describe the situation
any further.

He consulted the prison medical officer, and found Dr Karl Wilhelm
Liesching, Physician and Surgeon to the Court of Justice, a conscientious
man, but hard-pressed and frustrated by resistance from the top. Both
Liesching and his father (also a respected medical man) had reported
several times on Elliot's condition and requested that he be moved to
hospital. The person at the top of the system, to whom they made their
requests, was the Fiscal, who was responsible for all law-enforcement and
judicial process in the Cape. The Fiscal, Daniel Denyssen, had informed
Dr Liesching that 'the Government would not suffer any expenses to be
incurred for Prisoners'.[7]

Immediately after his inspection, James reported to Lord Charles,
who was told by the Fiscal that Dr Barry's claims were exaggerated.
James replied that if Lord Charles 'could afford the time to walk to the
Tronk, you could satisfy yourself as to the facts and be convinced that I
did not in the least exaggerate'.[8] The Governor decreed that the Colonial
Medical Inspector would henceforth be making visits to both the Tronk
and the Somerset Hospital; Mr Denyssen was instructed that 'you will
cause separate accommodation to be provided for the Sick at the Prison
and thereby secure to them that comfort which in their helpless condition
they so much require'.[9]

From a humanitarian point of view, it seemed an auspicious beginning.
But James would find that in ruffling the Fiscal's feathers he was making
a powerful enemy.

James's first inspection had exposed only a glimpse of the abuses going
on at the Tronk. In July he visited again, and discovered thirty male prisoners crammed into two small rooms beside the privy, in a 'very filthy,
& unwholesome state', without beds or bedding.[10] The Tronk possessed

only seven mattresses, which were reserved for the sick. Food was served in communal tubs, without spoons or cups, forcing the prisoners to 'feed like Pigs' so that 'the Strongest, or the Greediest necessarily get the most if not all'.[11] James was particularly distressed by the plight of the women prisoners – 'I saw six confined in one Room, without a Bed, & in a very dirty & wretched state'. They were given neither air nor exercise, only leaving their cell to attend church. In all, the Tronk 'exhibits a most disgusting scene'.[12] These efforts to improve health and welfare at the prison would go on for some time, seemingly in vain and in the midst of increasingly acrimonious arguments with Denyssen.

There was good news for James on 6 May 1824 when, after two years on half-pay, the Army returned him to the full list (on which he would remain for the rest of his career). He was subjected to the formality of an examination by three Army colleagues, who decided – without actually questioning him – that he was properly qualified 'from the high reputation he has acquired as a Physician in this Colony'.[13]

It was almost the only bright spot that year. By the middle of June, James's life had taken a strange, alarming turn. He'd become closer than ever to the Somerset family and to Lord Charles in particular. In April he had attended to the birth of Lady Mary's third child, a daughter called Augusta – born five weeks premature while the Somersets were holidaying at Camp's Bay[14] – and after the couple moved back to Newlands, James was in frequent attendance. However, if a certain strand of gossip was to be believed, there was tension building in the Somerset marriage – a tension focused around James Barry.

Cape Town: Tuesday 1 June 1824

Thomas Kift Deane rose from his bed in his lodgings in the Heerengracht. An Irishman by birth and a clerk by training, for the past two years he'd been secretary to the Colonial Medical Inspector, Dr James Barry. As Mr Deane opened the window he looked out on the cold wintry street, which the rising sun was just bringing to life.[15] Opposite, he saw two slave boys and a man in a grey cloak gathered near the little wooden bridge opposite. They were looking at a notice on the post of the bridge and talking excitedly. Mr Deane made out the words 'Barry' and 'Lord Charles'. He hurriedly dressed and went down, but the people were gone, as was the notice, leaving nothing but a few adhesive gum wafers. He glimpsed the man in the grey cloak walking away across the parade ground, but then lost sight of him through the trees. Mr Deane shrugged and went back to his room.

A few hours later, he bumped into his neighbour, John Findlay, a sea captain who lived with his wife in a house at the bottom of Heerengracht, and fell into conversation. At sunrise, Captain Findlay had come out onto his veranda and noticed some youths – one black, the other Asian – looking at a paper attached to the bridge post.[16] As Findlay approached, the Asian boy, who apparently didn't read well, said it was something about Lord Charles. Captain Findlay looked at the placard, which read:

> A person, living at Newlands, makes it known, or takes this method of making it known, to the Public authorities of this Colony that on the 5th [May] he detected Lord Charles buggering Dr Barry.[17]

Captain Findlay could scarcely credit his senses. He read on:

> Her Ladyship had her suspicions, or saw something that led her to sus-picion, which had caused a general quarrel and which was the reason ... [illegible] ... The person is ready to come and make oath to the above.[18]

There was more, but this was all Findlay would recall later; at that point he was called back to the house by his servant, having come out in his stockinged feet. When he returned in his shoes he found the placard gone. He believed he'd seen a stranger pass by on horseback, arriving from the parade ground at a gallop, crossing the bridge and passing away south along Heerengracht. Whether the horseman had taken the placard Captain Findlay couldn't tell.

It would transpire that Captain Findlay was the only person who had read the placard and would admit to it. Yet the contents spread through Cape Town with all the rapidity of the juiciest gossip.

James himself heard of it that morning, walking through the Heerengracht just as the story was beginning to spread. The shock was worse than a physical blow. He retreated blindly, and instead of going home he went into a nearby shop – perhaps some childhood homing instinct guiding Margaret's feet. James confessed to the shopkeeper's wife what he had just heard, and as the kind woman tried uselessly to comfort him, he broke down and cried.[19]

'A most diabolical Placard has been stuck up accusing His Excellency Lord Charles Somerset with unnatural practices with Dr Barry,' wrote Cape Town resident Samuel Eusebius Hudson, his scratchy nib racing eagerly, scarcely legibly, across the page of his diary; 'it has thrown the whole Cape into consternation. If true, it is pregnant with infamy to the parties. If false, it is a most convincing proof of what length the malignant will go to smear the character of this disgraceful man.' (Samuel Hudson had come out from England in 1796 on the staff of Lord Macartney, the first Governor, and had found all the subsequent governors wanting.) 'How galling it must be to the friends of Lord Charles and Dr Barry,' Hudson went on, torn between glee and impartiality; 'There are many who will enjoy to see these Arrogants humbled but if innocent the scheme is a diabolical one.'[20]

Large rewards for the apprehension of the culprit were offered – 6000 rixdollars by Lord Charles, 1000 by Dr Barry (a hefty portion of his annual salary) and 14,000 by a subscription from the town's merchant class.

Meanwhile, the Somersets presented a united front to Cape society. The day after the explosion of the scandal – an appropriately foul, rainy night – Lord Charles and Lady Mary went to the theatre, and pointedly took James with them. When they appeared in their box they were greeted by resounding applause from the audience. Yet some observers believed this was a smokescreen; Samuel Hudson, now more than half-convinced that the libel was true, lamented the shame that had been brought on Lady Mary: 'She is unfortunate in so bad a connection. A sacrifice of youth and beauty to age and haughtiness was in itself enough to encounter but when Infamy and Infidelity is added to the catalogue the prospects must be appalling and truly heart breaking.'[21]

Within three days the Fiscal, Daniel Denyssen, launched a court of inquiry into what had become known as 'the Placard' (*plakaat* in Dutch), the effect of which had been, in the Fiscal's words, 'to wound the heart' of Lord Charles and 'to create the most abominable suspicions in the hearts of the inhabitants'.[22] Clearly Samuel Hudson wasn't alone in wondering about the truth of the allegation. Concerned only with the Governor's position, Mr Denyssen made no reference to Dr Barry, nor of what wounds it had inflicted on *his* heart – not to mention his professional and social standing. Lord Charles was a son and brother of dukes; he could weather a good deal of scandal, whereas James might be ruined by it.

The Fiscal's inquiry ran for over a week, called a host of witnesses, and produced several suspects. On the very first day, James received an unsigned letter from an informant acting on his instructions; it suggested that there was a conspiracy afoot, and named three men.[23] The first was printer and newspaper proprietor George Grcig, a Scotsman recently arrived in Cape Town who the previous year had been given permission to set up a newspaper to rival the government-backed *Cape Town Gazette and African Advertiser*.[24] Mr Greig's *South African Commercial Advertiser* was a much more sensational organ that instantly upset the government with its political radicalism, allegedly misreporting trials, among other scurrilous practices. In May, the Fiscal had formally gagged the *Commercial Advertiser* and shut it down on grounds of 'deviation from the prospectus' originally submitted by Greig.[25]

The second possible conspirator was Greig's clerk, Joseph Green, while the third was a much shadier character. William Edwards was an Englishman, also recently arrived at the Cape. He had set up as a notary and lawyer and within weeks had become a stone in the boot of the government. He continually brought frivolous libel cases against the Governor and the Fiscal, and acquired a reputation for aggressiveness and showmanship in court, with interminable addresses that drew large crowds. Edwards himself had been variously charged with libel and contempt of court, and upon investigation was proved a fraud with no qualifications whatsoever to practise law – the closest he had come to certification had been working in Chester as a prothonotary* and marrying his principal's daughter. By March 1824 he was awaiting trial and repeatedly bothering Lord Charles and Earl Bathurst with letters complaining about his mistreatment while on remand in the Tronk (in fact he lived quite comfortably thanks to his wealth, and wasn't subject to the privations of other prisoners).[26] His trial had occurred in May, he was sentenced to transportation to New South Wales,[27] and was now appealing against his conviction.

William Edwards was clearly unbalanced, dishonest, and had an addiction to perceiving and perpetrating libels involving Lord Charles. One

---

* court clerk

of the black marks against George Greig was his sympathetic reporting of Edwards's trial. This was enough to convince the Fiscal that Greig and Edwards were responsible for the Placard. Undoubtedly they had a proven record of anti-government libel, but then again they were the very men the Fiscal most wanted to pin a crime upon, and he needed a quick resolution.

A fourth conspirator was added to the picture – a man with the unusual name of Bishop Burnett, a former naval lieutenant turned farmer with a record of wild, violent behaviour and a vicious temper. He came into the picture at the public inquiry when William Edwards's servant, Daniel Lee, was put on the stand. He confessed that in May he had delivered a package of papers from Burnett to his master; upon receiving it, Edwards opened it, took out the Placard and read it, and 'he laughed so loudly as to make me take particular notice of what he read'.[28] He cast some doubt on his reliability as a witness by referring to the libel as 'concerning Lord Charles and Dr Barry's wife', but it was seen as strong evidence against Edwards.

The homes of the suspects were thoroughly searched, but apart from a few satirical notes, no evidence of their guilt – or even complicity – could be found. And despite the succession of closely questioned witnesses, no conclusive evidence was uncovered. With deep regret, the Fiscal marked the case unsolved and hoped that more evidence would come to light in the future.

It did not. The author of the Placard was never identified with certainty, and it became part of the minutiae of Cape folklore. And yet there were many questions never asked – let alone answered – by the inquiry. One was the peculiar wording of the Placard, particularly its central claim – that a witness 'detected Lord Charles buggering Dr Barry'. That coarse term would be an odd choice for literate men such as Burnett, Greig and Edwards, who were passably educated and keenly interested in the law – surely they would more likely have written 'sodomising', which was not only a more literate expression but also a legal term (denoting an act that in the armed forces was punishable by death). The word sat strangely with the otherwise legalistic phrasing ('A person, living at Newlands, makes it known, or takes this method of making it known, to the Public authorities of this Colony ...'). It might well be taken as indicating that this was a genuine witness claim written down verbatim and embedded in legal phrasing.

Another question: if this was a calculated libel against the Governor, why didn't Greig, who had the equipment to hand, print up dozens of copies and, instead of flimsily wafering one to a bridge post, paste them to walls around the town, or scatter them about as handbills? And who was it that removed the Placard, and why? Thomas Deane's man in a grey cloak and Captain Findlay's horseman were never identified. The cloaked man had apparently crossed the bridge in the direction of the parade ground after looking at the Placard, so shortly before its disappearance that he must have taken it (unless the two slaves were responsible). Findlay's rider crossed the bridge *from* the parade ground – so might have met the cloaked man – arriving at a gallop and then riding away south, towards the centre of town.

Even if Burnett did originally pass the Placard to Edwards, was he or Greig necessarily the author? Possession did not prove authorship; it might be stolen property. Burnett himself appeared outraged at being implicated, and published a lengthy denial of the allegations against him – including Daniel Lee's claim to have passed the Placard from him to Edwards, which he called 'one monstrous falsehood', adding: 'What is meant by Doctor Barry's wife is best known to the conspirators, as he is, ever has been, and, if *rumour* speaks truth, ever will keep single.'[29] This comment alone indicates that while Burnett knew the gossip about Dr Barry's gender, he wasn't very familiar with the actual content of the Placard (which of course alleged a sexual act between Lord Charles and James, not James's non-existent wife). He claimed to have first heard of the Placard at the same time as the rest of Cape Town.

The scandalous incident at Newlands that the Placard claimed to report coincided with Lord Charles's residence there and Dr Barry's frequent presence in the weeks after the birth of the Somersets' new child. It fitted uncomfortably well. A stray fact, which may or may not be relevant, is that the incident was alleged to have occurred on Wednesday 5 May, the day before James was returned to full pay – a step probably assisted by Lord Charles's influence.

All this leads to an ultimate question. When James broke down in front of the shopkeeper's wife on the morning of the Placard's appearance, was it the distress of an innocent person slandered or of a guilty one exposed? And a further observation: if a witness really did see Lord Charles in the full act of adultery, was it not strange that they didn't simultaneously discover that Dr Barry was a woman? Of course, that could depend on many things – not least the witness's viewpoint and the couple's state of undress and position of the guilty couple. Catching a fleeting glimpse of physical lovemaking *in flagrante delicto* between two people believed to be male, one might simply assume it to be homosexual.

If the allegation was a lie, it was peculiarly well chosen and well timed. As Samuel Hudson indicated, Lord Charles's marriage was believed by some to be a regrettable one for his wife; also, she was at the end of a pregnancy, a time when a sex-starved husband with Lord Charles's proven appetites might turn elsewhere. And he and James were extraordinarily close – James was almost one of the family, protected and promoted by Lord Charles to an astonishing degree. The bond between them could only be described as love. But love of what kind?

Clearly it was of a deep, sincere and durable kind. In Lord Charles's place, many men would have saved their own skin by putting up a defensive show of unity with their wife and publicly shunning Dr Barry. On the contrary, Lord Charles stood by James, even at the risk to his own reputation, with the steadfastness of real love.

17

Dr Barry's Nemesis

We have reason to think that he would have been more successful in his applications for a correction of the abuses of which he complained ... if his representations both written and verbal had not been mixed up with reflections upon the motives of Individuals that led the Government to doubt whether his object was not rather to expose their conduct than to point out the errors of the system that they conducted.

Report of the Commissioners of Inquiry upon the Case of Dr Barry
14 March 1826[1]

Cape Town: Tuesday 10 August 1824

Karl Friedrich Liesching approached the door of Dr Barry's cottage and knocked hesitantly. The interview that was about to take place would not be a comfortable one. Karl Friedrich was a sprig of a large medical family. His older brother, Karl Wilhelm (medical attendant to the Court of Justice), had taken his MD at Göttingen and now practised in Cape Town. Their father, Friedrich Liesching, a German immigrant, himself the son of a physician, had been an Army surgeon and now ran an apothecary's shop in addition to his practice. Now young Karl Friedrich, who had trained locally as an apothecary, was ready to join the family business, and needed the proper licence to practise from the Colonial Medical Inspector. However, Karl Liesching and James Barry were not on good terms. Dr Barry had recently told Liesching that he 'would employ every possible means to resist the attainment' of his ambition.[2]

Their enmity dated back some months, its origin lost to history. Liesching, afraid to approach Barry directly, had applied in person to the Governor, hoping that he would use his influence; Lord Charles reassured the young man that private differences would not sway Dr Barry.[3] Privately Lord Charles must have known James better than this; officially he kept quiet. Two months then went by, and Liesching was told that his application had been referred to the Colonial Medical Inspector. More time passed.

The problem for Liesching was that, having trained in Cape Town, he didn't possess the European qualification required under Cape law. However, the law was murky; while a diploma from a European university was a *sine qua non* for physicians, it was different for surgeons and apothecaries – the law vaguely stipulated 'such Certificate as is usually required for these Arts'.[4] This law, which James had helped to draft, gave him leeway to exercise his mysterious grudge against Liesching.[5]

In August, Dr Barry was finally *ordered* to interview Karl Liesching.[6] He delayed a week, then told Thomas Deane to invite Mr Liesching for interview the following day. Liesching was admitted to the cottage by a servant and eventually shown into Dr Barry's office. James was not in a happy state. It was only two months since the infamous Placard, which was still the subject of official investigation and public gossip, and the hurt was still livid. On a professional level, after two years in his post he was still having to buy his own stationery,[7] and was increasingly irritated at having to use his home as his office. He had been lobbying the Governor on this matter, arguing that he should have 'a reasonable allowance made to me to provide the same', without success so far.

Therefore the unlucky Liesching found him unusually ill-disposed. The interview was brutally abrupt. Dr Barry asked coldly: 'Have you ever been in Europe?' Aside from having been born there, Liesching had to admit that he had not. 'Have you ever been in India?' Again, no. Dr Barry demanded Liesching's certificate, and that was the end of the interview.

'Staggered by this proceeding', Liesching went to the Colonial Office, and was astonished to be told by Acting Secretary Mr Brink that Dr Barry's report had already been received – indeed, it had already been signed off by the Governor. Dr Barry had refused to issue a licence. On pressing Mr Brink, who was a kindly gentleman and a good friend of Dr Barry, Liesching discovered that the report had been submitted and signed days before the interview. The entire thing had been a sham. 'I now plainly saw that I had been called for Mockery!'[8]

It was a shameful episode. James was acting on a sincere professional conviction, but motivated by a personal grudge. He pointed out that with the modelling of Cape standards on English law, 'the Medical Profession is at this period become tolerably respectable'; however, the Cape did not possess a medical school; 'neither Chemistry, Pharmacy, Botany, Anatomy, nor in short any of the necessary Sciences are taught in the Schools here, in fact there are no professional acquirements emanating from the Cape Instructions'; therefore it was 'absolutely impossible for any person to procure a Medical Education at the Cape'.[9] He believed that it was wrong to regard the apothecary's trade as less exacting and requiring less thorough training: 'The Physician, the Surgeon and the Patient, are totally at the mercy of the Apothecary, Chemist and Druggist,' James wrote. 'Therefore the English Medical Profession is guided by the most rigid Laws, and these Laws positively exclude Mr Liesching.'[10]

Yet his behaviour had been vindictive, and after years of training, the young man was left with no hope of taking over the apothecary business and thereby supporting his wife and child. Liesching forced himself into the presence of the Governor to protest, but was shouldered aside by a lackey and informed that His Excellency would receive any protests in writing.

Torn between personal loyalty and his sense of justice, Lord Charles put pressure on James to change his mind. In September he instructed him to examine Liesching again. James declined to do that, but convened a board made up of three professional friends: Samuel Bailey, the founder of the Somerset Hospital; Pieter Heinrich Polemann, a prominent Cape Town apothecary and botanist; and John Harfield Tredgold, a young English chemist and apothecary. They found that Mr Liesching's certificate 'by no means entitles him to an examination to practise as an Apothecary, Chemist and Druggist'.[11]

The battle between Barry and Liesching now drove a wedge between patron and favourite; in November Lord Charles brought in the Fiscal (who already had a dislike for James over the Tronk), and asked for his legal opinion. Denyssen confirmed that Liesching's qualifications were acceptable under Cape law, having been issued by a doctor and a licensed apothecary.[12] James, affronted that a lawyer should presume to judge a medical matter, remained obdurate. But he was growing isolated. His genial friend Mr Brink had now been replaced by a new man (styled Secretary to Government), just arrived from England.

Sir Richard Plasket was a much harder individual – as irritable as James himself – and James instantly got on his wrong side. Plasket instructed him again to examine Liesching, stating that it was the Governor's opinion, 'borne out by the concurrence of the legal advisers', that Liesching's qualifications were of the required kind.[13] More lawyers! And now Lord Charles was officially joining his voice to theirs.

Like his namesake uncle, James Barry was not a person to be emollient when his temper was up, no matter what the cost. This had gone beyond a mere technicality and petty personal spat, growing in James's mind into a single-handed defence of the medical profession, its standards, its ethics and his own professional standing. Was he to be gainsaid by lawyers? Absolutely not – no more than he would serve as a tooth-drawer to ignorant parsons. Indignation was now added to James's motives. He wrote to Plasket in a cold fury that 'I still feel it to be totally inconsistent with a sense of right in the conscientious discharge of my Professional Duty' to grant a licence to Karl Liesching, and threw the whole case into Lord Charles's lap, leaving it to him 'to dispense with the same' and grant a licence 'or otherwise, as shall seem meet to His Excellency'.[14]

Reluctantly, the Governor did exactly that. He convened his own medical board, composed of men from the Army medical staff – including James's military superior, the Principal Medical Officer. They subjected Liesching to a proper examination, in Latin, on pharmacy and chemistry, in which 'he acquitted himself very creditably', and pronounced him 'fully competent and qualified'.[15] Karl Liesching was licensed and his livelihood saved, after eight months of anguish.

If Liesching had learned the cost of tangling with Dr Barry, at the same time James was learning the cost of allowing himself to exercise his ill temper and arrogance. But he didn't change – once James Barry had taken a moral stand on any matter, he was constitutionally incapable of backing down.

While the Liesching affair was lumbering towards its conclusion, James had been monitoring conditions at the Tronk, increasingly dissatisfied with the lack of progress. In November 1824 he complained that 'notwithstanding the many Reports and remonstrances, made by me respecting the shameful state of the Tronk, nothing has yet been effected'.

The place was dirty, the food unwholesome, and 'the Females in particular suffer from a want of Fresh Air, Exercise and Bedding', while a prisoner with 'a severe disease of the thigh' who had been sent to hospital had been returned without proper treatment; 'that he may not be an Expence to the Government'.[16] Two convicts in heavy irons, 'sick and with bad, Sore Legs, were exposed to damp and cold without a Bed and certainly without Medical Advice – I also found the Female Prisoner Theresa, in Solitary Confinement on Bread and Water, ill & in an unfit state to bear her Punishment.' James discovered that a ten-year-old boy – one of the 'prize negroes' and slaves sent to the Tronk for punishment – had been set on the treadmill 'at the risk of being Ruptured'.[17]

Regarding both the Tronk and the Somerset Hospital (which was still in a bad state), James concluded angrily: 'I am of the opinion, nothing but the positive interference of Government, which no doubt must produce total change, can ever put any or either upon a proper or respectable footing.'[18] Two months later, on the last day of the year, he delivered another report on the Tronk, another catalogue of misery.[19]

One prisoner, John Carnall, a retired sea captain, kept a journal of life in the gaol. (Carnall was a friend of the notorious William Edwards; following the Placard affair, Edwards had escaped while en route to be put aboard a convict ship, and Carnall had been convicted of aiding and abetting him.) In his journal, Carnall recorded the privations, the regular round of floggings and the cries of the beaten; 'a Hottentot boy was flogged in front of my door, lashed to the post',[20] and almost every day he recorded 'flogging as usual'. One day he overheard a curious conversation between Dr Barry and the prisoner in the next cell, Stillwell, a former under-sheriff who had also been convicted of helping Edwards. It appeared that Stillwell had been complaining of his plight and hoping to gain the doctor's usually sympathetic ear. 'I cannot help thinking what a damned fool you were to let Edwards run away,' said James, still aggrieved at the man he believed responsible for the Placard. 'I always thought what a very unfit man you were to be a sheriff's officer. If you had been a soldier, you would have been shot for it. You ought to think yourself damned well off that you were not a soldier.'

'I do not think you have a right to accuse me of neglect of duty,' Stillwell protested; 'that remains for the court to decide on.' (In fact the court had already decided, and sentenced him to three months; he was now waiting for the result of an appeal.) James turned and walked away, 'apparently very much disappointed'. Perhaps he had hoped to provoke some revelation from Stillwell about the Placard.[21]

More months went by, still nothing was done about the Tronk, and James's increasingly desperate reports began to take on an ironic, taunting tone. Complaining of the lack of spiritual care in the prison, since the Colonial Chaplain didn't bother with the place aside from attending executions, James pointed out with a sneer that 'should our Pious Chaplain only succeed in reclaiming one Sinner; in making one Sober, Honest Christian, he might exclaim in the words of the New Testament "I say unto you that Joy shall be in Heaven over one Sinner that repenteth" &c., &c., &c.' The Fiscal was singled out for a sarcastic swipe: 'I need only to suggest this much, to excite the well-known Humanity of His Majesty's Fiscal, to be immediately attended to.'[22]

In March, James inspected the prison at Rondebosch, between Cape Town and Newlands, where he met stiff opposition from the gaoler, Mr Locke; he and his assistant 'evinced a great unwillingness to answer the most simple but necessary Questions' about diet, exercise, fresh air and medical care. When James questioned the black prisoners on these issues, Locke interjected, 'Why ask Questions from Blacks, when White Christians are present to answer?' along with 'many other such coarse and unwilling Observations, which I forbear to report'.[23]

Looking back on this period, James would write:

It requires nothing short of ocular demonstration to credit the very lamentable state of these institutions. I made many and various reports thereon to Government, and I regret to say, too often without effect; however as I now and then gained some little point, I felt it my bounden duty to persevere.[24]

That letter, written in December 1825, marked the culmination of a truly dreadful year for James Barry, worse than any before, in which his zeal and impatience with authority – and his downright insubordination – brought him to a crisis. The critical turn had begun quite unexpectedly one evening in August, the depth of the Cape winter.

On Thursday 18 August, after sundown, a sailor named Aaron Smith, well soaked in drink, decided to try his hand at housebreaking. By unlucky chance the property he selected was 11 Strandstraat, which happened to be the private home of Daniel Denyssen, the formidable Fiscal.

The burglar was immediately caught and taken to the Tronk, where under normal circumstances he would have been allowed to sober up and be released in the morning. But shortly after arriving, Smith attempted to escape, and was caught by one of the prison *dienaars*.*

The dienaars of Cape Town had a terrible reputation; both the prison warders and the *Justitie Dienaaren*, the town police, were noted for violent behaviour. One contemporary recorded that they had once been armed with swords, 'but they were found to be "swords in the hands of madmen"' and they were now restricted to carrying staves. 'These men are the refuse of the Cape population,' said this observer, 'drunken, worthless and inhuman, frequently selected from the convicts banished to Robben Island.'[25]

Aaron Smith was stopped near the Tronk's entrance and during the struggle was allegedly beaten with a stave on his wrists and elsewhere on his body. That evening he was examined by Dr Liesching, who declared him 'deranged in his mind' and recommended moving him to the Somerset Hospital's lunatic wards.[26] The Fiscal requested that very evening that the Governor order the transfer, 'there to be maintained at the expence of the Government on the same terms as the other Lunatics'.[27]

Before this could happen, the prisoner had to be seen by the Colonial Medical Inspector, and it was a week before he was able to do so. When James examined 'the supposed Lunatic' in the presence of Dr Liesching and Sheriff Mills, he was certain that 'Aaron Smith is perfectly Sane in Mind'; moreover, Dr Liesching now seemed to think the same.[28] James considered Smith's 'insanity' to have been no more than the effect of heavy drinking, and couldn't resist aiming another barb at the Fiscal: 'probably His Majesty's Fiscal's application for Aaron Smith's admission ... has been in the spirit of pure charity, for the benevolent purpose of having the Wounds inflicted upon this poor Man (on the day of his Admission into the Tronk) by the Dienaar, professionally attended to'. Growing angrier as he wrote, and abandoning professional detachment entirely, James described how 'the Dienaar exercised his brutality to the horror and dismay of many of the Prisoners who loudly exclaimed against it', and added that 'I beg leave here to say, that it is by no means an uncommon event to find Prisoners beat in the most savage Manner by these good People the Dienaars.'[29]

---

* *dienaar*: servant or officer (Dutch)

This was an impression confirmed by the diary of Captain Carnall and by the general view of the Fiscal's enforcers, but it shouldn't have distracted a good medical practitioner from conducting a thorough forensic examination of Smith's injuries. James apparently did not make such an examination – a terrible mistake, with dire consequences.

James Barry, it seemed, was intent on making himself the firm enemy of the Fiscal. A Dutchman born and bred, Daniel Denyssen had no love for the British, whom he saw as having usurped his country's territory; he certainly had no reason to like Dr Barry, seeing him as a busybody with no regard for correct procedure, no respect for officialdom, and most especially none for Denyssen himself. The Fiscal was an important and powerful personage; he knew it, and expected to be accorded due deference and respect. In setting himself against this man, James saw himself as the enemy of oppression and brutality. Others – a small but powerful few – viewed him as a troublemaker.

Lord Charles Somerset took his reports very seriously, and commanded Sir Richard Plasket to write to the Fiscal, 'to call your most serious attention to the facts stated by Dr Barry and to desire that a strict inquiry and investigation be made by you into the whole of this apparently disgraceful Business'.[30]

The Fiscal's investigation (into his own department, it should be remembered) consisted initially of a visit to the Tronk by Dr Liesching, who reported that the prisoners were nearly all in good health, well fed, and the cells were in a 'proper State of cleanliness'. (Unless a transformation had been wrought in the past week or so, this was a whitewash.) Dr Liesching regretted to report that Aaron Smith was certainly 'raving mad' and ought to be transferred to the Somerset.[31]

Dr Barry hurried immediately to the gaol. He'd been seeing Liesching almost every day for the past couple of weeks, yet the man had made no mention of a change in Smith's condition; neither had he mentioned the treatment he'd been administering, including a bleed. James was astonished that Smith was still being detained at all; he should have been discharged long ago, as the charge against him was trivial and in James's opinion it was 'highly improper to keep him longer confined; it being a well known fact, that persons who have once laboured under temporary insanity (whatever the cause may be) are subject to relapses if exposed to continual irritation'. Had Smith been released he would be in a better state, his 'situation in the Tronk being of itself sufficient to induce Madness in any person whose Mind has ever before been affected';[32] he was now 'ill and weak with his Mind partially deranged, and consequently a proper Subject for the professional Treatment of an Hospital ... altho' not for a Lunatic Asylum unless he shall hereafter evince Symptoms of permanent derangement'. Dr Barry had observed no such symptoms.

Again Lord Charles instructed the Fiscal to have Smith moved to the Somerset Hospital, and have him 'Confined in some secure place' within it.[33] Aaron Smith was almost certainly a chronic alcoholic, and therefore probably a sufferer from delirium tremens, brought on by having no access to alcohol while in the Tronk; this might well cause his 'raving madness'. Other cerebral and neurological disorders associated with chronic alcohol abuse, which had not been characterised at that time, could account for his weakness, illness and deranged mind.[34] In short, Dr Barry's view of the case was spot-on – as close to the truth as the limited medical understanding of the time would allow.

A few days after Lord Charles's order, James's professional career, driven along by his righteous ardour, ran headlong into a ditch. The Fiscal, stung beyond endurance by this latest instruction – with its implication that he and his officials had been neglecting or abusing their duty – and smarting from the Colonial Medical Inspector's ironic, sneering references to his 'spirit of pure charity' – raised the ante. He had James summoned before the Court of Justice to answer questions on his reports. James indignantly refused to cooperate with an interrogation on an official report written on the Governor's instructions, on the grounds that it would set a dangerous precedent, effectively providing the Fiscal with a power of veto on government reports.

The court (which happened to be one of the organs of the Fiscal's department) saw it differently; since this was a case that could result in a criminal prosecution against the dienaar, it was an offence to refuse an interrogation. On the Fiscal's direction, the sitting commissioner charged Dr Barry with contempt of court and passed a sentence of civil imprisonment.[35]

The court was not in full session, so James wasn't remanded in custody immediately. He was allowed to go free until a full session confirmed the sentence. He left the court with his mind whirling, but kept a hold on his wits. He needed legal advice.

Outside the building he met George Kekewich, his colleague in the inspection of the Tronk, who was astonished by James's tale.[36] James begged Kekewich to come with him to see John Bigge, a lawyer and important British government official. James desired both these men's advice, 'in order to prevent if possible my being (as I considered) further disgraced'.[37]

Bigge was an important man, one of two Commissioners of Inquiry who had been sent out by the home government to report on the administration and general state of the Cape Colony, Mauritius and Ceylon; they'd been at the Cape for just over two years now, with a specific brief to examine the British and Dutch legal structures and the situation of the black populations (particularly the slaves). Mr Bigge – who had been a patient of Dr Barry – listened sympathetically to his story. He didn't think James had broken the law; moreover, he had a poor opinion of the Court of Justice and disliked the Fiscal's influence upon it.[38] Mr Kekewich agreed, and they recommended that James apply to Lord Charles for help.[39]

In extreme haste, James wrote a letter summarising the situation, his pen scrawling wildly across the paper.[40] Carrying it in his pocket, he went straight to Government House, accompanied by Kekewich:

> After being detained some time, we were admitted, and I found Sir Richard Plasket with Lord Charles. I presented my letter and begged him to read it; he did so, but said he was not sure whether His Majesty's Fiscal was justified in his proceedings or not; upon which observation Mr Kekewich delivered his legal sentiments, adding, that they were those of Mr Bigge &c., &c. Sir Richard Plasket appeared perfectly of the same way of thinking.[41]

Lord Charles said he would talk to the Fiscal but, despite his power, the Governor couldn't command the Fiscal in a matter like this. It was a tricky situation. What James apparently took little account of was that there was a background to all of this; everybody in the Cape administration and judiciary was under review by the Commissioners of Inquiry, and many of them were watching their backs anxiously – particularly the Governor and the Fiscal. Lord Charles had long desired to trim the Fiscal's horns, and it seemed that the Commissioners might be on his side; however, in general they were not his allies; they were the agents of Westminster,

which was not friendly to Lord Charles Somerset. He could not afford
a war within his administration.

Denyssen was immensely powerful. His authority made him an unpopular man, especially feared by the black population over whom he and
his dienaars had terrifying powers of corporal punishment. Moreover,
his privilege in court cases was indefensible – as prosecutor in smuggling
cases he was entitled to a share of the spoils if he secured a conviction;
and in all criminal trials, 'even in those in which he is personally engaged'
(one of the Commissioners had reported), 'he assumes a seat on the bench,
next to the chief justice; and it arouses indignation to see the public
prosecutor in a situation where he can privately converse with … the
first magistrate', a practice 'so odious as to attract the notice and censure
of all'; it was 'strange that a sense of proper feeling has not taught him
to abstain from such a pretension'.[42]

James's exposure of abuses in the prison, and his barbs about Denyssen's
character, must have deeply stung a man who was acutely conscious of
the official scrutiny he was under. He may well have seen Dr Barry as the
cat's-paw of a Governor who was hoping to emasculate him. Lord Charles
had to take all this into account in handling the case, not to mention his
personal feelings about James.

The Fiscal was persuaded by Lord Charles not to act on Dr Barry's
imprisonment – at least not immediately.[43] However, Denyssen kept his
teeth firmly in James's hide; he chose to infer from Dr Barry's refusal to
answer questions that his report on the Tronk, 'however positive the same
may be, is devoid of any foundation', and described several incidents of
Aaron Smith's insane rages, blandly ignoring James's opinion that it was
incarceration that caused them.[44]

The threat of imprisonment still hung over James's head, and he
found it unbearable, especially once it became a subject for gossip in the
town. On the way back to Government House to consult Sir Richard
Plasket, he bumped into his old friend Colonel Bird, who called out,
'I'm astonished to find you at liberty. I was just on my way to the Tronk
to leave my card!'[45]

James's meeting with Plasket was a difficult one. Sir Richard 'had one
of his *headaches*', was in an irritable mood, and didn't want to be troubled
unless it was 'something particular'.[46] It was. James described what had
happened, and 'Sir Richard was pleased to say that for once I was right',
that he himself had originally suggested that Barry and Kekewich report

on the Tronk – and for good reason. Encouraged, James suggested that he might lay all the details of the case – especially the Fiscal's part in it – before the Commissioners of Inquiry. Both Kekewich and Colonel Bird had advised this. Sir Richard (who detested Bird) exclaimed irritably, 'You are always quoting Bird, or Bigge, or Kekewich!' James persevered, proposing to acquire all the documents from the Court of Justice and place them before the Commissioners. Sir Richard, turning suddenly hostile, replied, 'If you do, you shall be dismissed from your situation, and I will recommend it.'

'Indeed sir,' James answered, 'now you have threatened I will do so, not as a matter of complaint, but for their opinion and investigation, as well as for my own edification; it is a public concern.' He reminded Sir Richard again that he and Mr Kekewich had been ordered to report on the Tronk, that they had done so honestly, and that the final report 'may probably not be so mild'. Sir Richard called James's report thus far 'improper', but when challenged with the truth that James was 'working for the Public Good', he couldn't dispute it. Working himself into a passion, James declared, 'If I had had my sword on when Mr Fiscal proposed sending me to the Tronk, I should most certainly have cut off both his ears ... to make him look smart.'[47] Sir Richard laughed, but his peculiar hostility remained.

Plasket's involvement was deep and delicate. It seems that he was orchestrating a plan to reduce the Fiscal's power, and was using James's investigation of the Tronk to provide ammunition. But James had gone too far, arousing hostility and suspicion in the Fiscal. If this continued, the Fiscal could defend himself from any move to reform his department by accusing Lord Charles's government of vindictiveness and pointing to their support of the wayward Barry as favouritism and incompetence. Now that James was bringing in the Commissioners – who despite their dislike of the Fiscal were no friends to the Somerset administration – the situation was growing desperate.

Calling on the Commissioners of Inquiry James found both the principals at home: John Bigge and his colleague Major William Macbean Colebrooke, formerly of the Royal Artillery and now a civil servant and political agent (a combination of diplomat and intelligence officer). James repeated his conversation with Sir Richard to them 'without reserve'.[48] From that time on, he was convinced that the Secretary to Government had a personal grudge against him, and he told all his acquaintances about it at length – even rehearsing it to friends at a levée given by Lord Charles at Government House (despite the furious politicking, the social whirl went on).[49]

When Mr Bigge and Major Colebrooke queried Sir Richard about the alleged threat of dismissal and its circumstances, 'A conversation of a very unpleasant nature took place ... relative to the difference ... between his and Dr Barry's recollection', and 'the terms in which Sir Richard Plasket conducted his correspondence led to a suspension of the amicable intercourse that till then had subsisted between us.'[50] He alleged that Dr Barry was 'making his memory of such a convenient nature as just to meet and suit his own views and purposes'. James Barry was clearly not the only hot-tempered correspondent in the Cape government, nor the only one to speculate, in writing, on people's character.

On 29 September the Fiscal sent in his report on his investigation into the Smith case. It rebutted, in general and in detail, every allegation contained in James Barry's reports. Crucially, Aaron Smith himself now claimed that the bruises on his wrists were received a few days after his incarceration, and the prisoner who claimed to have witnessed the beating had apparently been discovered to harbour a grudge against the dienaar involved. Denyssen cited a report by two doctors of his own choosing, Laing and Abercrombie, who had examined Smith thoroughly and gave their opinion that his injuries (which included a previously unreported wrist fracture) had occurred prior to his imprisonment (which tended to contradict Smith's own revised testimony). Significantly, nothing substantive was produced to challenge James's medical opinion that Smith should not have been in prison at all. Had James given Smith a thorough physical examination in the first place, either he would now be armed with evidence to confound the Fiscal's doctors, or, if what they said was true, would not have made his accusation against the dienaar. It was a terrible mistake.

Having cleared himself and his department to his own satisfaction, the Fiscal dwelt on Dr Barry's conduct in making insinuations about the cruelty of the dienaars and about the Fiscal's character and motives. He savaged James, tearing apart his credibility, his professional judgement and his conduct.[51]

His Excellency Lord Charles Somerset – astonishingly and devastatingly – appeared to side with the Fiscal. Despite his abiding loyalty to James, with the prevailing political climate at home, in which his own position was precarious, he could not afford to look as if he were creating discord in his administration, and had no choice but diplomatic bargaining. There was no gainsaying the facts (or what purported to be facts) laid out in the Fiscal's report, and what was needed now was a statement of contrition from Dr Barry and a retraction of his allegations. 'His Excellency cannot refrain from remarking,' wrote Plasket to James, 'on the very great impropriety of your indulging yourself in reflexions on the Character of His Majesty's Fiscal – reflexions which were quite irrelevant to the Investigation you were desired to make in your Professional Character, and totally unconnected with your Official Duties.'[52]

James, alerted by this warning shot, gave a response that was unusually calm and measured, but hardly met Lord Charles's needs. He stated simply: 'In the discharge of an Office imposed upon me by His Excellency I deemed it necessary in my Report to state the appearances that manifested themselves.'[53] And he restated those appearances – Smith's bruises, his claim that they had been inflicted by the dienaar, and so on. He blandly denied that any 'uncandid or injurious reference' to the conduct of the Fiscal had been contained in his report and insisted that he was 'not aware of having attacked the Character, or reflected upon any neglect of duty on the part of His Majesty's Fiscal'. On the other hand, he would have 'esteemed myself unfit for my Station' had he not submitted a full and frank report. He pointed out again that it had been wrong for the court to presume to interrogate him on his official report; since he had never interfered with the duties of His Majesty's Fiscal, he begged to be excused from having his reports to government queried by that gentleman.

What he was saying – if one chose to see it – was that Denyssen's reaction to the report was hysterical, paranoid and unnecessary. Having provoked him into a personal battle, James was assuming an air of irreproachable rectitude. It might have gained him the moral high ground if it hadn't been so transparently disingenuous; the Fiscal seemed to be spoiling for a fight, but having goaded him into belligerence, James loftily declined to put up his fists. And he was certainly not about to apologise.

Lord Charles, caught between loyalty, duty and the politics of the scheme to reform the Fiscal's department, had been hoping for something better than this. A Colonial Medical Inspector needed to be a politician and a civil servant; a maverick, no matter how professionally gifted, would not be tolerated by the system. The measure resorted to by the Governor and his Secretary was an extreme one, a sacrificial move that would remove Denyssen's enemy at a stroke and at the same time prevent Denyssen defending himself by accusing the Governor of favouritism. James Barry had served Plasket's purpose in bringing evidence against the Fiscal, but hadn't behaved as a good political tool ought to. That very day, Lord Charles took a decision that had evidently been on the table for some time, placed there by Plasket. On 4 October 1825 the Governor instructed Sir Richard to write to Dr Barry:

> The Contents of your Letter of Yesterday's date, added to other Circumstances which have lately passed with reference to your Duties as Colonial Medical Inspector, have impressed upon His Excellency the Governor the impropriety of any One Individual being entrusted with the Sole Management and Control of the Colonial Medical Department here, and he has therefore felt it necessary to propose to Council, that the Duties of that Department be henceforth carried on by a Committee according to the original Intention of the Colonial Government in 1807 – when the Supreme Medical Committee was appointed.[54]

In the most civil manner possible, James was not only being dismissed from his post, but having it knocked out from under him.

18

'Blighting My Fair Prospects'

The Colonial Medical Inspector's office: Monday 10 October 1825

A dusty, clock-ticking quiet lay over the room. A copy of *The Times* – nearly four months old but only just arrived at the Cape – lay face-down on the desk, an item on the back page having caught Dr Barry's particular attention.

CORONER'S INQUEST.

[On] Wednesday an inquest was held at the Hare and Hounds, Buckbridge-street, St Giles's, before THOMAS STIRLING, Esq., coroner, on the body of Mr Redmond Barry, aged 66.

The following document will explain a great part of the previous life and circumstances of the unfortunate man:–

'Subscription for the relief of the brother of the late James Barry, Esq., historical painter ...

'Redmond Barry, a native of Ireland, the only surviving brother of the late James Barry, whose paintings adorn the great room of the Society for the Encouragement of Arts, &c, in the Adelphi, is, at the age of 66, blind and destitute ...'[1]

After serving his seven-year sentence for grand larceny (not mentioned in the subscription notice), Redmond had gone back to the Navy. He had taken part in more actions at sea and was wounded yet again, and in 1819 was blinded by a lightning strike. He returned to London and lived in his accustomed poverty. The subscription had raised £40, which had been quickly exhausted; 'after which he was as much embarrassed as ever, and was obliged to resort to his former means of support; living in a hovel of the most miserable and filthy description in Maynard-street, and actually starving'.[2] The inquest, which 'operated most powerfully upon the feelings of the Coroner, the jury, and all present', ended in a verdict of death 'by the visitation of God'.[3]

As a reminder of where Margaret Bulkley had come from, and of the imperative that had driven her to conjure Dr James Barry into existence, her uncle's death could not have come at a more poignant time. Dead in a garret in the Rookery – the pit of the world. For those who have fought their way from the deeps to the sunlit uplands by their own talents and exertions, there is an abiding dread of losing hold, of slipping back down. And what a depth to fall. Margaret's mother had been within an ace of a debtor's prison during that winter in Southwark in 1812, and James had been thoroughly entangled in the crisis. Now, having attained, through talent, charm and ceaseless hard work, a position no man of his age could normally expect, James was having it all torn from his grasp.

Also lying on the desk was that last, stunning letter from Plasket announcing the proposal to dissolve the Colonial Medical Inspectorship; it had lain there now for nearly a week and James had not responded. At last he took up his quill, dipped it, and began writing calmly and neatly:

> Colonial Medical Inspector's Office
> 10th October 1825
>
> Sir,
>   I have duly received the letter you did me the honor to address to
> me, dated the 4th inst. in which I am informed that …[4]

He reiterated the entire contents of the letter, almost verbatim, as if trying to uncover some previously unnoticed fault or misunderstanding that would make all this go away. There was none; it was as clear as could be. He added:

> In reply to which; I beg you to do me the favor most respectfully
> to assure His Excellency of my entire willingness to conform to any
> arrangements which are deemed requisite for the Conduct of the
> Department of Colonial Medical Inspector.

He signed off, 'I have the honor to be Sir, your Obedient Servant, James Barry MD, Colonial Medical Inspector.' It would be the last letter he would sign in that way; no amount of conformity now could prevent the outcome, and all he had left was the forbearance of Lord Charles.

A few days later James met Sir Richard,[5] who confirmed the decision to revive the Supreme Medical Committee, and offered Dr Barry membership of it. James was already resigned to this fate and willing to serve. Given his prior standing, he naturally assumed that he should take the presidency. Sir Richard hesitated. Actually, it had been decided to appoint Staff Physician John Arthur MD, the garrison's Principal Medical Officer. As he and Dr Barry both held Army commissions, and as Dr Arthur's was significantly senior, he must take the presidency. Bewildered and overwhelmed, James let his temper give way; he suggested that Sir Richard was motivated by personal hostility, and that the whole thing had been his idea.

James wrote to Lord Charles, his penstrokes growing more jittery with each paragraph:

> It will be impossible for me to reconcile to my feelings the acceptance of any subordinate place in the proposed Establishment, should it have received your Lordship's approval that such a place should be tendered to me.
>
> In this Event I beg respectfully to tender my resignation to [all] of the Civil Situations that I hold under your Lordship's appointment and I request to be honored with an early communication of your Lordship's final Intentions, and before they are made Public.[6]

There was a coded threat here: 'all the civil situations' included that as the Somersets' personal physician.

Lord Charles parted from convention by replying personally to James rather than through Plasket. He was in an awkward position, trapped between the official and the private, and the letter was an odd mix of formality and tenderness. He reminded James:

> The very improper Language in which you couched your Official Communications, and the imputations you unsparingly and unreservedly call upon Officers of this Government, so greatly Embarrassed the Government, that Sir Richard Plasket felt it his duty to submit to me the Expediency of restoring the Medical Committee.[7]

So there it was: the impetus had come from Plasket, as James had guessed. And Lord Charles was coming as close as he could to saying that he hadn't wanted to act on it. He certainly knew James's secret, even if not Margaret's true identity, and whether or not there had been any sexual relationship between them he must have recognised her courage and understood the extraordinary pressures on her. Whatever he knew, Charles Henry Somerset loved this woman. The briefest glimpse of his emotions slipped into his letter when he admitted that 'the only obstacle' to the revival of the committee 'was my Apprehensions, that it might hurt your feelings'.[8]

What Margaret felt could only be imagined. Neither she nor her alter ego was the kind to give up the fight. The matter still hadn't been formally agreed by the Council, and the next day James requested that he be allowed to attend in person to explain himself. But no – it was out of the question for individuals to make such representations.[9]

On 28 October the Council approved the reinstatement of the Supreme Medical Committee, and the following day Sir Richard wrote to James inviting him again to accept a place. Not only would James not be its premier, he wouldn't even be its second. Below Dr Arthur would be local physician and accoucheur Dr Johann Wehr (a former German military surgeon, now with a practice in Strandstraat); and below him Staff Surgeon John Murray. In *fourth place* would be Dr Barry, and finally Dr Louis Liesching – yet another member of that far-reaching medical dynasty.[10]

It was an opening, but it wasn't enough to overcome James's formidable pride. He wrote back the same day: 'I have the honor to state, for His Excellency's information, that I beg to decline accepting the Situation of Member of the Supreme Medical Committee about to be re-established.'[11]

On the first day of November 1825, the abolition of the office of Colonial Medical Inspector was publicly proclaimed.[12] James's place on the committee had been taken by his old colleague from the Vaccine Institution, William Lys, and his long-serving secretary, Thomas Deane, would now serve the committee.

It was a good set of men, including several who were James's friends (John Murray had presided over the board that had approved his return to full pay the year before),[13] but none of them individually could out-match him for medical skill, nor first-hand knowledge of the Cape's military and civil institutions, and none could equal him for wholehearted devotion to duty, zeal for improvement and determination to alleviate the plight of the Colony's most vulnerable people. Even together, as it transpired, they would struggle to manage the workload that James had handled alone.

His nemesis, the Fiscal, didn't escape unscathed. On the same day the proclamation was made, the Governor wrote to Lord Bathurst enclosing a copy of another proclamation that had passed in Council but not yet been made public, removing the Fiscal's authority over the police – the Justitie Dienaaren – and creating a new office for that role. 'I have no doubt,' wrote Lord Charles, 'that this arrangement (which is one that I have long wished to accomplish) will prove highly beneficial to the Colony.'[14] The stated reason was a familiar one – that the duties of the Fiscal were too many and too great for one individual – as well as the fact that the Fiscal's department had always aroused 'an ill feeling in the minds of the public and particularly of the British Residents'.

A Pyrrhic victory for James, whose case had undoubtedly aided the impetus for abridging the Fiscal's power. Even though his medical reports had had nothing to do with the police, the signal was clear – Mr Denyssen was not able to give all his duties sufficient care.

James Barry and Daniel Denyssen were not the only officials affected. Lord Charles Somerset himself was experiencing pressure from above; the Cape Colony was huge, its population and economy rapidly growing, and it was felt – according to the familiar refrain – that it was too much for one man.

The final opinion on James's case came far too late to affect it; the Commissioners of Inquiry combed through all the complexities of Dr Barry's period as Colonial Medical Inspector, and although they censured him for some aspects of his conduct and gave qualified support to the decision to abolish his office, they severely criticised the way in which it had been done:

> If the removal of Dr Barry however was the object, it would have become the Government to have paused before it resorted to a measure that was in its operation more severe and galling to his feelings than that of positive dismissal ... or to have endeavoured to make an arrangement that would have remedied the objection to the nature and quality of his duties.[15]

Dr Barry should have remained as Colonial Medical Inspector, they said, but with the requirement that he be answerable to a committee for matters of policy and judgement. In other words, in the view of His Majesty's Commissioners, Lord Charles Somerset and Sir Richard Plasket had not only done the wrong thing but done it in an ungentlemanly manner. They asked Sir Richard some questions about the grounds on which the office had been abolished, but he refused to answer them.[16] The Commissioners believed – but couldn't prove – that the Secretary to Government had forced the Governor to remove Dr Barry from his post. They agreed with James that there was a grudge, and they had 'much reason to complain that Sir Richard Plasket (whatever he may think of Dr Barry)' had used his correspondence with the Commissioners as 'a vehicle for imputations which, if they were known to Dr Barry, he would be bound as a gentleman to resent'.[17] No doubt they had heard of the tempestuous doctor's history as a duellist and thought Plasket had got off lightly.

By the time the Commissioners wrote their report, James had already gone down in the world, back to living in lodgings in the Heerengracht (probably with the Widow Sandenberg again), having given up his grace-and-favour residence upon resigning his civil appointments.[18]

In the immediate aftermath of his fall, James wrote directly to Lord Bathurst in London, rehearsing the whole sorry episode and lamenting his loss:

> And thus was the turn of an expression in my Report, and which Report, I contend, was absolutely necessary for the Public good inasmuch as it tended ... to ensure the safety of Prisoners from wanton brutality ... made the pretence for abolishing my Office, and totally destroying my hardly earned and hitherto highly estimated professional character, and blighting my fair prospects in life ...
>
> As to the temporary inconvenience of pecuniary matters, I have not, I do not give them a thought. I had indeed flattered myself that I was bartering my time, my health and my talents (such as they are) to the Public Benefit for honest Fame, not sacrificing them to infamy.[19]

On falling from office, James Barry left behind him a great legacy; through his efforts and initiative the cause of public health in the Cape of Good Hope had been significantly advanced. The Somerset Hospital had evolved from a hell-hole into a more or less functioning institution. It continued to improve, undergoing several rebuildings and expansions, and, a century on, it would become the University of Cape Town's first teaching hospital.[20] Hemel en Aarde had likewise been set in order, and the public benefited from stricter regulation of drugs and medicines. The water supply was good, as were the sanitary facilities, following one of Dr Barry's last acts as Inspector, replacing open sewers with iron pipes. Recollections of these improvements, and of the strange little Army doctor who brought them about, endured down the years in the collective memory of Cape Town.

But in his own time, in the rising summer of late 1825, James was faced with resuming the professional life ordained by his low rank – acting as a general practitioner to the Cape garrison's 2400 officers and men, their wives and children. He still had an elevated circle of friends, and his private patients helped fill out his life (if not his purse, for he still wouldn't take fees), but compared to what he'd lost, it was an empty shell. His world grew bleaker still when the new year got under way and the time came for Lord Charles to leave the Cape.

Cape Town: Sunday 5 March 1826

Heerengracht was wearing its Sunday best – the verges lined with an honour guard of troops from the garrison, townspeople gathered under the trees. At Government House a party had gathered – senior military officers, civil servants and a large number of personal friends, come to take leave of Lord Charles Somerset and his family.

It had been clear for months that the end was in sight. The attacks on his governorship were increasing, ranging from the scandalous (Bishop Burnett was publishing voluminously on the subject)[21] to the political (largely from Sir Rufane Donkin). Leader of the political charge in England was Henry Brougham, who was growing prominent among the Whig faction in Parliament and leapt upon anything scandalous concerning the Cape and its Tory Governor.

There was plenty to leap upon. The state of the colonial government was notoriously dire. Sir Richard Plasket had written about it frequently (and extremely disloyally) to a friend who was under-secretary to Lord Bathurst, remarking that 'every day that passes confirms me more and more in my opinion of the perfect incompetence of the present Establishment to carry on the Government with energy or with advantage' and that the Colony 'is at present at its very lowest ebb'.[22] Interestingly, although Plasket condemned the departments of government root and branch – including the Fiscal's – he made no mention of the Colonial Medical Inspector, despite this being at the height of the Barry–Denyssen clash, confirming that the sacrifice of Dr Barry was a hastily contrived devil's bargain to resolve a political stand-off between the Governor and the Fiscal, not a response to an actual problem.

By November 1825 it had been decided that Lord Charles must return to England to face the criticisms in person. He'd been persuaded to go by Sir Richard who, despite his contempt for the government, esteemed Lord Charles personally.[23]

Within the Colony the Governor was generally liked and admired, and most of the enemies he had there were fellow Britons. One, Dudley Perceval, had come to the Cape severely prejudiced against Lord Charles, but was quickly won round, observing: 'in all the mass of abuse that has been raked up against him, not one single Dutch name has appeared as an accuser'; they were 'universally attached to his person and indignant at the idea of his removal'.[24] Perceval had come expecting to find an arrogant, cold, unpleasant, all-round bad egg 'dreaded by his inferiors, shunned by his equals and detested by both. This I verily believe, is the opinion which his enemies have contrived to render very general in England … The fact is that Lord Charles Somerset is the most popular man in the Colony – *most astonishingly popular*.'[25]

Nonetheless, it had been decided at home that the Cape of Good Hope was too large to be governed by one man, and in February 1826, Lord Charles's old friend Major General Richard Bourke had arrived to take up the brand-new post of Lieutenant Governor of the Eastern District.

When the time came, the farewell procession left Government House. Lord Charles led on horseback, with the ladies following in a carriage; he was flanked by the Commissioners of Inquiry (representing the British government) and Major General Bourke (now Acting Governor). A sharp-featured man with a high-domed forehead, scarlet coat and vast gold epaulettes, Bourke contrasted vividly with the dark, modest and pleasant-looking Commissioners. Dr James Barry rode inconspicuously behind. The procession passed through the Company's Garden and along Heerengracht between the lines of troops and crowds of spectators, past the Tronk and the Custom House to the little jetty where the government barge was tied.

Here the Governor gave his farewells and salutes, and then, accompanied only by his family and a handful of close friends, he boarded the barge. The friends included James Barry – still, in spite of everything, the closest friend of all.[26] The crowds gathered on the beach and clinging to the housetops watched the barge cross the water to where the East Indiaman *Atlas* was anchored. All the ships in the bay were dressed in their best colours and gave rousing cheers, and HMS *Helicon* fired a thirteen-gun salute.

Aboard, the Somersets said their final goodbyes to their friends. James's attachment to Lord Charles had been lampooned by a local wag who claimed that on entering church one Sunday and finding the Governor's pew empty, Dr Barry had immediately left:

> With courteous devotion inspired
> Barry came to the temple of prayer
> But quickly turned round and retired
> When he found that HIS Lord was not there.[27]

Now the pew would always be empty, and James's life would have an irreparable hole at its centre. Again Margaret was trapped – she might have defied authority and followed Lord Charles to England, but that would cause embarrassment to him and personal ruin for James. Margaret, who had sacrificed so much already, would now have to do without her best friend, her love, her father figure.

The friends left the ship and went back to the shore. *Atlas* crowded on her canvas and was away with the breeze. The *South African Chronicle* wrote:

> At that hour the sun which had been obscured during the earlier part of the morning, shone forth with more than usual brightness, like the fair fame of an upright man which the fleeting breath of calumny may dim but cannot tarnish.[28]

That was how they saw it at the Cape; in London it would be different. Notionally, Lord Charles Somerset was on a mission to answer his critics in person, with the intention of returning to resume his governorship. But in reality, as everyone secretly guessed, he was never coming back.

Yet James did not give up on him.

19

A New Life

Wintry rain spattered against the windows, but Wilhelmina Munnik was oblivious; the curtains were tightly drawn, a fire hissed in the grate, and Wilhelmina's whole being was turned in on herself, upon the endless cycle of pain and the life of her unborn child. The labour had been going on all day and throughout the night. She took no notice of anxious relatives or the soft-footed, whispering servants, or of her anguished husband. As for the midwife – the one person upon whom she depended – she could do nothing to bring Wilhelmina's ordeal to an end. She probed and prodded and found that there could be no persuading this child out into the world; in the early hours, the desperate woman consulted the husband: the baby, she assured him, would die, and take its mother with it.

Thomas Frederick Munnik wasn't accustomed to this kind of crisis at all; he was a snuff dealer, with a thriving shop in Burg Street, Cape Town. He and Wilhelmina, who both came from long-established Cape families, had been married for ten years, and this was her second pregnancy; the first had produced a son who had died in infancy.[1] Ten years without children or even the hope of children – aside from that brief tragedy – and now this. The midwife had done all she could; they needed a doctor, not an accoucheur but a proper physician and surgeon who knew midwifery. Everyone's mind flew straight to Dr Barry, who lodged with Wilhelmina's widowed sister, Catherina Sandenberg.

A messenger was sent to ride the nine wet miles to Cape Town, and in the dead watches his hammering on the door woke the whole lodging house. James was accustomed to being called in the dead of night (a well-named passage of time, when the body and spirit were at their low ebb, illness came and worsened, and many slipped into death). While Danzer ran for a chaise, James dressed and gathered his obstetrical instruments – a small set of half a dozen or so pieces including scissors, specula and forceps in a soft leather roll, as well as his bulky surgical case and medicine bag – all the time extracting details of the case from the dripping messenger in the Dutch pidgin used by slaves and servants.

It was evidently an unusual emergency – perhaps even medically interesting. There was precious little of interest in the regular life of a common military doctor on the staff of a garrison. He'd almost forgotten what military duties were like during the past nine years; while he held government appointments, his military life had consisted largely of mess dinners and regimental balls, with rare visits to the Military Hospital. Now it was an endless parade of boils, carbuncles, fractures, venereal disease and an occasional hernia or amputation. No military surgery was required; the infrequent assegai or gunshot wounds sustained in frontier skirmishes would be treated by regimental surgeons; what James encountered instead was the depressing succession of injuries from fights among drunken troops and lacerations inflicted by floggings.

In Wynberg, James's chaise drew up outside the house on Waterloo Green. Waiting at the door were Thomas Munnik and his spinster sister; Dr Barry made straight for the midwife, interrogating her as he went briskly to the marital bedroom.

Wilhelmina's labour pains were draining the last reserves of her strength. An examination showed that the foetus was alive, but also that it would not pass through the cervix. Even the forceps – the obstetrician's wonder instrument – would be no help here. Cases this bad were rare, and there was only one way to bring out the child alive – a caesarean operation.

This was a decision no doctor wanted to make – a caesarean, while usually resulting in a live child, was almost invariably fatal to the mother. A tiny handful of cases were known in which the mother had survived – occurrences so rare that they made the medical journals – and in some of those it was the infant that died while the mother survived. There were three verified cases of both mother and baby surviving, and not a single one of them in Britain or anywhere in the Empire. Statistically, the chance of survival was negligible; typically there would be a brief interlude following the procedure, and then the surgical fever set in, and within days the patient would be dead. There was another option, a terrible one that the doctor was obliged to consider – perforation and dismemberment of the foetus to remove it. This still carried a risk to the mother, and was only done if the foetus could not be saved.

James spoke quietly to the midwife, and then to Wilhelmina, explaining to her what needed to be done, and the risk attached. Despite being famously ill-tempered, James Barry was known equally for his marvellously comforting bedside manner. And aside from his expertise in midwifery,[2] he had a secret advantage – there was not another practising physician or surgeon in the world who knew from personal experience what it was like to bear a child. Wilhelmina, in so much pain that death would be a release, consented to the operation.[3] The room was cleared of family members, leaving only the midwife to assist and a couple of female servants to help hold the patient. James prepared his instruments.

There had been an account published eight years earlier by a physician in Zurich called Locher, who had delivered a child successfully by the caesarean method while preserving the life of the mother. The case had been a sensation, translated and reported in the British journals, and James would have known it well – searching it, like other physicians and accoucheurs, for clues about procedure and treatment. Dr Locher hadn't really done anything obviously out of the ordinary. After failing to insert both blades of his forceps, he'd decided to operate. Once an enema had been given and the bowels and bladder emptied, he had the patient put in 'the position usual in herniotomy,* in which the weight of the abdomen presses more against the diaphragm'; then, with instruments ready, he ordered her to be secured.[4] James had no proper assistants, so he needed the midwife and servants to help – two holding down an arm each and one holding on to Wilhelmina's ankles.[5] The patient was given a leather strap to bite on. Dr Locher's description of his own operation was fairly standard, and James, having some practical experience of the procedure on deceased subjects, must have followed it closely. Locher had written:

Having performed before a similar operation, I was induced to make the incision immediately upon the linea alba,† as not a single blood-vessel of any importance had been injured on that occasion. Immediately beneath the navel the skin was pinched up in to a fold, both it and the

---

* head slightly lowered, pelvis elevated
† vertical structure forming the midline of the abdomen, formed mainly of strong fibrous tissue

adipous [sic] membrane cut through, and the cut continued downwards
to the length of from eight to ten inches. The sphere of the uterus, now
appearing, extended the fat edges of the incision, so that there appeared
a considerable vaulted surface of the womb. There protruded also a
portion of small intestine, which, however, was easily kept back by
means of linen anointed with fat. In order not to cut through the uterus
exactly in a place where the placenta might accidentally be situated,
and thus excite a violent bleeding, I chose a somewhat uneven part of
its surface, and there made a little incision, so that I could introduce
the index of the left-hand, to serve as a guide for the progress of the
knife. The uterus was then cut open from six to eight inches along
the finger. Immediately the child presented itself, together with its
membranes, yet without any water. The hemorrhage till then was a
mere nothing. The nearest part of the child was an arm. This, as there
was room enough, was disengaged first from the uterus, and after it
carefully one part of the child after the other in succession, and last
of all the head. Already before the head was freed from the womb,
the infant moved its limbs, and on the development of the head, to
the greatest joy of the mother and all the attendants, it proved its life
by loud cries.[6]

Mr and Mrs Munnik had a son, alive and healthy. Once the umbilical cord
had been cut he was passed to the midwife while James got on with the
rest of the procedure; the placenta was removed, and the wound sponged
and closed. Dr Locher had chosen not to suture the uterus, as he had seen
in dissections of deceased caesarean patients that it contracted and closed
up of its own accord; 'I therefore joined the external integuments with
five sutures, covered the wound with lint, and applied some adhesive
plasters, confining the whole with a couple of compresses and a broad
bandage.'[7] The baby was placed with the mother and an emulsion of
laudanum and tincture of cinnamon prescribed.

James remained with the patient for much of that day, and called
regularly over the next several days. The soreness of Wilhelmina's
wound faded somewhat, and then the critical period began. In the case
of Dr Locher's patient, three days went by placidly, with a seeming
improvement, but on the fourth his patient fell suddenly ill, with
violent spasms, cold extremities and cold sweat, incontinent in her
bladder and confused in her mind, scarcely able to breathe; her life was

despaired of. Treated with enemas and external friction, the patient was better within a day. By the tenth day after the operation the stitches could be removed. With good food and wine, the patient returned fully to health.

No record was left of the precise course of Wilhelmina Munnik's condition after her operation (other than that she was unable to feed the child, which had to be put to a wet nurse chosen from among the slaves), but it cannot have been very different. Miraculously, Wilhelmina made it through the crisis – mother and son lived.

At the time there was no way of knowing precisely what the magical factor was that distinguished Dr Barry and Dr Locher from the thousands of other practitioners who had performed caesareans; since surgical fever was caused by bacterial infection, it was probably hygiene – clean hands, clean instruments – rather than technique. Yet if so, the hygiene must have been fortuitous, since no practitioner anywhere had any inkling of what bacterial infection was, nor of how it came about. Certainly Dr Locher didn't mention hygiene in his report. James Barry was devoted to general cleanliness, and no doubt this helped. Perhaps Dr Locher was similarly inclined. They may both have been helped by unusual skill as physicians in treating their patient afterwards.

Thomas and Wilhelmina Munnik's gratitude was immense. James was offered a large fee, but refused it, saying that if they wished to thank him they could do so by naming the boy after him. Possibly he was joking, but the parents were in earnest, and a few weeks later, on 20 August 1826 at the Lutheran church on Strandstraat in Cape Town, James Barry Munnik was baptised, with Dr James Barry as godfather.[8] In return, James gave the family the miniature portrait he'd had made when he was newly commissioned, fresh and youthful in red coatee and that now terribly old-fashioned Roman hairstyle.

The portrait became one of the Munniks' most treasured heirlooms, and such was the impression that James had made, they preserved the name too; when James Barry Munnik grew up he had a son, who in turn named *his* son James Barry Munnik, and so on into the next century. The name branched out too – a cousin, Albertus Hertzog, who grew up with the first James Barry Munnik, named his son James Barry Munnik Hertzog. It was almost as if fate, having once conjured a fictional James Barry into existence, was trying to balance the books with a multitude of natural-born James Barrys.[9] The miracle of Wynberg was just one of the many tales that caused the original, not entirely fictional, James Barry to become a part of Cape legend.

The case clearly touched James deeply. Margaret might have given a thought to her own child, born in a different world, a different life-time. Juliana Bulkley was a grown woman now, still living in the city of Cork, unmarried and earning her bread by her needle.[10] How much knowledge she had of her mother is unknown, but she must have been told something by her Bulkley and Barry relations; perhaps they told her Margaret was dead – she would certainly have no idea that her mother was living as an Army doctor at the bottom end of the globe, working miracles.

Meanwhile, Margaret was obscuring James's origins still further. It was now ten years since Dr Barry had arrived at the Cape; Margaret was thirty-seven years old, approaching middle age, and James's appearance could no longer be ascribed to youth. There were few now at the Cape (among English upper society, at least) who had known James for long, and fewer still who would remember his first arrival. So it was around this time that James began to suggest – in the vaguest possible terms – that his odd physical characteristics were due to his having been born prematurely, claiming that his mother had died in childbirth, his father also dying around the same time. He'd been adopted by an influential family, and they continued to take an interest in him and provide protection and support.[11] He began to elaborate his name, calling himself James Miranda Steuart Barry, discreetly acknowledging his debt to his two early patrons, and allowing those who knew the family names of the Earl of Buchan to infer some connection.

Although rumour still had it that Dr Barry was really a female, he had remained so firmly in his role that the idea began to waver, and some medical men privately theorised that he was asexual, that he'd been con-ceived a male 'in whom sexual development had been arrested about the sixth month of foetal life'.[12] Most people, though, simply accepted him as a small, mercurial and decidedly peculiar man.

Without Lord Charles, James was lonely, adrift, almost purposeless. The abolition of his office continued to prey on his mind, the odour of shame unbearable. A year had passed since his appeal to Lord Bathurst, and no reply had come, so he sat down and wrote again, rehearsing the story and his grievance one more time. 'I have waited,' he wrote; 'nothing has been done':

> I have only further to say: that my silence hitherto on this subject
> arose (and my present backwardness arises) from my ardent wish to do
> nothing that can in any way injure Lord Charles Somerset, but solely
> to rescue my good name from dishonor.[13]

Shortly after posting this second letter, James received Bathurst's reply to the first one. The Secretary of State saw no reason to doubt the propriety of what had been done, and had no intention of issuing any sanctions or inquiries, or of reinstating Dr Barry's position. James was aghast that the Secretary of State thought he was begging for his job back, and wrote again to disclaim that notion:

> But I do complain of the precedent, and to me injurious and disgraceful
> manner in which it was done ... and also, I contend, the injustice of
> my not being placed at the Head of that Board, after the arduous and
> zealous professional labour in which I had been engaged for a series
> of years ...
>   It is perhaps ... needless for me to enforce how dear, how very dear
> to me, my good name is, and how very anxious I am to make every
> human effort in order to avert the heavy calamities consequent to the
> loss of it.
>   I therefore deem it my bounden Duty to vindicate my integrity and
> to rescue it as soon as possible from the unworthy imputation which
> has been heaped upon it – and to manifest my honourable transac-
> tions to the World:– without which, even my claims to and anxious
> Expectations of Military Promotion may continue to be obstructed,
> if not totally annihilated.[14]

In fact, James's character and professional standing had not been materi-ally harmed. When people wanted the best doctor in the Cape of Good Hope, they generally came to Dr Barry, and he had many influential friends still, including the Commissioners of Inquiry.[15]

James found stimulation for his active mind in botany and pharma-cology, and began writing a paper on the properties of *Arctopus echinatus*, which was used in native medicine and which he was convinced was effective in treating venereal disease – the perennial curse of all garrisons. At the end of 1826, Principal Medical Officer Dr John Arthur produced his annual report on the health of the garrison troops (he had by this time resigned his position as chairman of the Supreme Medical Committee; in fact all its members had been astonished at the amount of work it involved, and that Dr Barry had previously done it all alone). He reported that while health in the garrison was generally good, 'Our efforts to prevent the propagation of Venereal Complaints have been less successful than we would have wished' despite the efforts of the dienaars to rid the town of 'those loose, abandoned, idle Characters that usually communicate the Complaint to the Soldiery'.[16]

Treatment of venereal disease was ugly, uncomfortable and often painful. Gonorrhoea was treated by applying local decongestant measures to a painful and swollen penis (in severe cases), with sedatives, local dressings to catch the purulent discharge, and the administration of extract of cubebs (a variety of Indonesian pepper) or balsam of copaiba (from a South American tree) or even turpentine. Direct instillation into the urethra was recommended, using a variety of solutions of metallic salts, including silver nitrate, for their antiseptic properties. The men themselves practised the more radical measure of instilling gunpowder into the urethra.[17]

Syphilis wasn't always clinically distinguished from gonorrhoea. Both were so common that concurrent infection with both was always a possibility. Preparations of calomel (mercury or mercurous chloride) were generally prescribed for syphilis for prolonged periods – a treatment that became a byword: 'Two minutes with Venus, two years with Mercury.'[18]

These treatments – none of which had any real clinical benefit – fell to the more junior medical officers, including Dr Barry, and this, combined with his love of botany, induced him to write a paper on the subject:

> In examining into the Natural History of the Cape, its Vegetable Kingdom will be discovered to abound in many rare and valuable medicinal productions, and the Arctopus ... which I now propose to offer to the consideration of the Profession will, I trust, be deemed neither unimportant nor uninteresting.[19]

Some years earlier a surgeon with the 21st Dragoons had found it useful in treating syphilis, but the samples he sent back to England had proved useless. James thought he knew the reason: it had been 'unfortunately exhibited only in the form of a Decoction,* on which occasion the Gum Resin, that important principle wherein a peculiarly antisyphilitic virtue apparently resides ... was completely lost'. James went on to describe the botany and pharmacology of *Arctopus* in great detail, as well as its usage: 'the Gum Resin should be administered under the form of Pills from 8 to 12 grains, gradually increased ... each dose followed up by one-fourth of a pint of Decoction, to which a drachm of the Tincture may be added with benefit.' Beyond the specifics of this medicine, he expanded upon the full treatment:

> A warm bath ... taken once in 6 to 8 days, affords great relief to the patient; a sea-water bath, or some brandy, or vinegar, added to the fresh water, will be found to increase the efficacy. Any ulcers or blotches should be washed and dressed once or twice daily with the Decoction ... The state of the bowels must of course be attended to; any saline bitter purgative, or turpentine, castor oil ... answer well. The diet should be plain and nutritious in almost equal proportions of animal and vegetable food, a moderate quantity of old wine may be allowed ... During the use of the Arctopus, fresh air should be freely admitted; and where it is practicable the patient ought to take gentle and regular exercise, as the body is by no means so susceptible of the variations of atmosphere as when under the influence of Mercury.[20]

Dr Arthur was impressed, and included a copy with his annual report: 'I can say nothing as yet from my own knowledge,' he commented, 'but after perusing his paper I have sent it to the Hospitals to be copied – I intend to obtain for them a supply of the Medicine and to direct trials to be made of it.'[21]

The following year, on 22 November 1827, James was promoted from assistant to full staff surgeon,[22] a rank equivalent to that of major. Overnight his salary doubled to 15 shillings a day and his status within the Army Medical Department was finally on a properly sound footing.

During these years, James was essentially marking time, although probably not conscious of it. He still had friends and a working life, but was

---

* concentration of liquid by heating or boiling

fundamentally alone and unchallenged for the first time in his existence, with nobody to act as his support and patron.

He could hardly even keep his manservant. In June 1827, five years after his previous attempt, Danzer ran away again. He'd been staying in Wynberg at the home of Valentinus Schönberg, a former landdrost and retired government sequestrator* (quite why James had left Danzer there isn't clear from the records). Danzer was left in the house alone for two hours one evening; homesick for his family in Graaff Reinet, he seized his chance, took a fine brown stallion from the stable and rode off.

He got as far as Worcester on the far side of the mountains before he was caught. Brought back to Cape Town in August he was put on trial for horse theft, and pleaded guilty; in mitigation he said that he missed his parents, and insisted that he had intended to return after visiting them. The court had no sympathy – 'such a crime, in a country with good Justice, cannot be condoned but requires rigorous punishment in accordance with the Law.' Danzer was sentenced 'to be bound to a whipping post, and given a severe lashing on his bare back, and then to be put in irons and sent to Robben Island for Twelve consecutive months' labour without remuneration'.[23]

James was powerless to help. Danzer appealed, claiming that Dr Barry had given him permission to go away, and that he hadn't known it was a crime to take Mr Schönberg's horse.[24] About a week later, General Bourke – now full Governor – took pity on the young man and remitted his sentence, instructing the landdrost of the Cape District accordingly.[25] But the landdrost failed to act, and before either James Barry or the Governor knew what was happening, Danzer was in chains bound for Robben Island. It took until February 1828 – a full six months – for James to secure his release and have him returned to his service.[26]

In August 1828 new orders came through from the Army Medical Department. After nearly twelve years, James Barry's posting at the Cape of Good Hope was at an end. He was to pack up and proceed to the island of Mauritius to join the medical staff there.

The Cape had become home. Almost one-third of Margaret's life had been spent here, and four-fifths of James's professional career. The

---

* official in charge of civil sentences and liquidating insolvent estates

only place Margaret knew better was Cork, and even that was a distant memory. But Dr Barry was now a full staff surgeon, and the department had no room for a man with that rank in the Cape garrison; it was time to move him on.

Danzer, just returned to service after the horror of Robben Island, was upset; he wanted to stay with the doctor. But as he wasn't quite eighteen and his six-year indenture was still in force, he couldn't leave the Cape. James applied to the Governor to have the indenture replaced with a new one, under special terms.[27] The request was granted.

On Monday 8 September 1828, a farewell party was thrown for James:

> The friends of Dr Barry with a view to marking their high opinion of his merit, and of their regret at his departure for Mauritius on promotion, invited him to a Dinner at George's Hotel on Monday last. Amongst the company might be seen many distinguished Civil, Military and Mercantile Gentlemen, and the evening passed harmoniously; the Dinner and Wines were excellent. Health and prosperity to Dr Barry was repeatedly drunk with enthusiasm, and the impression excited on Dr Barry was evident. He returned his acknowledgement for these last marks of attention with great taste and feeling, and the party separated at a late hour.[28]

He was leaving behind a Cape Colony whose government was still struggling with the radical review and reforms in whose backdraft he and Lord Charles had been caught. James had changed a lot and learned a great deal in twelve years. He'd acquired a small measure of the serenity needed to accept the things he couldn't change, and had more than enough courage to change the things he could, but the wisdom to tell the difference would always elude his grasp.

On 26 September 1828, the little Indiaman *Eliza Jane* raised anchor in Table Bay. On board, taking a last view of the beach and the town, and the spectacular mountainous backdrop, was Dr James Barry, and with him were Danzer and Dr Barry's orderly, Private John Smith. With the wind on her port quarter, *Eliza Jane* passed the peninsula, heading south to round the Cape for the Indian Ocean.[29]

20

A Precipitate Departure

Mauritius had put behind it the cholera epidemic of nine years earlier, as well as the great fire that had preceded it, yet Port Louis had developed little, and if anything it had declined. A lady-friend of James's described a depressing place of 'narrow ill-disposed streets'; the houses were 'low, dark, dirty and inconvenient – a medley of French, English, and Indian taste and contrivance', which her husband thought 'not much better than Indian stables'.[1] There were mansions for the better off, in the style of Indian bungalows, but when Dr Barry was rowed ashore with his servants on 9 October 1828,[2] he found a town whose character sat ill with the mountainous green paradise that surrounded it.

Culturally it was an uncomfortable place; the French population resented the British far more than the Cape Dutch did, and were even more resistant to Britain's attempts to reform the conditions of the island's thousands of slaves. The military presence had been strengthened, with two battalions of infantry, along with units of artillery and engineers, all under the new Governor and Commander in Chief, Lieutenant General Sir Charles Colville,[3] a veteran of the Napoleonic Wars, now in semi-retirement. The medical staff was seriously undermanned – hence James's posting. Aside from the regimental surgeons, the staff had no inspector, and just one assistant surgeon, one apothecary and a single hospital assistant.

Colville, having heard rumours of Dr Barry's behaviour at the Cape, took a thorough dislike to him, and it didn't help that James was friendly with the Commissioners of Inquiry, who were now here and disturbing the Governor's peace of mind. Insultingly, Colville turned his nose up at James and appointed Dr Shanks, an assistant surgeon with the 82nd Foot, as the island's Principal Medical Officer, on the grounds that Dr Barry did not speak French (which wasn't true), an equally false claim that Barry had absented himself from his post on first arriving at the Cape in 1816, and that he was not familiar with the island – also false.[4] The situation was finally resolved when, four months after James's arrival, a senior staff surgeon called Charles Collier stopped at Mauritius en route from Ceylon to England, and was persuaded to stay and join the staff.[5] James was made superintending surgeon under him, and went on with the routine garrison medical duties he'd become accustomed to.

There were about fifteen hundred men and officers in the garrison, plus around five hundred wives and children. Dysentery was endemic, along with the ubiquitous soldierly problems of venereal infection and lacerated backs from floggings.[6] Medicine was progressing – Mr Collier noted that the use of the innovative stethoscope at Mauritius, 'although not so constant as a zealous conviction of its utility could desire, is more frequent than it was'; surgeons in the 29th Foot were using them, but few others.[7]

If it appeared that James had settled calmly into his new life in Mauritius, it didn't remain that way for long. Within just a few months of arriving, James Barry managed to run athwart the establishment.

It began with a friendship. Early in 1829, he became acquainted with Mrs Elizabeth Fenton, the wife of a captain who'd recently resigned his commission with the intention of settling in Australia; she was pregnant and had been unwell, and the couple had stopped at Mauritius, where the birth would be safer than aboard ship. James Barry and Bessie Fenton became particularly close friends; yet what James did not know was that Bessie Fenton was aware of his secret – and had known it before she even met him.

In Calcutta, while staying with a sick friend, she had become acquainted with the lady's nurse. This woman told the story of how she had moved to Calcutta after being driven out of the Cape of Good Hope by a Dr James Barry. She had burst in on him one night and discovered that 'the nominal Dr Barry *was* and *is a woman*'.[8] Arriving at Mauritius and discovering that Barry was here, Mrs Fenton was keen to meet him, and was won over by him. Although she never admitted to him that she knew his secret, she became closer to him than would normally be considered proper with a gentleman friend.

It may have been this friendship – and an associated jealousy – that led to James's clash with the establishment. When Mrs Fenton went into labour, she sent for her medical man, Dr Shanks of the 82nd; he couldn't be found, so instead her nurse went to the mess of the 29th Foot and came back with one of the assistant regimental surgeons, a very junior man named Robertson who was a complete stranger. 'After the progress of some dreadful hours,' Mrs Fenton wrote, 'I saw, evidently by his manner, he was alarmed for the result, and I had full time to feel I stood on the verge of eternity.'[9] Robertson decided that she needed one of the more experienced staff surgeons, and suggested Dr Henry Hart, an assistant surgeon who was believed to be in town. At no point, apparently, was Dr Barry's name mentioned, despite his being known for his skill in midwifery and being a more senior surgeon.[10] However, Mrs Fenton's baby was born and she was satisfied with her doctor.

James took umbrage at the whole business, and whether from jealousy or professional disapproval or some lingering offence from the contretemps over seniority with Governor Colville and Dr Shanks, he brought charges against both Hart and Robertson for engaging in private practice to the detriment of their military medical duties. It was a charge laden with personal spite; Mrs Fenton had the impression that he had 'been long at war' with the two men and had been waiting for an opportunity to attack them.[11]

It was proven that Robertson and Hart had been off-duty when they were called out, and that Dr Hart's continued attendance afterwards was necessary, 'making it apparent that the charge was instigated by malice, not public zeal'.[12] Governor Colville, chairing the court of inquiry, acquitted both doctors, and added that as Mrs Fenton was the wife of a former officer she was entitled to be attended by a military surgeon. James was officially censured for bringing the case and temporarily suspended from duty.[13] A report was sent home describing Staff Surgeon Barry as 'somewhat unfortunate in manner, lacking in tact and impatient of control'.[14]

His friendship with Bessie Fenton was apparently unaffected by all this, and since they both found themselves at a loose end in June (her passage to Australia had been delayed), they planned to take a holiday together with the baby; 'I shall just put Flora in a basket, and set off on a pedestrian tour through the island with my friend Dr Barry,' she wrote in her diary.[15] Perhaps, with her privileged insight, she understood James better than most; she certainly valued him, and when she left Mauritius,

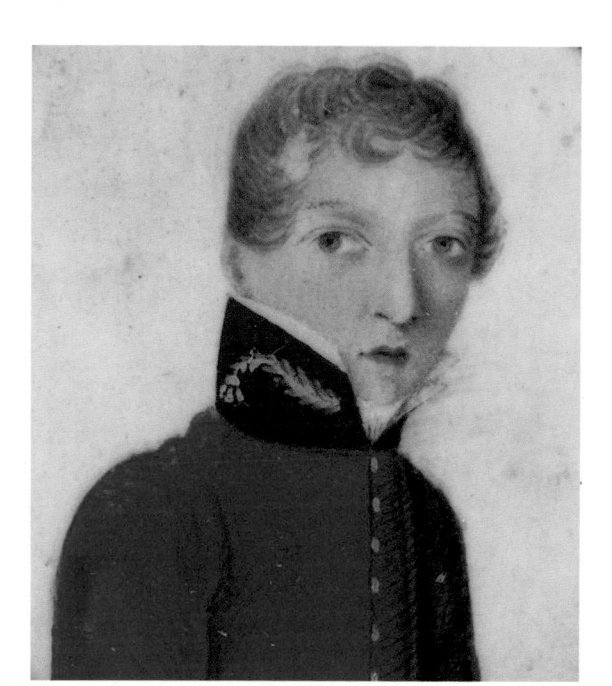

Dr James Barry, Assistant Staff Surgeon, miniature portrait, c. 1815. *Photo by Michael du Preez*

James Barry's commission as Assistant Staff Surgeon, 1815. *Museum Afrika*

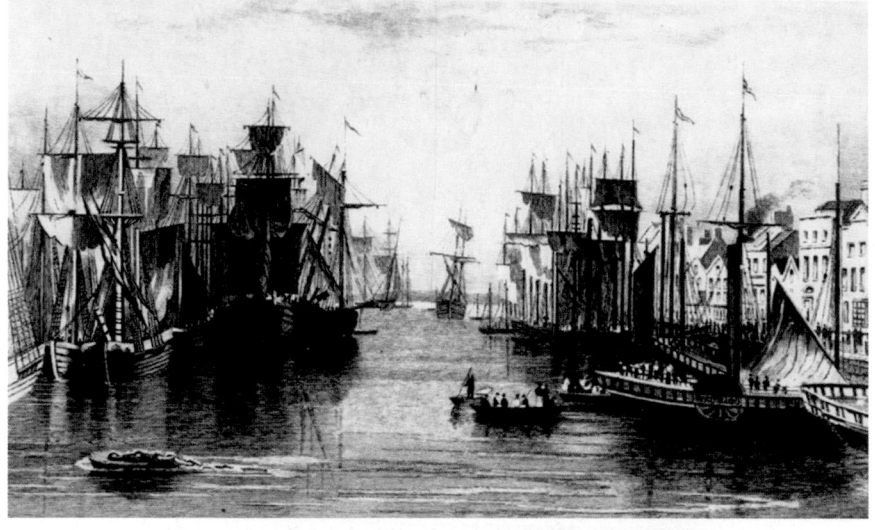

Merchant's Quay, Cork, early 19th century. *Cork City Libraries*

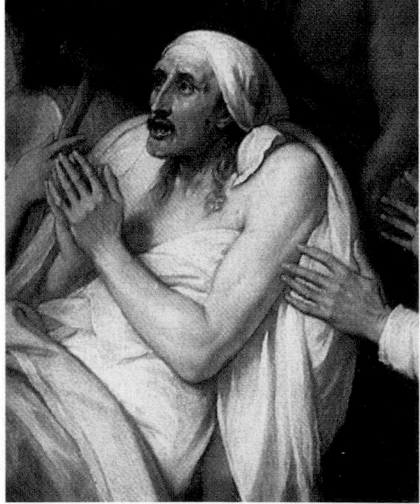

Redmond Barry in a detail from *Christ Healing the Sick* by Benjamin West, c. 1811. *Pennsylvania Hospital collection*

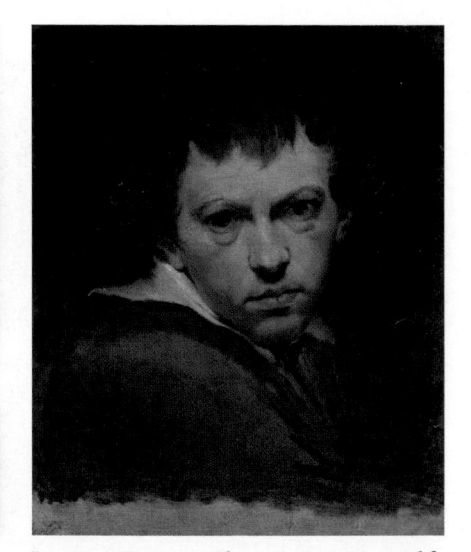

James Barry the painter, self-portrait, c. 1777. *V&A*

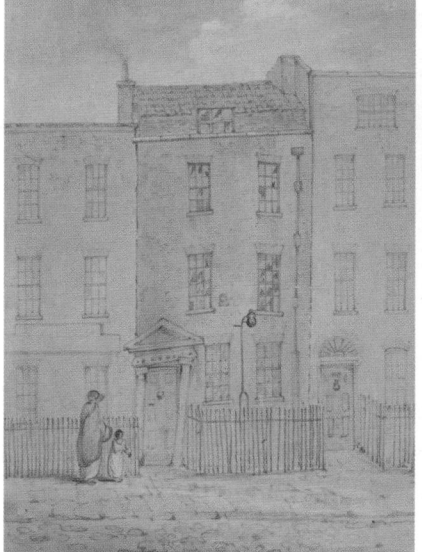

The house of James Barry RA, London, c. 1805. *Yale Center for British Art*

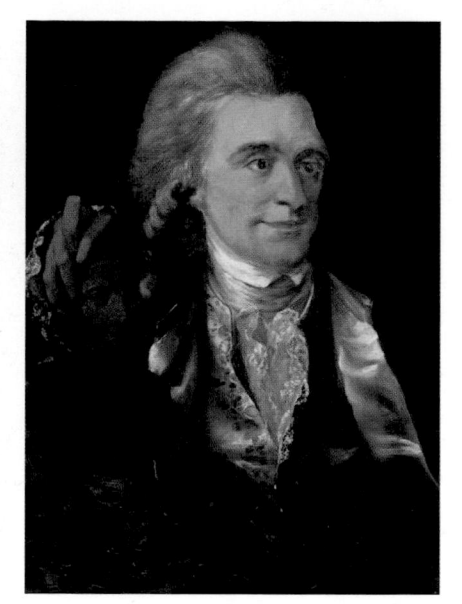

David Steuart Erskine, 11th Earl of Buchan. *Perth Museum and Art Gallery*

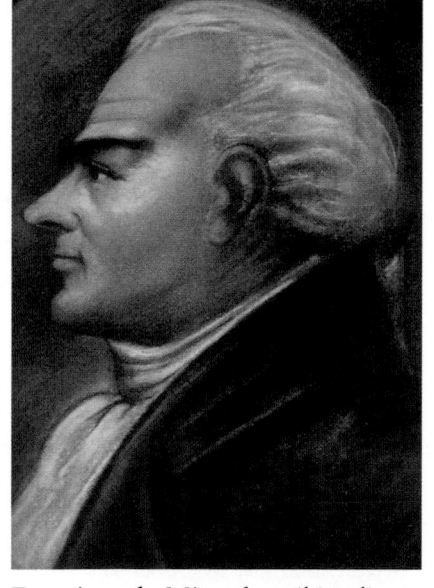

Francisco de Miranda. *wikimedia.org*

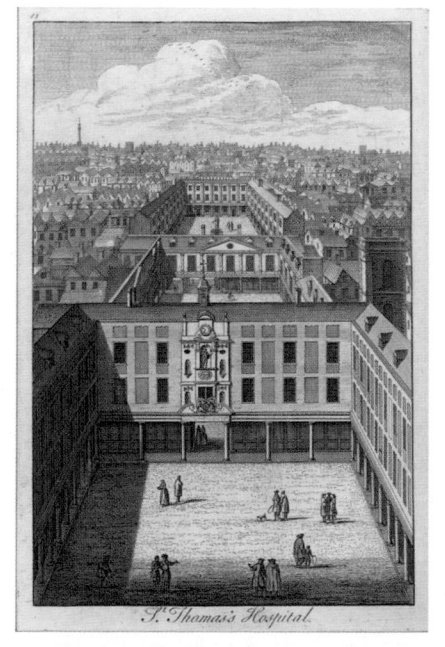

St Thomas's Hospital, mid–18th century. *King's College, London*

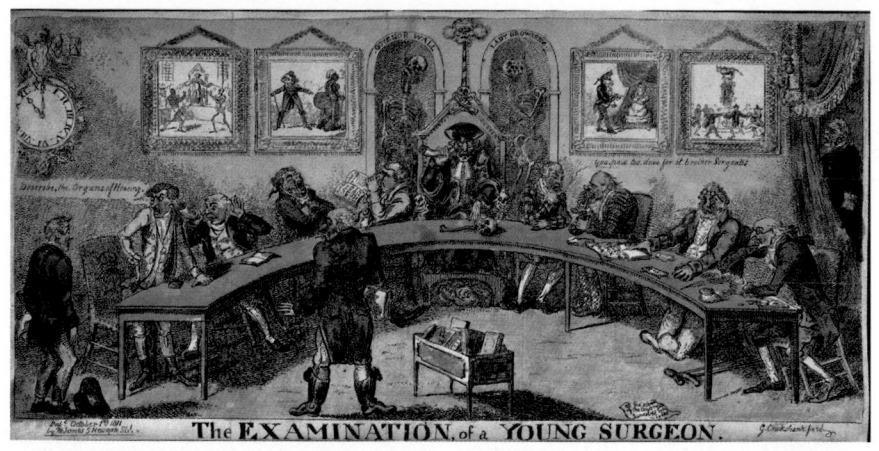

An examination at the Royal College of Surgeons: cartoon by George Cruikshank, 1811. Henry Cline is seated third from right, taking snuff. *RCS*

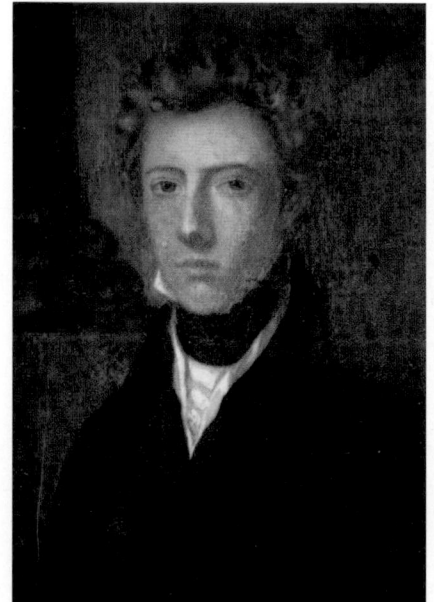

Portrait claimed to be of Dr James Barry, c. 1820s. *Museum Afrika*

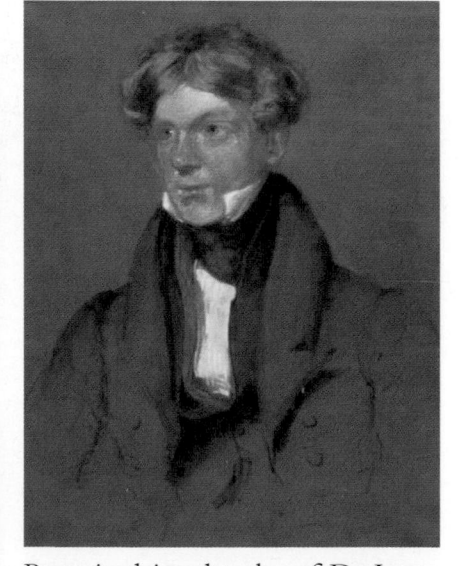

Portrait claimed to be of Dr James Barry, c. 1830s, attributed to George Richmond RA. *Artware Fine Art*

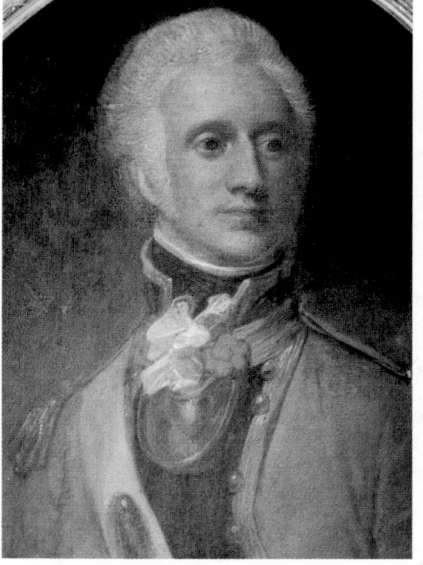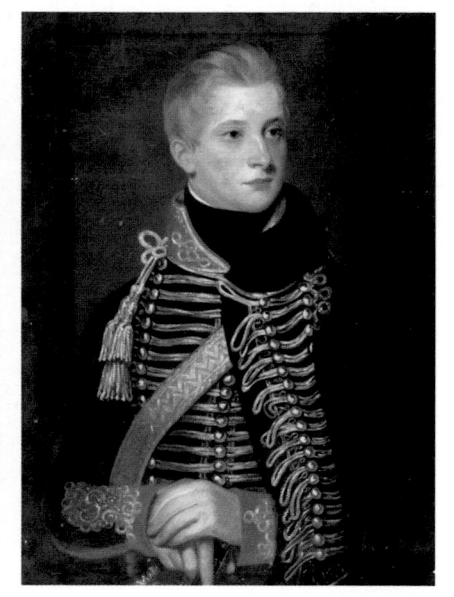

Lord Charles Henry Somerset. *Earl of Devon's collection*

Captain Abraham Josias Cloete by George Koberwein. *Museum Afrika*

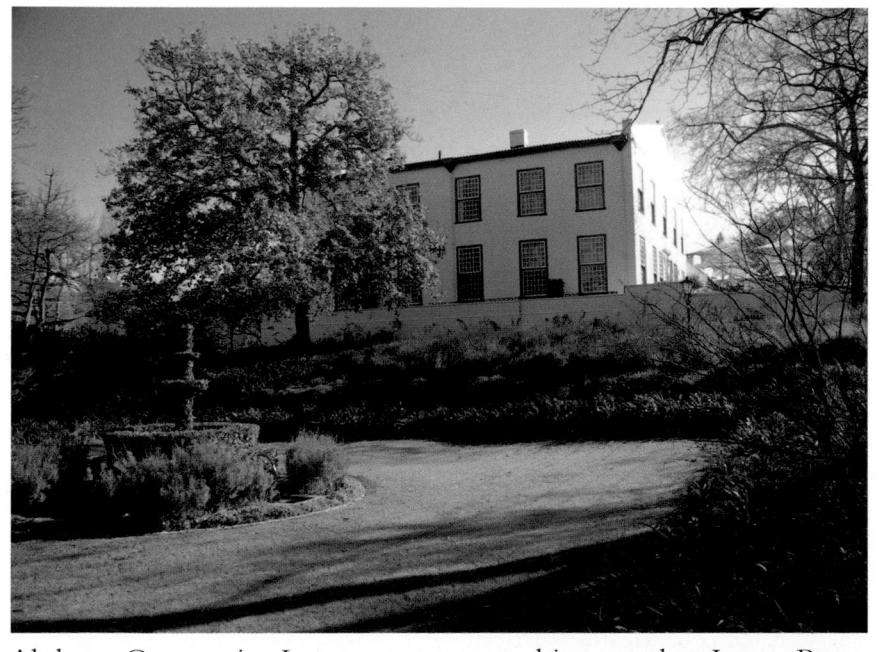

Alphen, Constantia. It was on or near this spot that James Barry fought his duel with Captain Cloete. *Photo by Michael du Preez*

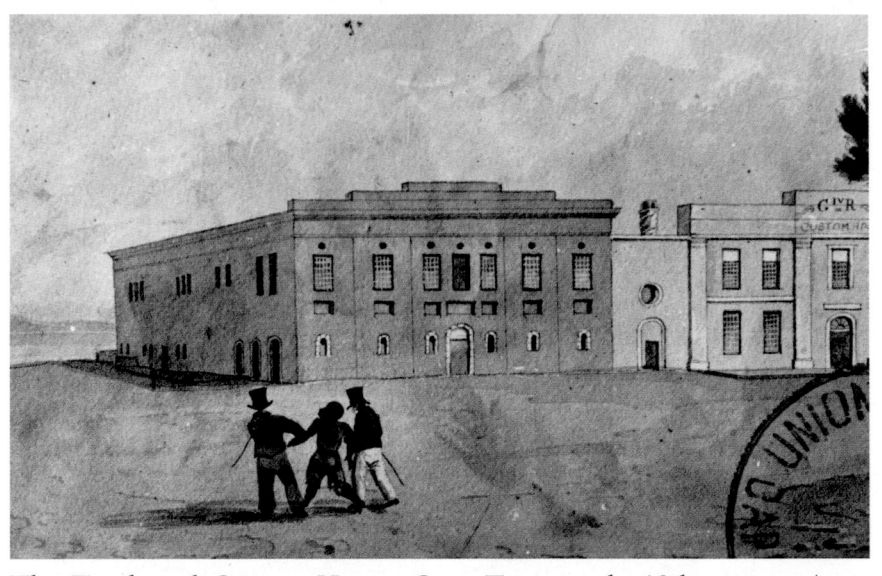

The Tronk and Custom House, Cape Town, early 19th century (note dienaars and prisoner in foreground). *Western Cape Archives*

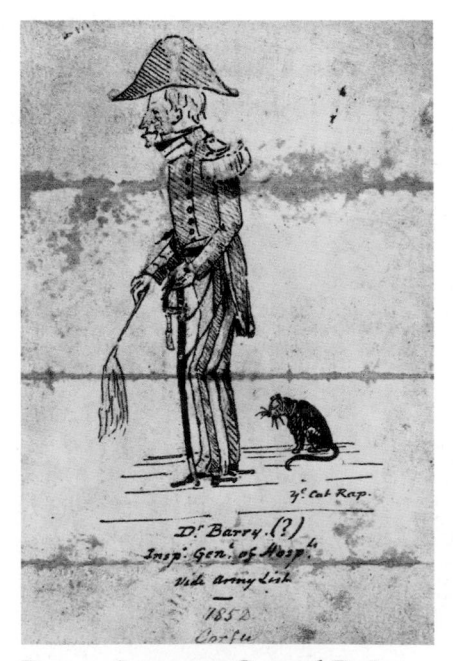

Deputy Inspector General Dr James Barry, c. 1852: caricature attributed to Edward Lear. *Army Medical Services Museum*

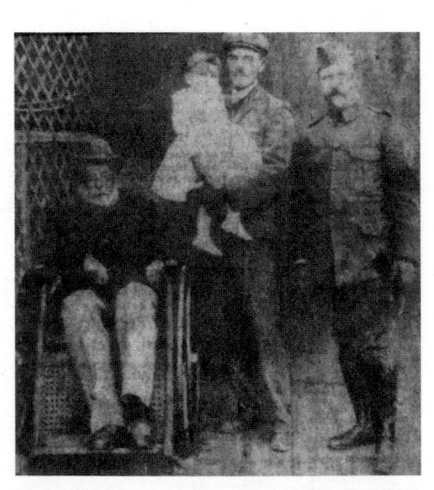

James Barry Munnik (left) in old age. *Argus*

James Barry's house in St Helena.
Photo by Barbara George

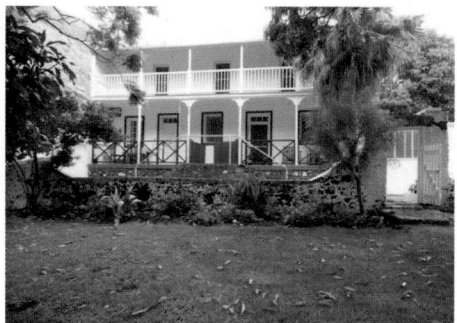

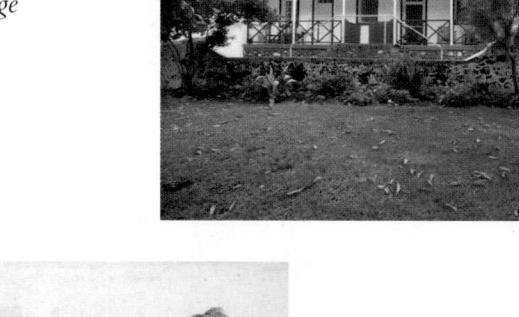

Newlands House, early
19th century. *Western Cape
Archives*

Kingston, Jamaica, early
19th century. *archive.org*

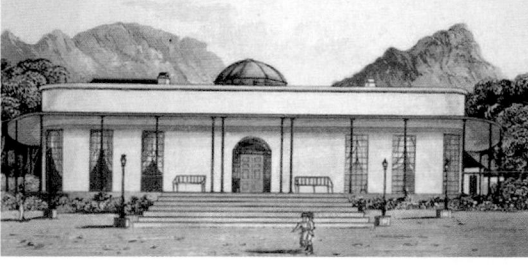

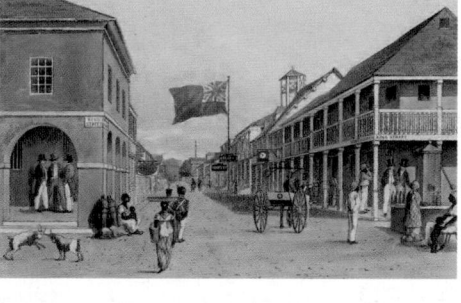

Selimiye (Scutari) Barracks, 1856; military funeral underway in foreground. *National Army Museum*

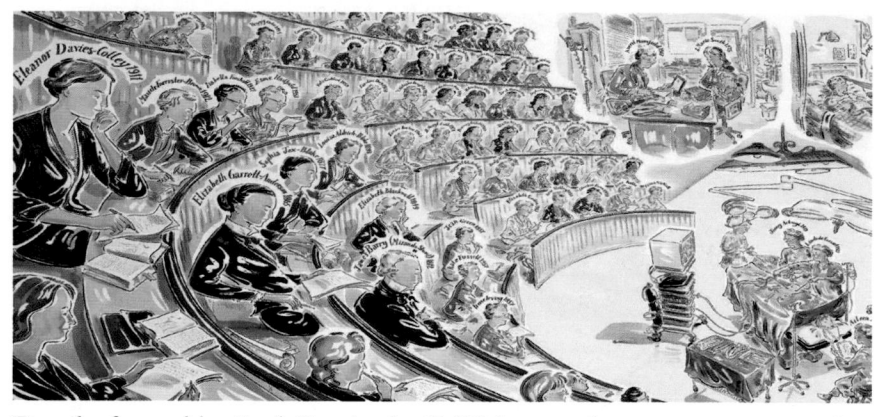

Detail of mural by Paul Cox in the RCS lecture theatre, commemorating pioneering women members. James Barry (front, left of centre) is the earliest. *RCS*

Dr James Barry's commission as Inspector General of Hospitals, 1857. This was the first ever promotion of a woman to general rank in the British Army. *National Archives*

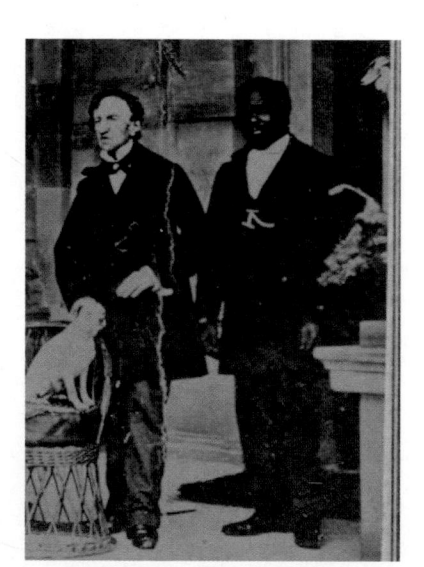

Dr James Barry with John and Psyche in Jamaica, 1862. *Army Medical Services Museum*

Mrs Fenton took Dr Barry's secret with her, and apparently kept it for the rest of her life.

There was one member of the medical establishment for whom James had a very high regard indeed. Mr Montgomery, a naval surgeon at the Civil Hospital in Port Louis, was an advanced thinker. When news came of a new procedure for operating on carotid aneurysms, developed by James Wardrop – an eminent Scottish surgeon practising in London – both Dr Barry and Mr Montgomery were keen to try it, and it was Montgomery who had the opportunity, with James in attendance.

It was a tricky operation; Astley Cooper had attempted it before Wardrop, but it had eluded even his skill.[16] An aneurysm is the abnormal widening of an artery; with the widening comes weakness of the arterial wall, and then, with the constant pulsating pressure of the blood, the vessel widens, until the weakened wall is unable to take the strain any longer and ruptures, with dire results. Prior to the late 1820s, the orthodox technique – pioneered by Astley Cooper – was proximal ligation, in which the vessel was tied on the 'upstream' side of the aneurysm, reducing the flow of blood into it. However, this was not possible with aneurysms in which the proximal end was inaccessible. Wardrop's radical new method – first suggested, but not implemented, by the French surgeon Pierre Brasdor – was the much more difficult distal ligation, where a ligature was applied 'downstream'.

The subject of Montgomery's trial was 'a free black, tall, rather of a spare habit of body, but emaciated and debilitated'.[17] He had an aneurysm in a carotid artery, probably the result of syphilis. The aneurysm was huge, triangular in shape with its base under the inner side of the collar bone, and extending four inches to the angle of the jaw, leaving very little space for operating. To perform any operation on a vessel as vital as a carotid artery in a fully conscious patient required an exceedingly skilled touch.

With James watching keenly and taking notes (which he later turned into a detailed paper), Montgomery made a precise incision and cautious dissection – rendered doubly difficult by the patient's restlessness, 'it being impossible to steady his head for two minutes'. When the carotid was exposed, James laid a finger on it and 'could distinguish no pulsation whatever'. 'Immediately after this,' he wrote, 'Mr Montgomery passed a crude needle (made here for the occasion), armed with a double ligature,

underneath the artery, and took it up with great skill and facility.' Once
the wound was sutured and dressed, the patient was given diluted wine
and put to bed. Four days later he was doing well, the swelling having
diminished and the other symptoms – pain, palpitation, cough – having
subsided. James was full of admiration:

> The surgical paraphernalia was unusually clumsy, and the patient
> in many points of view a bad subject for operation. Yet, under all
> these circumstances, it was impossible to perform any operation in
> a more masterly or scientific manner, and in no one process did Mr
> Montgomery lose either his presence of mind or steadiness of hand;
> scarcely one drop of blood was lost, except that which came from the
> minute vessels of the integuments and muscles. The operation was
> performed in about twenty-five minutes.[18]

High praise indeed from James Barry.

Such interludes were rare, and with Bessie Fenton gone, James's life in
Mauritius muddled on in a state of hostile relations with the Governor
and certain of his fellow practitioners. It was hardly a satisfactory state
in which to spend one's fortieth year. Margaret was now crossing the
threshold into middle age, and James's life and career showed no sign of
becoming settled.

Then, in August 1829, came two items of news that changed
everything. The first was not unexpected. In April that year, David
Steuart Erskine, 11th Earl of Buchan, had died at the age of eighty-six.
Both of James's early father figures, whose names he had incorporated
into his own, were now dead. On the heels of that news, James received a
message from England that threw him into a panic; Lord Charles Somerset
was dangerously ill.

Knowing Lord Charles's medical condition intimately, James was
afraid for his life. The message had taken months to reach Mauritius,
and it might already be too late. Without warning or permission, James
abandoned his post; accompanied by his two servants and his hurriedly
packed belongings, on 27 August he boarded the brig *Rifleman*, bound
for England.[19]

21

An Indefatigable Friend

London: Saturday 12 December 1829

Done up against the savage cold of an English winter, James Barry stood on *Rifleman*'s deck, looking out across the smoky, strange-familiar London skyline. He'd arrived alone; the ship had called at the Cape after its two-week voyage from Mauritius, and his two servants had disembarked there.[1] It was a sad parting, particularly for Danzer, who would never see his friend and master again; but he'd been homesick in Cape Town, so what would he have been like in England?

James took a hackney coach into town. If anything could remind a person of this city, it would be that smell of leather, horse and mustiness peculiar to hackney coaches. The metropolis was changing rapidly, growing and altering. Had James taken a boat upriver instead, he would have noticed the new St Katharine's Dock at Wapping, that there were now two London Bridges – the new one a hundred feet upstream of the ancient one, which was awaiting demolition, the lodgings he had shared with Mrs Bulkley in the Borough High Street having been pulled down to make way for the diverted road. In the north, Brook Street, which had once ended in fields, was now swamped by the growth of suburbs between London and Camden Town.

The coach clattered and heaved through the packed streets, making its way haltingly westward. The sea voyage had been a mercifully short one – less than four months all told from Mauritius, in which he'd had little to do but fret about the state in which he would find Lord Charles Somerset, and the trouble he might be in with the Army. Lord Charles might already be beyond help, although this was improbable; the out-of-date British newspapers at Madeira and the Canaries had shown that he had still been active on the social scene throughout that year – particularly the races, where his name cropped up again and again alongside the rest of the sporting nobility.[2]

If His Lordship's health was precarious, his public standing was another matter altogether; the newspapers from any time in the past couple of years revealed that Lord Charles Somerset was in thoroughly bad odour with the press – the *Morning Chronicle* professed a reluctance even to write about the Cape because 'the mal-administration of Lord Charles Somerset has made the subject but too familiar to the public'.[3] The allegations made by people like Donkin and Bishop Burnett had stuck, despite his attempts to defend himself. On the other hand, Henry Brougham – now climbing high politically, with the Whigs gaining ground over the Tory government – had reversed his opinion; as a Whig politician he had been one of Somerset's most hostile detractors, and had put Burnett's allegations before Parliament; but in an extraordinary development he had now – as a private lawyer – taken Lord Charles *as a client*. One newspaper, loathing the entire Somerset clan, commented that Brougham's advocacy for the former Governor proved 'the professional morality which holds regard for truth and justice to be utterly set aside by a fee'.[4] There followed the spectacle of Brougham performing verbal backward somersaults as he tried to explain away this conflict of interests as a matter of professional detachment.

Quite possibly it was an act of calculated cunning on Lord Charles's part, choosing his greatest enemy as his legal advocate. The arrangement worked to both their advantages in the end. Lord Charles, keeping to the background, grew more and more ill but also less and less vilified, while Brougham, studying the huge collection of official papers to which his new professional relationship with Lord Charles gave him access, began to doubt the justice of the charges against the man. Evidently someone – or everyone – had been telling libellous falsehoods.

Having settled himself in lodgings, James paid a call on his friend at his residence in Piccadilly. They hadn't seen each other since their parting on the deck of HMS *Hyperion*. Those four years had aged and debilitated Lord Charles visibly. That Saturday – the day of James's arrival in England – had been his sixty-second birthday, but he seemed much older. Although he still rode, he was unable to walk either as briskly or for as long as hitherto, due largely to shortness of breath. There was also a tendency to breathlessness at night, and he had taken to sleeping propped up by a heap of pillows. His feet and lower legs were inclined to swell, especially as the day wore on.

James was satisfied that his friend's condition was serious but stable. That was the first worry taken care of; now came the second: facing up to the Army. Dressed in his finest, James took himself off to 5 Berkeley Street, the Army Medical Department headquarters, to report to the Director General. According to legend – which apparently had its roots in James Barry's own telling – he faced the interview with a shameless swagger, undaunted by authority. After a wait, he was shown in to the great man's office.

Sir James McGrigor MD was a Scotsman who had started his Army career as a regimental surgeon with the Connaught Rangers, had served in India and as Wellington's Surgeon General in the Peninsular War, and had since been the chief force in shaping the modern, reformed Army Medical Department. Having already been knighted he was now waiting on his baronetcy. One might expect such a man to be a tartar, but in fact he was a pleasant-looking fellow with an unruly mop of silver hair and a dimple in his chin, and hooded, baggy eyes. The story of James's interview with him may be apocryphal, but James apparently dined out on it for decades; as Charles Dickens later related it:

'Sir,' said the director, 'I do not understand your reporting yourself in this fashion. You admit you have returned without leave of absence. May I ask how this is?'

'Well,' said James, coolly running his long white fingers through his crisp sandy curls, 'I have come home to have my hair cut.'[5]

It did him no harm; now that he was in England, he had the influence not only of Lord Charles on his side but of other members of the Somerset family, several of whom were in positions of influence in the Army – none higher than Lord Charles's much younger brother, Major General Lord FitzRoy Somerset, a protégé of the Duke of Wellington and now Military Secretary to Wellington's successor, General Lord Hill, Commander in Chief of the Forces. Like his mentor, FitzRoy had an enormous curved beak of a nose, but that was the only point of resemblance; he had large, gentle blue eyes, and his mouth seemed permanently set in a mild, pleasant smile that sat oddly with his heavy jaw, and he was generous and sparing of people's feelings. He wore his empty right sleeve pinned by a loop to his tunic button, the arm having been left behind in a surgeon's bucket at Waterloo. At forty-one, he was only a year older than Margaret (although officially James was more than a decade younger).

Lord FitzRoy took a liking to James, possibly for his brother's sake, and his power at Horse Guards ensured that the wrinkles were all smoothed out. In January 1830, a month on from his precipitate return, instead of a reprimand Dr Barry was issued a new posting: this time to Jamaica.[6] However, he had no intention of taking it up; he couldn't leave England while Lord Charles needed his care. Resuming his position as personal physician, James devoted himself, with far fewer distractions this time, to attending his friend.

James's diagnosis wasn't recorded, but from letters written later by Lord Charles himself, describing his symptoms and Dr Barry's treatment, it is almost certain that he was suffering from congestive heart failure, a condition in which the heart is too weak to adequately pump blood to the body; its symptoms include shortness of breath, fatigue and swelling of the legs. Heart failure was not understood in 1830, and all a physician could do was treat the signs and symptoms he saw (based on a detailed but limited understanding of physiology and the wisdom of experience) as they followed their insidious course.[7]

Not all his time was devoted to his patient; he also presented his paper on Montgomery's aneurysm operation to pioneer James Wardrop, in recognition of 'your ingenious and successful operation'; Wardrop was so pleased and impressed that he arranged for the paper – including Dr Barry's covering letter – to be published in *The Lancet*: James's first professional publication.[8]

Through the following year, Lord Charles Somerset continued his usual life as well as he was able, attracting little stabs of hostile press as he went. In February, in consequence of his rank as a general (retired), he succeeded to the honorary colonelcy of the 33rd First Yorkshire West Riding Regiment of Foot (thereby resigning the less prestigious colonelcy of the 1st West India Regiment); at the same time his son obtained the lieutenant-colonelcy of the 1st Royal Dragoons. This caused ire in military circles; regimental colonelcies were intended as honours for generals with significant war service behind them, and it was held a shame that they should be given to men with no battle service. The Somersets seemed to have a particular stranglehold on the system, what with Lord

Charles's brothers Edward and FitzRoy (who *were* war veterans) having position and influence in the Army.[9]

In April Lord Charles went to Newmarket for the races (as always) and in midsummer took a tour of the country; then came Ascot and in August Goodwood.[10] Some newspapers were friendly; in May the *Berkshire Chronicle* reported in its 'Comicalities and Queerisms' column a dinner-table conversation in which 'Lord Charles Somerset was telling a long story about his walking one day in the woods at the Cape, and coming plump upon a huge shaggy lion. "Thinking to frighten him," said the noble lord, "I ran at him with all my *might*," "Whereupon," said a wag, interrupting him, "I suppose he ran away with all his *main*" (mane). "Just so," said his lordship.'[11] In the autumn he took a house at Newmarket, where he found the air beneficial and felt content in the heart of the world he most loved – the world of horses and racing.

But he was growing more and more seriously ill. When James travelled down to visit him, he found him suffering still from shortness of breath, which had 'obtained a sort of *freehold property* on my Lungs', he told his brother Henry, Duke of Beaufort, and was now keeping him awake most of the night.[12] James administered an expectorant that initially put him to sleep; he woke after an hour with 'one of my most violent fits of coughing', but once this had passed, 'I fell asleep again & slept for 3 hours which is what I have not done for upwards of a month before'.

In November he went to stay with the Earl of Darlington, who had rented Snettisham Hall, an ancient estate near Hunstanton on the Norfolk coast.[13] For five weeks he had been getting episodes of extreme lassitude and debility; he wasn't happy with the 'tonic' he had been given and had abstained from medicines – and his cough was 'certainly quite as bad as ever'.[14] However, he was able to ride on the local beaches for nearly two hours every day. It was a perfect place, with miles of flat sandy beaches from Heacham to Holme, and he was so pleased with the place that he 'made an arrangement for Sea Water to be brought in fresh every Morning for my Shower Bath. I wish I had thought of it sooner – as I hope it will do me good.'

While Lord Charles settled in at Snettisham, James went up to London, where he had been invited to a grand levée given by the new King at St James's Palace on 17 November.[15] It was a magnificent affair, with a guard of honour and a detachment of Horse Guards in the courtyard, each with its band trumpeting splendidly. While William IV – only a few months on the throne – gave audiences to a succession of grandees, beginning with the Duke of Wellington and Sir Robert Peel, dozens of dukes, earls, viscounts, lords, generals and admirals stood about, drinking and prosing at high volume. Dr James Barry, Surgeon to the Forces, was second in line to be presented to the King, accompanied and sponsored by another of the Somerset brothers – Lord Edward. Between FitzRoy and Charles in age, Edward had fought at Salamanca, charged at Talavera and commanded the Household Cavalry Brigade at Waterloo.

There were some interesting people among the guests; one was Major General Sir Willoughby Cotton, who had just been appointed to the lieutenant-governorship and command of the forces in Jamaica.[16] As James had been appointed to Jamaica (albeit in abeyance since January), Lord Edward would certainly have taken care to introduce them. Cotton was a genial man, stolid with a pouchy face that appeared to be sliding down his skull, only held in place by his spike of a nose; in his youth he had been infamous as ringleader of the great Rugby School rebellion of 1797, in which the boys mutinied against the headmaster, blew in his classroom door with gunpowder and had to be suppressed by the local militia. Among the other officers, honourables and reverends was a fair smattering of medical men being presented by their sponsors: another staff surgeon and an inspector general of hospitals, as well as the newly appointed Physician Extraordinary to the Queen. This was the first royal presentation of James Barry's career, and a vastly important step, constituting the Somerset family's public confirmation that James Barry was their man.

This was just as well, because things were about to get heated. It had been proposed by Lord FitzRoy that perhaps a second physician should be engaged for his brother – not as a replacement but a supplement, yet still a dangerous suggestion where Dr Barry was concerned. The doctor settled on was Sir Henry Halford, a man who had been eminent in the profession when Margaret Bulkley was just a small child, and pre-eminent – as physician to the King and the Prince Regent – while James Barry was still a student. Since 1820 Halford had been President of the Royal College of Physicians. He had been at the King's levée, and possibly this had prompted the notion of consulting him, now he and James were at least on a shared social footing. Since they were intended to work in conjunction, Lord FitzRoy arranged a meeting between them in London just before Christmas to discuss the case.[17]

Now in his mid-sixties, Sir Henry Halford was a trim, bantam-sized hive of earnest professional energy, with sharp eyes, silver hair brushed flat to his scalp, and a brow ridge that might have been drawn with a ruler. Despite his eminence, Halford's professional expertise was in fact not of the best; he had relied heavily on his bedside manner in establishing himself, while his scientific understanding had fossilised some decades earlier. James Wardrop particularly disliked Halford, calling him 'the eel-backed baronet', while the surgeon J. F. Clarke – who detested both men ('Jemmy' Wardrop was 'vain, self-opinionated, and scurrilous' in his view)[18] – considered Halford a 'thorough courtier' and 'vain ... cringing to superiors, haughty to inferiors'; 'fussy, superficial, and time-serving', he 'contributed little to the art and science of Medicine; he was proud of his "Latinity", and delivered the Harveian Oration in a style which commended itself to the *literati*, but not to the *practitioners* of the age'.[19] Halford later aroused censure by allegedly leaving a travelling companion to die of an apoplexy without treatment while he carried on home to attend a dinner party.[20] *The Lancet* said of him that 'he is all tact and nothing else. He is ignorant of recent discoveries ... he has never written a line that is worthy of perusal on any scientific subject.'[21]

And this was the man with whom the prickly, thoroughly intolerant, scientifically progressive Dr James Barry would have to cooperate. In fact, cooperation was rarely feasible in the upper social reaches of the medical profession, which was a web of jealousies and backbiting. The only man for whom everyone had unalloyed liking and respect was Astley Cooper – now Sir Astley, having been raised to a baronetcy after removing a cyst from King George IV's head.

Lord FitzRoy's idea proved an unwise one; the disagreement between Halford and Barry came instantly, and the stress added to Lord Charles's suffering. Halford advised that the patient (who was back in Newmarket for the Christmas season) should repair to Bath to take the waters, in view of their time-honoured reputation. James disagreed vehemently with this antiquated recommendation but was overruled by Halford.

The patient was reluctant – 'it is a sad routing of self, servants and horses', he wrote to his brother the Duke; '170 miles and living in a lodging house (which of all things I detest) instead of one's comfortable nest'.[22] He hated leaving Newmarket – 'No place in this Island agrees with me as the air of this place', although it was more likely the sporting society he would miss. 'However as waters are a specific in my Case there is a chance that the drinking of the Bath waters may have some Influence over my Cough – the thing I dread is the Atmosphere there and I have written to Sir Henry to request him to say in what part of Bath he so recommends me to reside for I think it of material consequence.' Wherever he chose to live, he would need a carriage, 'as I am now totally unable to walk & wd be hard set to get to the Pump Room'.

By early January, Lord Charles was lodging, reluctantly and in ill humour, at 24 Bennett Street, a typical thoroughfare of handsome three-storey townhouses round the corner from the Assembly Rooms, the hub of Bath society. James travelled down from London at the beginning of the first week, arriving on Tuesday evening. He was finding it extremely difficult to tolerate collaborating with Sir Henry Halford, and Lord Charles found the situation rather trying too; he had come to think of James as a kind of mad genius (or at least affected to regard him that way, since he surely knew that at least some of James's quirks had grown from being a woman in a man's guise), and when James arrived that evening, His Lordship found him to be 'in tolerable sane mind'. This lasted until the following day, when 'I mentioned Sir Henry Halford & then he went off in a strain so I shall not mention that again.'[23] In fact he did mention Halford again and decided that James was 'quite as mad as ever'.[24]

While Lord Charles obeyed Sir Henry by swallowing quantities of the cloudy, sulphurous water, Dr Barry sniffed disdainfully and set about treating the lung condition, which was severe: 'On Tuesday night I cough'd in the most violent manner for 6½ hours with an intensification of 3 minutes,' wrote Lord Charles:

Of course I got no repose I was dreadfully feeble and since yesterday – last night he gave me something to check the quantity and glutinousness of the Phlegm and it certainly had some effect and procured me some sleep – It is to me (who could never swallow an onion) the most nauseous thing I ever took – being the juice of onions in syrup of Roses – so bad, I taste, smell – breathe onions. I took a few spoonsful 3 times during the night.[25]

James would certainly have also prescribed digitalis, which was then considered almost a wonder drug for heart conditions. Lord Charles disliked all Dr Barry's medicines but was thoroughly pleased with the

Bath waters, believing after four days that he was experiencing 'all the favourable effects that they say evince that it agrees with one'. It upset him that 'Dr Barry chose to say after I left London that he was always agst my drinking the water (the very purpose for which I came this long journey) & of course he has not yet admitted that the water agrees with me.'[26] Lord Charles and his wife were both rash enough to tell James that the waters seemed to be working, and he was so cross that Lord Charles was 'quite sure that he had come here predetermined that I wd *not* drink the water' for a set period, so that 'he should then be the Judge and *he could make up his mind* (which mind he had made up before he left London).'[27]

Patient and physician clashed again when Lord Charles learned (through FitzRoy) that James had written to Halford reporting that the waters could not safely be drunk by the patient, and omitted to mention the great benefit he felt from them. Deprived of the waters for a single day on James's orders, Lord Charles was 'in a State of Torpor all day & had no appetite whatsoever ... What to do I know not.'[28] He claimed that he had discovered Dr Barry falsifying his pulse rate while he was off the water – stating it to be perfectly normal when in fact (according to Lord Charles's own measurement) it was dangerously fast.

With the benefit of hindsight, it is certain that if Lord Charles was getting any benefit from the Bath water, it was a placebo effect. In fact, Dr Barry was absolutely right in his opinion – more right, in fact, than he could have known. Bath water would be decidedly unhealthy for a patient with heart failure; containing a very high level of sodium ions combined with chloride ions, it would provide the individual with an excess of salt. This would inevitably lead to the retention of more fluid in a cardiac patient and aggravate the existing fluid retention, placing yet more strain upon the heart. Both pulmonary and peripheral circulation would be affected, making the breathing worse and exacerbating the swelling of the lower legs. As for the discrepancy in their pulse measurements, the individual beats of a weakened heart would not always be clearly palpable to an expert, let alone to an unskilled touch, and Lord Charles was probably miscounting, feeling beats that were not there.

Nonetheless, Lord Charles was absolutely convinced of his and Sir Henry's rightness, and with James barring him from drinking the water, he was miserable in Bath:

Staying here in this detestable Place is useless – as for the Air it wd
have been better & cheaper to have taken lodgings in Fleet Street or
Cheapside & I feel concerned that if Dr Barry had given an *honest*
opinion I shd be continuing the waters – with a Hope of recovery. I
am now brought 170 miles 2 be the victim of his Temper and Jealousy
of Sir Henry – I am in a sad State of Mind and Body – and … Know
not what to do or what to decide upon – I am having the greatest
discomfort at an enormous Expence and Without Hope of receiving
a Benefit.[29]

A fortnight later he left Bath. By the time he stopped at Marlborough
he was already feeling better, simply for being in fresher air. Dr
Barry desired that he should go to the seaside for the air and seawater
shower baths. Feeling that he had been reduced to death's door, Lord
Charles was exasperated with both his medical men – 'the Victim
of temper and Jealousy on one side & professional Complaisancy
on the other'.[30]

He made his way across England in stages, and by early February
was at Breckland Lodge near Thetford. James had taken to assuring him
that the illness would end favourably: compassion overcoming realism.
By now James would have known very well that his friend's days were
numbered and that there was nothing to be done for him other than ease
his symptoms. He was still capable of riding for whole hours at a time,
despite the discomfort of his swollen legs, which were so large now that
he had to wear the special oversized straw boots that were available for
such patients. He intended travelling to London and then on to Brighton;
the weather was mild for February, and he anticipated 'riding about 25
miles each Day's Journey which wd be better than sitting the whole day
in a carriage'.[31]

Since leaving the congestion of Bath he had felt so happy to be riding
in the fresh air that he overestimated his stamina; after pausing for a week
in London (during which he saw Halford), he carried on to Brighton –
too soon in James's opinion – and instead of making the journey in two
stages as James had advised, he did the whole forty-six miles in one day,
arriving at the Bedford Hotel on St Valentine's Day.

Brighton – with its racier social scene and memories of his younger
days as one of the Prince of Wales's bucks – was perhaps his second
favourite place to stay, after Newmarket, while the Bedford Hotel, a new

place standing on the sea-front, was the *dernier cri* in style. Yet his health was now utterly broken. Lifelong he had pushed himself physically and mentally, but he had grown progressively frailer in the past few days – he managed to go out on horseback three days running, accompanied each time by James, but by the fourth day he was too weak to contemplate exercise. Yet he still drove himself socially; the King and Queen were in Brighton, staying at the Pavilion, and Lord Charles was among their visitors on the 19th.[32] The next day, Sunday 20 February 1831, he was unable to leave his bed, and there, in the company of his wife Lady Mary, his daughter Georgiana and James Barry, he breathed his last.

Brighton: Saturday 26 February 1831

The funeral procession drew away from the front of the Bedford Hotel: a hearse drawn by horses with sable plumes, with three mourning coaches following behind. According to the wishes of Lord Charles it was a very small, private funeral; he felt that he had experienced enough pomp in his life, and wished that his death be marked 'with the least possible expense and that my funeral may on no account be attended with any parade'.[33] The mourners included only close members of his family – Lady Mary Somerset, his sons and daughters, his brothers Lord Edward and Henry, Duke of Beaufort, and the Duke's son Henry, Marquess of Worcester; a handful of other relatives included George Wyndham, 3rd Earl of Egremont, father-in-law to Lord Charles's eldest daughter, Elizabeth, and Lady Mary's brother, Captain Poulett. The only mourner who was not a relative was Dr James Barry.

Hearse and coaches drove the short distance to the chapel of St Andrew's, a newly built Regency-style church close to the sea-front in the fashionable Brunswick Town district between Brighton and Hove. After the service, the remains of General Lord Charles Henry Somerset, 1767 to 1831, were interred in the brand-new, previously unused vault of the chapel.[34]

Lord Charles Somerset had lived the last few years of his life in ill health and public detestation, yet he died just as his reputation was being rehabilitated. The *Morning Post* obituary noted the proven 'falsehood and absurdity' of the charges against him over his governorship of the Cape, and the reversal of Henry Brougham's opinion of him:

The candour with which the present Lord Chancellor acknowledged
the futility of various allegations, on the faith of which he had arraigned
Lord Charles's conduct, must be fresh in the public recollection. His
Lordship subsequently received a more complete and signal vindication
on the return of papers moved for in the House of Commons ... In
them was found the most convincing evidence, not only of Lord Charles
Somerset's enlightened and comprehensive plans for the advancement
of the colonial interests, but of his truly patriotic spirit in sacrificing
the emoluments of his office to ... those financial regulations which
it was one of the earliest measures of his Government to introduce.
To the welfare of the Colony his time and faculties were uniformly
devoted.[35]

Most of the mourners left Brighton the day after the funeral.[36] Of them
all, not even Lady Mary was more bereft than James Barry; he had lost
not only a friend but a man who had been his protector, benefactor,
surrogate father, and perhaps – once – rather more than that.

James had received a letter of condolence from an old friend who
must have known how much Lord Charles had meant to him. Lady Mary
Fitzroy, the wife of Colonel Charles Fitzroy, who had been Military
Secretary and a dear friend to Lord Charles Somerset at the Cape, had
not been in Brighton and had last seen him in London; she asked James
to describe how it had all been. 'I have entered into detail as you wish,'
he wrote back, the day before the funeral, 'but I am unable of doing
justice to my more than father – my almost only friend.'[37] He continues:

> There is indeed a melancholy satisfaction in relating what took place
> during the last moments of poor Lord Charles who was to the last a
> kind, a sincere & an indefatigable friend, and had been so thro life to
> many, some of whom did not appreciate it.
>
> We who have known him for years and in other climes & under
> the most trying circumstances can conscientiously before God & man
> declare that he was a man more sinned against than sinning.
>
> Since my arrival in Europe (now about 14 months) I have been
> almost always with him & during the last few weeks, day & night I
> have been near him.
>
> Poor Lord Charles, during his sufferings, & he suffered much, he
> never for one minute forgot the interests of his friends.

James described how his wife and daughter 'closely watched him', Lady Mary spending weeks lying on a couch near him. For James, who knew that his patient was doomed, Lord Charles's comfort and the happiness he got from his friends had been the most important thing, and he had tried to dissuade him from leaving London for Brighton, 'alas before he ought to have done so. But it is not for man to say what ought to have been.' And James had to admit that Lord Charles was never happier than when riding, and they had ridden side by side – as had become their habit – all the way.[38]

Now, without his more-than father, his indefatigable, almost only friend, James had nothing to hold him in England. It was time to ride on alone.

PART III

Flagrant Breaches of Discipline
1831–1845

22

Fever Island

I own I am shock'd at the purchase of slaves,
And fear those who buy them and sell them are knaves;
What I hear of their hardships, their tortures, and groans
Is almost enough to draw pity from stones.

I pity them greatly, but I must be mum,
For how could we do without sugar and rum?

William Cowper, 'Pity for Poor Africans' (1788)

Jamaica: Christmas 1831

It began as a strike; then the strike became a rebellion; the rebellion became a war; and the war became a slaughter.

The wealth of Jamaica came from its huge sugar plantations, and from rum; and the sugar economy depended on slaves – three hundred thousand of them, now growing increasingly restless and impatient for emancipation; everybody knew that abolition must come, but when? The plantation owners were anxious too – the sugar trade, having peaked a decade earlier, was in decline through overworking the land, which reduced productivity, and since the abolition of the slave trade in 1807 slave labour had become more expensive to sustain. The lives of the enslaved in Britain's colonies had been improved by various 'amelioration' laws that encouraged marriage among slaves, allowed their evidence to be recognised in trials, abolished whipping of female slaves, let slaves receive bequests of money, provided for the appointment of a slave 'protector' to oversee their rights, and so on; but some colonial administrations dragged their feet, and the Jamaican Assembly was one of them.[1] With anger rising, the situation was in perpetual danger of catching fire, with order kept by the plantation drivers on the one hand and the British Army on the other.

A simple dispute over holidays was the eventual trigger. In 1831 Christmas Day fell on a Sunday, so with Boxing Day being Monday, the slaves naturally expected to have Tuesday off in lieu, or to be paid wages. The planters refused. Prompted by the influential slave and Baptist preacher Samuel 'Daddy' Sharpe, the slaves planned a strike for the Tuesday.

The strike was the spark; caught in the conflagration that followed was Dr James Barry.

James had been in Jamaica only six months. With Lord FitzRoy Somerset's influence, the Army Medical Department had allowed several postponements of his posting (on full pay) while he cared for Lord Charles. Once he had finished mourning, James made his preparations, renewed his kit, his clothes and his uniforms, and on 20 April 1831 his official posting began;[2] he boarded the merchant brig *Guardian* for Jamaica.

On Sunday 12 June, *Guardian* passed the headland of Port Royal – a town of ill repute whose name echoed through the pirate tales of the previous two centuries – lurking behind its fort at the end of the long neck of ground enclosing the great expanse of Kingston Harbour.[3] At Kingston, *Guardian* disembarked her only two passengers – a young Baptist minister and a middle-aged but youthful-looking, beautifully dressed and very diminutive military surgeon.

Kingston was quite unlike any of the settlements at the Cape; older than most, Spanish in character (even though it had been built under British rule), and despite the number of chapels and ministries, designed more for indulgence than for industry. Its hub was the junction of King Street and Harbour Street, a long, straight thoroughfare lined with low two-storey buildings in warm amber stucco with long colonnades and first-floor galleries; its Hispanic flavour contrasted with the British red-coats and the enormous blue ensign flying over Harty's tavern. It was a noisy, bustling place filled with traders and sailors, prostitutes, hawkers and respectable citizens, and the speech of every part of the globe: rather like a sweltering-hot version of Cork.

Two miles inland from Kingston lay Up Park Camp, the main base of the British Jamaican garrison, a huge palisaded enclosure of over two hundred acres.[4] The garrison was large for such a small colony, with several British infantry regiments as well as one of the colonial West India Regiments (of which there were eight in various postings, manned partly by local slaves who were freed upon enlistment). Passing the sentries outside the gates James recognised the facings and insignia of the 33rd Regiment, whose colonelcy Lord Charles Somerset had enjoyed briefly during his last year.

Up Park wasn't the only camp – there was Stoney Hill nine miles away, and troops were dispersed to outposts around the island. Presiding over the garrison was Lieutenant Governor and Commander in Chief Major General Sir Willoughby Cotton, who had only arrived two months before James.[5] Above him, at the very top of the hierarchy, was Governor Somerset Lowry-Corry, 2nd Earl of Belmore.

Despite the size of the garrison and the medical staff, James Barry was the only staff surgeon. Above him was Deputy Inspector General of Hospitals Thomas Draper and below him were four assistant surgeons, an apothecary and two hospital assistants; there was also a staff physician, Dr Weir.[6] In addition each regiment had its own surgeon and assistants.

The Up Park hospital – which served the whole garrison – contained an alarming number of soldiers suffering from fever of one kind or another. Fever was endemic in the West Indies and not helped by barrack conditions, which were damp and dirty, with unglazed windows allowing in the mosquitoes that infested the area around the large outdoor bathing tank. This was a fine breeding ground for the *Anopheles* mosquito, carrier of malaria, while the humid wooded country backing the camp was perfect for the *Aedes* mosquito, carrier of the yellow fever virus, the plague of the Indies. In consequence, the garrison suffered an annual mortality rate of over 300 men a year, twelve per cent of the command, of which over 250 were from fevers;[7] this was more than ten times the mortality rate James had known at the Cape. Black troops were more resistant to fever, and didn't drink as much alcohol as the whites, but were more susceptible to smallpox and tuberculosis.

During the worst season (starting in April), fever occurred 'in a much more aggravated form, attended with violent head ache, irritability of stomach, great prostration of strength, and usually with considerable yellowness of skin, running its course with celerity, most of the fatal cases terminating on the fourth day'.[8] The cause was not understood, and the unfortunate patients were subjected to a variety of centuries-old treatments – emetics, purgatives, diaphoretics, diuretics, bleeding and cold baths, along with strychnine,[9] which was used as a stimulant. Only the fortunate survived. James Barry was more than usually cautious with this type of aggressive treatment – particularly bleeding – while concentrating more on fresh air, nutritious diet and cleanliness. Simply keeping the patient comfortable, hydrated and well nourished would have been more effective and resulted in better outcomes.

Among the black population there were practitioners who shared Dr Barry's approach. Known as 'doctresses', these were local women, unqualified yet running small private institutions based on traditional healing and relying on nourishment and hydration. They were particularly popular among naval officers; one doctress, Cubah Cornwallis, a former slave, had become famous in the previous century for treating both the young Nelson and the future William IV when he was a midshipman. Another noted practitioner was Mary Seacole, who worked at Up Park and later achieved some renown (though considerably less than she deserved) in the Crimean War. Generally the doctresses had greater success in curing fevers than did the doctors.

Although James had his quarters initially at Up Park, he soon moved to Stoney Hill, whose officers' accommodation was much pleasanter – a two-storey building with a veranda facing south towards the sea. This came at the cost of a daily commute along the steep, winding road to Up Park in the brougham provided for his use (one of the perks of being a staff surgeon rather than a mere assistant).

Fever aside, it was a pleasant but not very secure station in which to live. Other than Up Park and Stoney Hill, there were more than twenty outposts around the island, ostensibly to defend it from external threat, but mostly to protect the white population from the slaves, who outnumbered their owners (most of whom lived in England and were represented by agents and deputies) twenty-six to one. The British Army served here as a police force, a job that should have belonged to the local Jamaica militia, who were too ill-trained and poorly led to perform it.

Throughout the 1820s Lord Bathurst had been exhorting local colonial powers to enact the amelioration measures. In the Crown Colonies, which were under the direct authority of Westminster, some degree of emancipation had been achieved. But Jamaica, despite having a colonial governor and garrison, was under the rule of its own elected Assembly, which was in lockstep with the plantation owners – the so-called 'plantocracy'. So disgusted were they by the amelioration proposals, they had considered seceding from the Empire and joining the United States. A plantocracy newspaper of 1831 described the Jamaican slaves as 'peasantry' who were 'idle, sensual, but cheerful, merry and contented'; the paper opposed banning the flogging of female slaves, as they were more unruly than the men.[10]

A slave rebellion was inevitable, and it came at Christmas 1831, with Samuel Sharpe's strike. Trouble began during the night of 27 December at the Kensington plantation in the parish of St James on the northwest coast, when the strike turned into a violent revolt. Property was torched, and the uprising instantly spread to other plantations and parishes, illuminating the night across the whole western end of Jamaica. In St James alone, over a hundred properties were fired, including over forty sugar works and dozens of planters' homes.

The military presence in the area was weak, the barracks at Montego Bay having fallen into disuse due to its unhealthy state. The militia were called out, under the command of a planter; they were poorly trained and ineffectually led, and were unequal to the task of riot control in hostile terrain. It was reported that 'the Negroes had attacked ... in considerable numbers, advancing in four columns. The Western Interior Regiment of Militia commenced a very brisk fire, which had the effect of dispersing them, after having killed ten and wounding twenty-five of their number.' Having slowed down the rebels, the militia quickly retreated towards the coast.[11]

On New Year's Day, Sir Willoughby Cotton sailed from Kingston to Montego Bay with a hundred men of the 84th Regiment, together with a troop of artillery and a rocket brigade.* The next day, the Royal Navy frigate *Blanche* arrived from Port Royal and landed two hundred men from the 77th Regiment and two more companies of the 84th. They formed up and moved inland. In the rear were the surgeons, including Dr James Barry who, after twenty-nine years as an Army surgeon, was about to gain his first experience of front-line military surgery.

---

* *rocket*: artillery weapon; an explosive incendiary device like a giant firework; originally pioneered by Tipu Sultan in India and used against the British, later improved in England by William Congreve

By this time the slaves had joined together in large, well-armed bodies; Montego Bay itself was under threat and people had begun to flee. Cotton's force made quick progress, pushing back the rebels (whose attacks had slowed that day due to Sabbath religious observance and meetings).

James had a little experience of looking after wounded soldiers in their convalescence, during his time at Greenwich and among the French prisoners of war from Waterloo who had been brought to Plymouth; but this was the first time he had set up a makeshift hospital in the field and put his instruments to work digging out musket balls and stitching sword cuts – or in this case machete cuts.

The British troops were not numerous, and suffered a total of ten fatal casualties and an unknown number of wounded, compared with hundreds of rebel slaves dead. They captured a number of the alleged ringleaders, who were rapidly tried and executed. It was discovered that the slaves believed slavery had been officially abolished but the Assembly was refusing to free them. General Cotton issued a proclamation:

NEGROES,

You have taken up arms against your masters, and have burnt and plundered their houses and buildings. Some wicked persons have told you that the King has made you free, and that your masters held your freedom from you. In the name of the King, I come amongst you, to tell you, that you are misled. I bring with me numerous forces to punish the guilty, and all who are found with the rebels, will be put to death without mercy. You cannot resist the King's Troops:– surrender yourselves and beg that your crime may be pardoned. All who yield themselves up at any Military Post, immediately, provided they are not principals or chiefs in the burnings that have been committed, will receive His Majesty's pardon: all who hold out will meet with certain death.[12]

(This the proclamation of a man with his own history of violent mutiny, but that had been in another century and another world.) By the end of the first week of January 1832 the rebellion had been suppressed and the manhunts, trials and executions got under way in earnest, carried out mainly by the civil authorities with the help of the militia; hundreds were rounded up and either whipped, transported or (in most cases) hanged.

In St James parish alone, the total number of slaves either killed in the rebellion or hanged was 237; throughout the western parishes there were reprisals, the militia destroying slave villages and killing their livestock.[13] The whole tragedy became known as the Baptist War, based on claims like those of the newspaper the *Watchman*:

> The manner in which the rebellion has been conducted affords abundant proof that it has been concocted and carried out by individuals possessing much more knowledge than negroes in general can be possessed of; and it is the opinion of almost every one here, that the Sectarians, especially the Baptists, are its principal source, as it is well-known that the ringleaders on every estate have been Baptists.[14]

These ringleaders were executed: among them the originator, the slave and Baptist preacher Samuel Sharpe, who became a legend among the black population and a national hero.

With the rebellion over, life in Jamaica gradually returned to normal. The following year, Westminster passed the Slavery Abolition Act, with emancipation reaching Jamaica in 1834, although it would take another four years for it to be fully enacted.

James Barry was there in the early years, settling into the military, medical and social life of the island. There were mess dinners, social calls, grand balls, horse racing outside Kingston, and regattas in the harbour, with the rival crews of frigates competing in their cutters and longboats. A fort adjutant called Wilson recalled that Dr Barry 'loved attending weddings, Christenings', and would frequently be encountered at General Cotton's dinners, where he amused the guests with 'outrageous stories' and portrayed himself as 'quite a lady-killer', always attaching himself to the 'finest and best-looking woman in the room'.[15]

Among the Jamaica garrison were James's old acquaintances from Mauritius, the 56th (West Essex) Regiment. One of the regiment's assistant surgeons, Edward Bradford, recalled of Dr Barry:

> I first met him in 1832, in Jamaica. His appearance and manners were then most singular. His stature scarcely reached five feet. He was quite destitute of all the characters of manhood. His voice was that of an aged woman. He sought every opportunity of making himself conspicuous,

and wore the longest sword and spurs he could obtain. He was always addicted to pet animals, dogs, monkeys, and parrots. His food consisted at this time of milk and fruit … He delighted in scandal and gossip … When travelling he carefully secluded himself from observation. When he was ill he invariably exacted from the officer who attended him a promise that, in the event of his death, strict precautions should be adopted to prevent any examination of his person. Through life his irritable and impatient temper brought him into constant collision with authority; he was, however, very capable of generous feeling, and of gratitude to those who were kind to him.[16]

His fondness for pets was remarked by everyone, and he had a little dog, called Psyche (one of a succession with the same name),[17] which followed him everywhere. Likewise his odd diet – which had turned vegetarian – was usually noticed.

In Jamaica he acquired a new manservant; not content with the men available as orderlies in the British regiments, he wanted someone to replace Danzer – not just a servant but a trusted companion. He heard that one of the regimental surgeons was about to return home on extended sick leave, and would be leaving behind his orderly, a young black soldier of the West India Regiment called John,[18] who was known to have given exemplary service. It was agreed that Dr Barry would take him on. Neither James nor John could have imagined that their relationship was to endure uninterrupted for the rest of James's life.

While James Barry's career in Jamaica continued on its routine way, significant political events were taking place elsewhere that would have a bearing on his life.

On the far side of the Atlantic, the island of St Helena was changing hands. Since 1658 it had been governed by the British East India Company (under a charter from Oliver Cromwell), with a six-year interlude when it came under Crown rule during Napoleon Bonaparte's captivity. After Bonaparte's death in 1821 it had reverted to the Company. However, that was now changing; the British government had grown increasingly unhappy with the Company's near total monopoly on eastern trade, which, combined with its powers of governance, its trading fleet and army, had made it into a monstrously powerful entity. In 1833 Parliament passed the Government of India Act, which entirely shut down the

Company as a commercial operation, although it retained its army and its administrative role in India. As part of the arrangement, St Helena came back under Crown control.

That meant it had to be garrisoned, and that in turn meant that a hospital and medical staff were required. Director General Sir James McGrigor cast his eyes over the list of surgeons and deputy inspectors, and settled on the name of James Barry MD, staff surgeon with seven years' seniority – still fairly junior, but he'd been in the Army for twenty years, and was a good friend of Lord FitzRoy Somerset. McGrigor despatched an order to Dr Barry, requiring him to transfer to St Helena, to take up the post of Principal Medical Officer.

It was the end of 1834 when James received the order. It was a significant advance in his career; a return to the kind of authority and power he had enjoyed for a time at the Cape. He ordered John to begin packing his things, and started saying his farewells to friends and colleagues. In February 1835 he boarded ship for England. Why he went there rather than straight to St Helena is the first of several mysteries arising in that year.

23

The Past Revisited

Merchant's Quay, Cork: May 1835

Mary Anne Bulkley stood on the waterfront amidst the bustle that had once been a part of her everyday life. It had been such a long time. Behind her stood the house where she and Jeremiah had kept their shop; it was in the hands of strangers nowadays, and had been these past twenty years and more. Cork was changing; the quays were less busy than they had been, now that Cobh had come into its own, and only vessels with very shallow drafts still came up the Lee to the city quays. Yet the place was expanding, new streets laid out, marshes reclaimed and built on.

Mrs Bulkley had turned seventy the previous year, carrying on decade after decade in spite of the nervous illnesses that had threatened to finish her off. She had once written her will and given out mourning rings, when she'd still had the means and a daughter to consider; now there was nothing to bequeath, and after years of struggle, circumstances had finally driven her back to the city of her birth.

In their own ways, each of her children had disappointed her. From Margaret there came nothing – she had parted from her mother after choosing to keep her disguise and join the Army, and after that … gone overseas, and no word.[1] Surprisingly, Margaret's hapless brother John had managed to survive the hell of the Royal York Rangers, the fevers and ferocious battles of the West Indian campaign of 1808–9, and had eventually made his way back to England. In middle age he had married (or at least set up home with) a London girl, Elizabeth, almost two decades younger than himself; they lived in Deptford in Kent, where there was a great naval dockyard. Elizabeth took his name, and just this previous year, in the spring of 1834, she'd given him a daughter, Esther.[2] Mary

Anne's husband, Jeremiah, was long gone – like Redmond Barry, in his desperation Jeremiah had committed some trivial crime, and in 1823 had been put aboard a convict ship bound for New South Wales.[3]

Mrs Bulkley turned her back on Merchant's Quay and crossed the river, passing south into the district where the city was expanding most rapidly: down Anglesey Road, past rows of little houses; on her right stood the Orphan Asylum, on her left the grim brick walls of a looming, sprawling building. She came to the entrance and looked up: there was the Lunatic Asylum, a long building stretching back from the road, and adjoining it the forbidding edifice of the House of Industry. The work-house. She forced herself to knock; the judas hole flipped open, she spoke to the man within, and the door swung open to admit her.

The House of Industry was a large institution, run jointly with the Lunatic Asylum; although old and showing the strain of the heavy demand upon it, it appeared on paper to be well appointed – one con-temporary described it:

> The House of Industry is an extensive building, affording accommo-dation to 1200 inmates, who are always under its roof, and of whom two-thirds are women; these are employed in household work, washing, spinning, plain work, weaving, and platting straw; and the males in picking oakum, weaving, quarrying and breaking stones for the roads, and in cleaning the streets. The establishment contains two medical and surgical hospitals … and there are three schools for boys and girls, each under a separate teacher. It is … conducted with the greatest regard to the comfort and moral improvement of the inmates.[4]

That is what the compiler of the directory was told; in fact, the situation was far bleaker. The institution might *hold* 1200 but could only accommo-date one-sixth of that number in reasonable conditions; the inmates were wretched, supplied with no clothing in which to perform their arduous work (so that those who arrived in rags were soon almost naked) and had to be provided for out of any surplus from donations to the Lunatic Asylum. The problem was sheer lack of funds and overcrowding, and the gross level of poverty in Ireland.[5] Like workhouses everywhere, the House of Industry was a place of suffering and shame.

Mary Anne Bulkley was known in Cork on account of her family connections. Her entry through that infamous door – and her purpose

there – became known, and within days an Irish newspaper carried a
short paragraph among its miscellany of minor news:

> Among the applicants for admission to the House of Industry, Cork,
> last week, was the sister of the well-known James Barry, the celebrated
> but unfortunate historical painter.[6]

Just a tiny notice, but the name caught people's attention, and the following week it was reproduced in papers across Ireland, from the *Waterford
Mail* to the *Belfast Commercial Chronicle*. It quickly hopped the Irish Sea –
by Thursday 28 May it was in the London *Morning Post* (which habitually
kept an eye on Irish news), on Saturday in *The Spectator*, and quickly spread
to the *Cambridge Chronicle*, the *Bristol Mirror*, the *Blackburn Standard*, and
on to Hereford, Devon, Yorkshire, Cumberland, Liverpool ... wherever there was a local newspaper, Mrs Bulkley's plight was announced.
If she was aware of this – and she would surely have heard – the shame
must have been unbearable; every person dreaded the workhouse, and
the dread was less about the slave labour than about the degradation
and humiliation it involved; yet few had their plight announced in
newspapers throughout the kingdom. It caught the eye of one art lover,
who – identifying himself only as 'An Admirer of Genius' – wrote in
protest to *The Times*:

> Will the Society of Arts suffer this? The sister of the great genius who
> developed the progress of civilization on the walls of their great room
> in want and unrelieved! Dr Johnson's and Burke's high estimation of
> this painter's great grasp of mind should alone awaken consideration
> for his unfortunate sister.[7]

If any subscription was raised, it left no trace. Charles Warren the
engraver, who had started the subscription for Redmond Barry in similar circumstances, was long dead; all Mary Anne's old friends were
dead and gone – Dr Fryer, Daniel Reardon, Joseph Bonomi; James and
Margaret's early sponsors had also long since passed on: General Miranda,
the Earl of Buchan ... Mary Anne Bulkley knew no one who would be
in a position to help.

Except for one person. A month or more prior to Mrs Bulkley's disgrace, Dr James Barry had returned to Britain from Jamaica, and cannot

have failed to be aware of the newspaper notices – particularly the letter in *The Times*.

No trace survives of James having been in touch since he joined the Army in 1813, nor any record of them establishing contact now. All that is known for certain is that at this point, in the middle of 1835, for the only time in his long career – or indeed in his or Margaret's life – Dr James Barry vanishes from the record. He continued to be in the Army and on full pay; but other than a note that he was 'At Home' for a year and two months – without apparent duties and not sick – he goes missing, during a change in postings that should not have involved his visiting England at all.[8]

Margaret had become more cautious than ever in obscuring James's past, shrouding it in vague allusions to dead parents and wealthy but anonymous relations. If she helped her mother, it would have been in strict secrecy – perhaps she even emerged from her disguise, became Margaret again for a while. Now that she was middle-aged she could travel alone without much difficulty (posing as a widow would suffice), and although James was far from rich, he had means.

After a year in mysterious obscurity, on 19 April 1836 Dr Barry emerged again into the light, when he and his manservant John took ship at last for their long-delayed voyage to St Helena. What happened to Mrs Bulkley is not clear, but she eventually found her way back to England and joined her son John's family. However it had come about, Mrs Bulkley was one of the few to escape the workhouse in old age, and lived on for many more years.

The East Indiaman *Lord William Bentinck* sailed from the Downs – the roadstead off the Kent coast where merchantmen and naval squadrons gathered before sailing – on 25 April, bound for St Helena, the Cape and Calcutta. On board was James Barry, along with an old acquaintance from the Cape. Andries Stockenström was a frontier worthy who had been landdrost of Graaff Reinet in James's day; he'd come to London the previous year to give evidence to Parliament about relations between frontier settlers and the Xhosa (which were exploding in violence again). He was now sailing back in triumph – the new Secretary of State for War and the Colonies had been sufficiently impressed to appoint him Lieutenant Governor of the Eastern Province (his appointment was perhaps intended to help mollify the increasingly anti-British Dutch population).

Lord William Bentinck tacked west-southwest down the English Channel and out into the Atlantic, heading for the trade winds. All went well at first. But then, about three weeks out, the first case of smallpox occurred on board, and with it the first intimation of terror.

A report by the ship's surgeon traced the infection to a Dr Batson, who had boarded at Gravesend on 20 April, apparently already with signs of feeling unwell. Between 8 and 14 May, he was decidedly sick, and the disease began to spread; a twenty-year-old woman called Lela was the first to catch it; she shared a cabin with Batson's *ayah** and had helped her make his bed. With the ship approaching the Equator and the coast of Brazil (where they would catch the trade wind southeast for St Helena and the Cape), Lela died; her body was wrapped in sailcloth, weighted and buried over the side.[9]

Batson weathered the disease, but not before it had spread to three more passengers and a crewman. The ship's surgeon worked to contain the infection – probably with the help of Dr Barry, who had extensive experience of it and had been immunised. With the ship approaching St Helena, the captain had no choice: he could not land with such a contagion on board, and so he bore away, passed the island and set a course for the nearest port with quarantine facilities.

Table Bay: Sunday 3 July 1836

The cable rushed out through the hawse hole, and *Lord William Bentinck*'s anchor plunged into the blue-green water of the bay. On deck, James Barry looked out at a sight he hadn't expected to see again. Seven years hadn't changed Cape Town visibly – there was the Castle dominating the beach, and the group of buildings with the threatening bulk of the Tronk on the right, then the bay sweeping round, and the spot where the Somerset Hospital sat, obscured by the nearer buildings. And over it all, the crest of the peninsula's mountainous spine. This was as close as James would get for the present; the Yellow Jack[†] was flying at the ship's masthead, and nobody would be allowed ashore.

A short distance west along the bay stood the Chavonnes Battery: a hexagonal fort with thick walls and embankments built into the rocks

---

* Indian nursemaid
[†] signal flag indicating contagion aboard

and jutting into the sea. Now stripped of its guns, it served as the Cape Colony's quarantine facility, and was cut off by a military cordon. Here the ship's passengers would be confined.

Later that day, the quarantine process began. It was thorough, and must have required some sharp practice on Dr Barry's part, since it involved stripping and being sponged with vinegar or a solution of sodium hypochlorite before putting on clothes fumigated with chlorine gas. Presumably, as a senior doctor, he was trusted to sponge and dress himself in private. The garments belonging to Lela, the dead woman, were destroyed, and all passengers' belongings – apart from their personal linen, bedding and anything they couldn't live without – had to be left aboard the ship.[10]

Then the passengers and infected crewmen were taken to the Chavonnes. Animals from the ship – including six donkeys and James's little dog, Psyche – were also treated with vinegar and were obliged to swim ashore by themselves. Psyche had to be kept under tight control, as any stray animals found within the *cordon sanitaire* would be put down. The only thing that came in and out was mail, and that was fumigated.

So their confinement began. Three days after their arrival, James watched in frustration and anger as *Lord William Bentinck* – cleared to proceed – replaced the Yellow Jack with the Blue Peter, raised anchor and sailed on for Calcutta, with everyone's belongings still on board. All James's uniforms, civilian clothes, boots, papers and personal effects were gone. (He would presumably have been allowed to take his medical equipment into quarantine.)

The passengers and crew were kept in the Chavonnes for just over three weeks. James suffered a further crisis during discharge, when everyone's body linen had to be steeped in chloride of lime and all bedding burned; included in this conflagration were some objects that James described as 'three pillows of a particular description', which he claimed were 'necessary to me under the peculiar circumstances into which severe accidents have placed me and which cost me 15 guineas each'.[11] Since James Barry had never had any 'severe accidents', had never shown any signs of injury, and since no pillows, however 'particular', would be likely to cost anything like that much, it is probable that these were prosthetics that Margaret used to enhance James's build and lend some masculine bulk to his frame; previously she had improvised with stuffing kapok in his lining, which was both inconvenient and imperfect. She had presumably had these special articles discreetly tailor-made by some London corsetiere or theatrical costumer; hence the staggering price of 45 guineas (about two months' pay) for what could only euphemistically be described as 'pillows'. When the Chavonnes warden demanded them, James protested that they were expensive and indispensable, but it was useless – they 'were wantonly and against my strongest remonstrances seized and destroyed'.[12] As if that weren't enough, his body linen – shirts and underwear – was so thoroughly steeped in chloride of lime that it 'fell to rags in the washing' and had to be thrown away.

James calculated his total loss from the quarantine at £142 16s, including – which was particularly galling – board and lodging for the period in confinement. This total was more than half a year's pay, not to mention what he'd lost in allowances due to the delay in his taking up his post. Moreover, he would now have to pay for his own passage back to St Helena. He wrote a strongly worded letter to the Cape Governor, Lieutenant General Sir Benjamin D'Urban, describing his losses, itemising the costs, and insisting that 'it is a duty I owe to myself to beg your Excellency to consider that if the Public required these sacrifices from me, the Public may be supposed to have been preserved by the arrangements entered into by your Excellency's Authority', and therefore the public should make good his losses; 'my Agents here are Messrs Dickson, Burnes & Co. who in my absence will receive … the amount which your Excellency may deem me entitled.'[13] It was a vain expectation; he was told that the Governor 'finds it certainly out of his power to award you any indemnification at the public expense'.[14]

James had to wait some weeks for a ship, so took the opportunity to look around the old familiar places – although there wasn't much sign of it in Cape Town, the Cape Colony was changing; the march of Anglicisation had accelerated, and the Dutch population was feeling increasingly alienated (being forced to give up their slaves had displeased many of them). There were moves among the farmers to leave, striking out northwards from the Eastern Province; only the previous year, the first marches of what would become known as the Great Trek had begun. At the same time, another war had broken out with the Xhosa on the eastern frontier – the first since 1819.

There was one happy event during James's stay; he was reunited with his godson and namesake, James Barry Munnik, now ten years old.

Unhappily, the boy no longer lived at home; his mother, Wilhelmina, had died in 1830 when he was four,[15] and little James had been put into the care of the Sandenberg family, who were Wilhelmina's relations. Her sister, Mrs Sandenberg (James's former landlady from the Heerengracht), had also died, and now her son Sebastian was helping to look after the boy, with help from his sister-in-law and his sweetheart (the latter apparently the daughter of James's old patient, Mrs Cloete – all these Cape families were connected in one way or another).[16] James and his godson struck up an affectionate friendship, and in the following years began a correspondence. James the elder wrote to his namesake:

> My Dear James Barry,
>   I was much pleased with your letter, it was well written and does you and your Master great credit – I have written to you before, but I hoped your watch would have arrived from England – I expect it daily – you have a young friend of mine – Mr Baker at your school. I hope you and he are friends – write to me by every opportunity – I shall always be glad to see your letters – remember me most kindly to your father & to Mrs Sandenberg & Bastian and his Lady – & to my Dear old friend his [sic – her] mother Mrs Cloete – I trust she is quite well – I have no time to say more than God bless my Dear Boy & prosper you.
>   Yours affectionately
>   James Barry[17]

Their correspondence continued for a while, but was unfortunately driven onto the rocks by the innocent candour of the young boy, who told his godfather that 'people are talking about you and saying that you look rather like a lady'.[18] The shutters came down, and no further communication between James Barry and James Barry Munnik took place.

It was callous – as was Margaret's separation from her mother – but the stakes had always been high and had been riding for too long and risen too steeply for James to bear even the slightest risk of exposure. It was an obsessive, almost neurotic aversion. Having these dangerous rumours brayed in his face by a leering jackanapes of a subaltern was one thing – and had been swiftly met by a well-aimed riding crop – but having them bruited about by an affectionate godson must be disturbing to an entirely different degree.

But all that lay in the future when, in late August 1836, after nearly two months trapped at the Cape, equipped with new linen and accoutrements but without his valuable padding, James said his farewells and boarded the brig *Lord Hobart*, bound for St Helena. His elevated heels never touched Cape soil again.

24

An Officer and a Gentleman

St Helena is one entire rock … There is only one landing place …
and this is strongly defended by batteries, the guns of which are level
with the sea. The island is infested with rats, which commit the most
dreadful destruction; otherwise it produces corn and fruit, and abounds
in game. By the possession of the Cape it is no longer visited by our
India ships, and but for this new visitor [Napoleon] it would have
fallen into total decay.

Morning Chronicle, 24 July 1815

According to James's friend the Comte de Las Cases, the best Napoleon could say of St Helena was: 'This rock … is wild and barren, no doubt; the climate is monotonous and unwholesome; but the temperature, it must be confessed, is mild and agreeable.'[1]

Twenty-one years on, it hadn't changed. Even Napoleon was still here, under a slab in the hills, his dying wish to be buried by the Seine denied.[2] From the deck of *Lord Hobart*, the island resembled an immense floating fortress, six miles from end to end, with near-vertical rock walls dropping into the roiling sea. Just two months earlier, HMS *Beagle* had called here with Charles Darwin aboard, on the homeward leg of his monumental voyage of discovery; he'd been impressed by its 'forbidding aspect' and struck by its unusual geology.[3]

Rounding the northern headland at a safe distance, a cleft was revealed in the continuous wall – James Bay, and within it Jamestown, the only port. Behind the battlemented waterfront rose a church tower, surrounded by low buildings; the town straggled away up the bottom of a rocky, scrubby valley so narrow it was like a corridor. All who approached it were depressed, dismayed and even intimidated by the sight.

As *Lord Hobart* dropped anchor, a launch came alongside and a young man clambered up the side, introducing himself as Dr Richard Hopkins of the Army Medical Department; it was his task to inspect the passengers and crew and issue pratique.* Dr Hopkins had to inspect every ship arriving in James Bay, on top of his duties at the hospital; he was very young, less than two years in his rank as assistant staff surgeon,[4] and it was a great responsibility. It was a relief to discover that the new Principal Medical Officer was among the passengers – considerably later than expected. There were tales told about Dr Barry in the service concerning his appearance (which lived up to the gossip in every way) as well as his conduct – but he was said to be a good doctor, and it was all hands to the pumps on St Helena.

James was put in the picture as they walked up through the town, his few belongings trundling behind under John's care. Since the Crown takeover, most of St Helena's wealthier inhabitants – including its civilian doctors – had cleared off. This had had a devastating effect on the life and economy of the place; wages were low and the poorer inhabitants were living on a diet of rice with small amounts of salt meat.[5] To cap the misery, slavery was still in force for the hundred or so slaves on the island, St Helena having been exempted from the Abolition Act of 1833.[6] As an outpost of fairly dubious value, the island wasn't a high priority to the government, which resented spending money on it. It quickly became apparent that being appointed its Principal Medical Officer was more of a challenge than an advancement.

James wasn't the only late arrival. It had taken nearly two years for His Majesty's Governor to get here and take over; Major General George Middlemore had arrived in February 1836, only seven months ahead of James. Middlemore's inaugural proclamation had promised that it was 'His Majesty's gracious disposition to make every necessary and proper Provision for the good Government of this Settlement'.[7] In fact, the British government was about to make swingeing financial cuts to services here, not least to the medical provision. St Helena was in need of an informed, decisive and imaginative governor, but Middlemore appeared to enjoy few of these qualities.[8]

---

* licence to enter port; clean bill of health

His Majesty's Commissioners of Inquiry – still on the case after more than a decade (though Bigge and Colebrooke had stood down) – had reviewed the medical provision for the civilian population, and realising that the Army would be obliged to take responsibility for it all, had recommended that:

> As long as the temporary arrangement lasted, by which civilians had to be treated at the military hospital, the hospital at Jamestown should be placed under charge of an establishment of medical officers composed of 1 Staff Surgeon paid £274-5-0 per annum, (with an allowance of £38-12 for forage), 1 Assistant Surgeon paid £182-12 per annum and 1 Apothecary to be paid £91-5.[9]

This meant that Dr Barry, with Hopkins to assist him, had to oversee the regimental surgeons, provide care to the rest of the garrison *and* attend to a population numbering nearly five thousand, as well as inspect (on average) two incoming ships a day.[10]

When Dr Barry made his first inspection of the St Helena facilities, he found good and bad. The 91st Highland Regiment's hospital (inherited from the East India Company) was 'clean and well arranged' with a low mortality rate, which James attributed to the assistant surgeon, William Cruickshank Eddie, whose 'zeal, ability and attention' James admired.[11] The Civil Hospital was a different matter; as he walked among the untidy beds, Dr Barry was disturbed to find a large number of women with venereal diseases, a result of the poverty left in the wake of the East India Company's withdrawal, which had forced many women into prostitution.

These conditions were utterly unacceptable. James decided that new accommodation was needed immediately, and wrote to Captain Alexander of the Royal Engineers about his dismay at finding venereal and fever patients mixed, and female and male patients crowded into adjacent wards, which was 'absolutely improper' both medically and morally, and asking that extra wards be created.[12]

Alexander jumped to it, suggesting to the Colonial Secretary, Mr W. H. Seale, that a disused brewery nearby could be adapted;[13] the Governor gave permission to investigate the costs. Two months went by and nothing was done, Middlemore being under pressure from Lord Glenelg, the Secretary of State for War and the Colonies, not to approve any additional expenses.[14] Running out of patience, in November James wrote to Middlemore:

> Sir … the number of females affected with venereal disease has greatly increased, and the hospital itself is now actually crowded with the Military and Civil population. So much so that we shall be at a loss to accommodate even the troops, in the event of an accident, or increase in disease in the garrison.
>
> Your Excellency was pleased in September last to sanction that accommodation for the Females (which it is always incorrect to treat in a Military hospital) should be fitted up by the Ordnance Department in a waste building near the hospital … And I beg to represent that it is of vital importance to the troops that this building is prepared.[15]

It was another two months before approval was given for conversion of a bakehouse.[16] It took another year before the project was approved by Whitehall, by which time the conversion had commenced. Long before that, James had begun irritating Mr Seale by unilaterally taking on more staff – including a ward master – for the hospital; the Colonial Secretary refused to pay him for the period in which he was employed without official sanction.[17] Dr Barry was already beginning to get under the skin of the administration.

James was also trying to tackle the immediate problem of 'the disgusting circumstances of male attendants on the female patients' (interestingly, he subscribed to the conventional view of male–female roles and relations); he wrote to Director General McGrigor that he had 'immediately hired a respectable woman of colour as Matron'.[18] The precise duties of this woman are not described, although they appear to have involved patient care, which was unusual; the term 'matron' had traditionally meant a woman responsible for the domestic running and general cleanliness of a hospital – a kind of housekeeper – often with responsibility for hiring nursing and ancillary staff, but during the period starting in the 1830s, with nursing becoming more skilled, the role began to evolve into the modern one of head nurse. James Barry appears to have been at the forefront of this development – especially in appointing a black matron, perhaps inspired by his experience of doctresses in Jamaica.

He forged ahead with his plans for the hospital, no doubt taking hints from two manuals McGrigor had sent him: *Instructions for Regimental and*

Detachment Hospitals, and a copy of *General Instructions for Medical Officers, Heads of Staff and Others in Charge of Departments*. Sir James, bearing in mind that this was Dr Barry's first command appointment, had helpfully underlined in red the passages he considered to be of most importance and accompanied the books with a letter rehearsing them further.[19]

Meanwhile, warnings were coming to the Governor from Lord Glenelg that he was reluctant to sanction any expense for the medical care of civilians in St Helena.[20] James seemed oblivious to the politics of the situation, and thought only of medicine, health, welfare and radical reform. This had happened before, and it hadn't ended well for him.

It probably didn't help that Middlemore had been forced to confess to Dr Barry that he'd been doing some unauthorised medical management prior to his arrival; since the medical staff had consisted solely of Dr Hopkins, and because he was overworked, the Governor had authorised extra pay for him.[21] Now, to Middlemore's embarrassment and the surgeon's dismay, Hopkins was required to refund the money. Even more embarrassingly, James himself was alleged to have received excess pay on the same scale during his first month (which he denied); each received an unnecessarily curt, unapologetic note from Mr Seale, demanding immediate repayment – in Hopkins's case amounting to £109, representing seven months' hard work.[22] Eventually, after months of argument, it was grudgingly conceded that they could keep the money.

Pay might be short, but work wasn't; James even had to step in occasionally to deal with the regimental surgeons' needs – particularly when there was an outbreak of dysentery among the NCOs and men of the 91st. It was decided that it was connected with diet, and the rations were improved, with more fresh meat.[23] Middlemore grumbled about the expense, but had to comply. The irritations were steadily building up; before long there would be another crisis in the career of Dr James Barry.

Jamestown: Sunday 20 November 1836

Margaret was enjoying a rare moment of freedom. The door was locked, and the paraphernalia of James Barry – clothes, linen, padding – lay neatly folded on a chair, while in front of the fire stood a steaming tub.[24] It was pleasant to have a moment away from the pressure of duty; the wrangling over the hospital had lately landed James in a dispute with the Assistant Commissary General over supplies, which had turned very unpleasant. Privacy and escape were invaluable.

James had settled in an attractive cottage at the upper end of Jamestown, with a bathhouse built onto it and a garden with a mango tree that he particularly admired.[25] The climate of St Helena was agreeable, and the interior, though small (the whole island was only forty-seven square miles), was much pleasanter than the coast led visitors to expect. There were green hills, trees and spectacular valleys. Charles Darwin had likened it to Wales, and noted the number of British plants that grew here, and the familiar look of the 'numerous cottages and small white houses; some buried at the bottom of the deepest valleys, and others mounted on the crests of the lofty hills'.[26]

Darwin had spent six days exploring the island's unique volcanic geology and its flora and fauna. He had departed only two months before James Barry arrived, having already nearly crossed paths at the Cape; HMS *Beagle* had reached Cape Town from the east just as James Barry's afflicted ship was approaching it from the northwest, and had travelled on to St Helena just as James went into quarantine;[27] had it not been for that unlucky chance, these two revolutionary figures would certainly have met on this island. The educated population was small, and James was an enthusiastic botanist; Darwin had also been a medical student at Edinburgh in the 1820s and studied anatomy under Munro.

The peace of Margaret's bath was interrupted by a thundering knock on the street door. She heard John answer it, and a moment later was surprised to hear the voice of George Barnes, a subaltern in the 91st who held the post of Town Major,* asking to see Dr Barry right away. Margaret called out to him to wait, got hurriedly out of the bath, wrapped a dressing gown around herself, along with a semblance of James, and opened the door.

'I'm sorry, Barry,' said Barnes, 'I have bad news for you.'[28]

James reported later that he was 'seized with agitation' by this, supposing that he was being dragged out – on a Sunday morning! – to inspect some newly arrived ship. But Barnes shook his head.

'No,' he said, producing a written order. 'I am come to put you in arrest.'

---

* officer in a garrison responsible for keeping order among troops in the town

James stared. 'I thought he was mad,' he recalled later, and 'spurned the idea of such a thing', declining to acknowledge Barnes's authority.

The cause of the attempted arrest was unbelievably trivial – his dispute with the Commissary. James had needed daily supplies for the patients in the Civil Hospital, and relied upon Assistant Commissary General Francis Edward Knowles, who was an awkward man to deal with. He was very sensitive about his rank – which despite having the word 'general' in it was only equivalent to a captain.[29] It appeared that he took a dislike to Dr Barry, and the very notion of cooperating seemed to grate. When James politely requested supplies, Knowles refused, and would not be persuaded.[30] Rather than going to General Middlemore (who was sure to object to the costs), James had taken the improper step of writing directly to Lord Glenelg in London, drawing his attention to the official regulations on managing hospitals and enclosing a copy of his correspondence with Mr Knowles; under the regulations the Commissariat was obliged to provide supplies. James drew attention to 'the total absence of all rational objections on the part of the Commissary here to further the ends of the Service … I shall therefore take the most efficient means in my power of obtaining the necessary supplies, until favoured by your Lordship's instructions.'[31]

James's clerk had made a copy of the letter for the records, and somehow it slipped out of the office and into circulation among the colonial officials. When Knowles saw the copy, he exploded with indignation. It was unseemly for a man in Dr Barry's position to write directly to the Secretary of State – especially with a complaint about a fellow officer. Knowles was particularly aggrieved at being reported in this way by a man he regarded as his junior (mistakenly thinking Dr Barry's rank, like his own, was equivalent to a captain, which would make Knowles senior due to time in-rank; in fact James ranked as a major). Knowles lodged a formal charge of misconduct against Dr Barry. It was upheld, and Town Major Barnes was sent to arrest him.

Standing there with a damp dressing gown barely concealing Margaret's form, James simply refused to be arrested. Was General Middlemore aware of this business? Apparently not. James dismissed the Town Major, then dressed carefully in his best uniform and, borrowing a carriage, set off in style to Plantation House, the Governor's residence.

He never got there. Barnes intercepted the carriage halfway; he'd seen Middlemore and received his authority for the arrest. Still James refused, and ordered the carriage to turn back, intending to go home and write a formal protest; but Barnes followed him, knocked again, and finally managed to place him under arrest.

Distraught, James asked Barnes what he should do; 'I had never been in arrest … I had patients of the greatest importance, one dying, two dead at the hospital.'[32] It made no difference – Dr Barry was to remain where he was, under house arrest and temporarily relieved of his office.

While Assistant Staff Surgeon Hopkins laboured alone under the burden of medical care and ship inspections, the government busied itself with the important business of inquiring into Assistant Commissary General Knowles's wounded dignity. James was summoned on the orders of His Excellency the Governor to appear before a general court martial on 24 November 1836. The hearing began, was postponed for a week, and eventually resumed on Saturday 3 December, with Lieutenant Colonel Hamelin Trelawney of the Royal Artillery presiding. The charge brought by Assistant Commissary General Knowles against Staff Surgeon Dr James Barry was:

> Conduct unbecoming the character of an Officer and a Gentleman, in having by a letter dated 14th November 1836 officially reported direct to the Rt Hon the Secretary at War, that the Asst Commissary-General had objected, or had interposed objections to comply with Article No 2 of the regulations of 28th February 1835, for the management of Hospitals on Foreign Stations, or words to that effect, which report is opposed to fact and tending greatly to prejudice the professional character of the Asst Commissary-General in the estimation of the authorities in England.[33]

James conducted his own defence, and there followed four days of argument in which every nuance of the regulations and the officers' conduct was picked over. Eventually Knowles had to admit that his case against Barry was wholly about wounded pride; he clung to his erroneous belief that they were equal in rank and that he therefore held seniority: 'I am the same rank as the prisoner … My Commission was in 1816. His was in 1827.'[34] The proceedings became decidedly personal, hingeing on Barry's and Knowles's delicate yet differing notions of gentlemanly conduct. James admitted having been shown a private note from Knowles to Middlemore, but not having read it because 'a gentleman ought not to do so',[35] while Knowles insisted that a gentleman ought not to direct complaints over the heads of one's immediate superiors. It emerged that as copies of James's letter to Glenelg were spread around, its contents had been altered and distorted, apparently making the offence seem graver. James accused Knowles of having 'a certain influence with the Governor' (apparently based on his glimpse of the private note). The fact that Middlemore had sanctioned this farcical court martial seemed to confirm that.

Eventually the court reached its decision:

> The Court having maturely weighed and considered the evidence in support of the charge against the prisoner, Dr James Barry, his Defence, and the evidence adduced in support of it, is of the opinion that Staff surgeon Dr James Barry is NOT GUILTY of the charge preferred against him.
>
> The Court finds that the prisoner wrote the letter upon which the charge was founded, but is of the opinion that he was justified in so doing and doth therefore fully and honorably acquit him.[36]

James commented: 'It was probably the first instance of an officer being brought to trial for the performance of his duty.'[37]

He eventually achieved full satisfaction; the Treasury Commissioners ordered the Commissariat Department to supply the Civil Hospital on the same basis as the Military, 'by which means the [colonial] Government saved considerably & the patients were better provided for'.[38]

But it wasn't over yet. Middlemore was sour about the whole thing – especially the claims and revelations that had come out about himself, and added a note to the record, regretting that 'so much extraneous and irrelevant matter has been introduced by permission of the Court', adding that he would be referring the whole matter to Horse Guards and the attention of Commander in Chief General Lord Hill.[39] He was principally worried that his own refusal to give evidence (he was called by both sides) might get him into trouble. Accordingly, that same day he wrote to General Lord FitzRoy Somerset:

> I could not approve the proceedings of this Court Martial because I was of the opinion that … the Court had permitted Dr J. Barry to introduce in his defence accusations which I consider disrespectful to

myself, holding the situation of Commanding Officer and Governor of this island …

I cannot recollect in the long period during which I have held H.M. Commission (above 40 years) a single instance of a General Officer situated as I am, being obliged to appear as evidence before a general Court Martial …

I therefore conceive that the summons was disrespectful and not authorised.[40]

Was General Middlemore aware that he was addressing a man who, besides his position as right hand to the Commander in Chief, was a personal friend and sponsor of James Barry? Probably not. James had been known to drop hints that he had influential family connections, but didn't usually talk about them explicitly.

Having begun it, it was Knowles who brought the sorry episode to a conclusion by appealing the court's decision – through Middlemore – to Lord FitzRoy Somerset.[41] Unsurprisingly, his appeal was denied.

25

Homeward Bound

Trouble came at James Barry from all directions. Even Margaret's bath was no longer a refuge. Gossip had run among the servant women of St Helena that Dr Barry might not be a man. They had discussed this extensively, until one day his laundress decided to resolve the question. The bathhouse built onto James's cottage was made of timber and not perfectly made. The laundress hid behind it one morning, intending to spy through a crack in the wall.

Margaret, preparing to take off her disguise, must have noticed something amiss – a noise, a shadow. Guessing instantly what was afoot, James rushed out, snatching up a crop, and ran to the back of the bathhouse, where he caught the laundress red-handed. Overcome by the rage that had seized him before when his disguise was threatened, he thrashed the woman severely. 'From the way he beat her,' said one of the laundress's friends, 'we all knew that the doctor could not have been a man.'[1] Yet they kept their gossip to themselves.

James maintained a rigorous clinical schedule at both the Military and Civil hospitals; he and Hopkins also provided care to all paupers, the homeless, prisoners, and sailors of all nations calling at the island.[2] With the heavy load of shipping – especially from faraway places in the East, where control of smallpox was non-existent – James established a vaccination service among the local population. It was a vital precaution; there had been an instance in 1802 when measles had been introduced from an unquarantined ship – it began an epidemic in which 160 islanders died (from a population of about 2,000).[3]

James was nothing if not energetic, and what time was left over from his medical duties he spent partly on humanitarian acts. He involved himself in the cases of two prisoners in the town gaol (evidently not discouraged by the disastrous Aaron Smith case). One, identified only as 'Caesar' (presumably a slave), had been sentenced to life imprisonment for committing 'an unnatural act'; in James's opinion he was 'partly an idiot' with 'all the appearance of labouring under Satyriasis,* consequently an extremely improper and dangerous subject to be loose among young lads or any other prisoners'. James urged that he be 'placed in some other position'.[4] Precisely what happened to Caesar is unknown.

The other prisoner was a Chinese labourer called Acho. He had been in gaol for years, having got involved with a gang of burglars; they were all sentenced to death, then had their sentences commuted to transportation for life – all except Acho. Yet his death sentence wasn't carried out, and he had been left languishing in prison. His case had been reviewed recently and was still awaiting a decision.[5] James was dismayed by Acho's plight; he'd come into contact with him at the Civil Hospital, where he'd been admitted several times with problems that were more mental than physical:

> On his last admission, I found him in so weak and desponding a state that I feared for his intellect and therefore thought it fit to remove him into my own residence close to the hospital, to have him more immediately under my own eye and to give him advantage of air and exercise in my little garden, I being personally responsible for his safety and also that he should be paraded or mustered when required by any of the authorities.[6]

All seemed well until a Friday morning in July 1837, when the Civil Provost† came to the hospital 'without any written authority and there insisted on having the patient delivered up to him'; since Dr Barry was not present, the order could not be complied with, which caused trouble. James wrote to the Colonial Secretary to plead that:

> This unfortunate man, being subjected to the taunts and observations of prisoners or even patients, will in my judgement drive him to despair or

---

* uncontrollable sexual desire
† law officer; civilian equivalent to Town Major

madness. I therefore earnestly and respectfully submit that the convict
patient Acho be permitted to remain under my professional superintendence until his case be finally decided, I being of course personally
responsible as I am for others.[7]

Given the silence that followed this letter, his wish must have been
granted, Acho continuing to live in the little cottage with its garden and
mango tree. In October, a judicial decision was reached: 'to grant him
a pardon under the Great Seal of the island upon condition that he be
transported for life'.[8] The wretched man, apparently incapable of doing
any harm, was taken from James's custody and put aboard a convict ship,
never to be seen again.

Despite his huge burden of work and the humanitarian cases he had
taken a personal interest in, James still somehow had time and energy for
another vendetta. The target of his ire this time was the newly arrived
Colonial Chaplain, Reverend William Helps.

He never made clear the nature of his problem with Reverend Helps;
perhaps he was irritated that the Chaplain, already in possession of a
good salary from the Army (and a well-paid parish living he still held
in England), was given a generous bonus for ministering to St Helena's
civilian population, bringing his earnings just from his chaplaincy to
£600 a year, more than double the pay received by the Principal Medical
Officer, who had been firmly and embarrassingly denied any supplement
for his extra duties.

Yet there was undoubtedly more to it than jealousy. James Barry was
very serious about religion, and about proper Christian observance; his
morality was stark, and he was harshly judgemental, especially of those
he considered privileged. To anyone with eyes to see it, the Reverend
William Helps certainly lacked the rectitude expected from a clergyman.
Now in his mid-sixties, he was in the autumn of a life of hopeless financial
chaos. Thirty years earlier, having lost the rectorship of one parish, he
had moved to another and opened a school that was used as a means of
chiselling money out of wealthy parents – boys were neglected, Helps and
his wife spent much of their time in London, and eventually the wayward
cleric found himself in a debtors' prison.[9] He gained another preferment
in the Church, but managed to end up bankrupt again in 1828, despite
having an income of £1,200 a year; his bishop had him released, and he

was given a new living in Nottinghamshire (which he held for the rest of his life).[10] Now, two decades on, he was presumably in such financial (or possibly legal) trouble that he had been compelled to join the Army chaplaincy and leave the country.

James must have known some of this (Helps's school venture and first imprisonment had taken place at the time when Margaret was trying to find work as a governess, so she may have read of the scandal). Alternatively Helps may have brought his misbehaviour to St Helena – certainly he ran up debts there that were still unsettled when he died eleven years later.[11] Perhaps there was something worse that went unrecorded.

Whatever the cause, James evidently saw the Chaplain as an overpaid, overprotected hypocrite, and took against him with a vengeance. His hostility was such that the Governor had to set up a court of inquiry into the case of Dr Barry vs Reverend Helps. However, according to Middlemore, despite James's antipathy he 'never reported to me in any one instance his reasons for accusing the Rev. Divine, but has thought fit to threaten him with officially denouncing him to the authorities at home without my knowledge or consent'; again the Governor wrote to Lord FitzRoy Somerset, complaining that 'Such conduct in a small community like St Helena creates perpetual jarrings and discontent.'[12]

Helps was not removed from his post, and whatever he had done, James apparently didn't carry out his threat to denounce him. Perhaps the cleric was persuaded to repent of whatever mysterious sin it was that James knew of – it can't have been his general indebtedness, which was public knowledge, reported in newspapers going back decades.

By this time, General Middlemore had developed a strong dislike for James Barry. He'd anticipated that the governorship of St Helena would be a quiet posting with which to bring his long military career to an end; instead, he had this increasingly irritating stone in his shoe. An opportunity to rid himself of it finally offered itself in May 1837.

In April, the Governor was approached by a surgeon, a Mr Reed, offering to take on indigent patients – mainly convicts and prisoners in the town gaol – for a fee of 15 shillings each (with medicines provided by the hospital or dispensary). Mr Reed was something of a mystery – he had quit St Helena when the government took over, but was now back and in need of work. But the rate of pay he was demanding was very high. At first, Barry and Middlemore were in agreement – the prisoners were already well cared for by the hospital, and the populace, rich and poor, were taken care of by Dr Hopkins and the assistant surgeons of the 91st; there was no need for Mr Reed. 'I beg here most distinctly to state,' wrote James to General Middlemore, 'that I am perfectly certain that no application for advice or medicine has been unattended since my arrival in this command'; and yet, on 1 May, when James paid a visit to the prison, 'I was peremptorily refused admission' because the churchwardens, who were responsible for funding prisoners' and paupers' welfare, had agreed to let Reed attend them, even though they had been getting the service free from Dr Barry and his assistant.[13]

Worried that the churchwardens were being taken advantage of (and resenting any encroachment on what he saw as his territory), James suggested that if they put £60 a year at his disposal, he would provide all the medical services the prison required. The Governor applied pressure by refusing their application to supply medicines (not included in Reed's 15 shilling fees) at government expense. The churchwardens accepted Dr Barry's offer and undertook to pay him £60 a year.

For that, James not only visited the sick and injured at the prison; he also undertook to visit the paupers at their homes – which would save the parish the ninepence a day it cost to have them treated at the hospital, and also 'enable me to direct health inspections, from time to time, of the poor, as by such means much illness may be prevented'.[14] Thus James began bringing to St Helena some of the public health improvements he had pioneered at the Cape.

Reed wrote a long, indignant letter to the Governor, complaining of the 'extreme hardship to which I am exposed … which must entail upon me very great inconvenience and injury … deprived of an income that I have hitherto derived from attending the Parochial poor of the island'.[15] It wasn't fair or proper, he argued, that military medical officers, salaried at government expense, should take on work that private practitioners depended on for their living. The Governor declined to get involved, but Reed went on and on protesting – claiming that he had agreed to provide the same service for £100 a year, with medicines found, but been turned down in favour of Dr Barry's lower bid. He also claimed – rather wildly and untruthfully – that he had 'never raised a fee' and 'never received one farthing although my attendance has been continually required and never refused'.[16]

He harped on the subject of Dr Barry having appropriated government money to support a practice that deprived others of making a living. This was a masterstroke: identifying Dr Barry's name with the appropriation of government funds. Middlemore decided that this was a good opportunity to take James Barry down a peg (despite the fact that financially it made no sense to let Reed do Barry's work, since the 'government funds' involved were Army salaries, not the island's funds). He studied the matter, and worked out a way to cut Barry out – and perhaps get rid of him altogether. A few days later, James received a letter from the Colonial Secretary:

> I am directed by H.E. to state that H.E. will not authorise the appointment of any person as Medical Practitioner on behalf of the Parish, who has not passed the legal and proper examinations in London … and that Dr Reed is found to be the only available M.O. whose services can be recognised in St Helena at present.[17]

Here was irony – an extreme version of the same argument that James had used to thwart Karl Liesching all those years ago, now used against him. But in this case it was not only unjust but grossly false, for of course James Barry *had* been qualified by the Royal College of Surgeons in London, and also possessed an MD from Edinburgh University – a qualification as sound and respected as any on earth – which was considerably more than that possessed by Mr Reed (who was only a surgeon, regardless of the Governor affording him the courtesy title 'Dr'). Demanding a London qualification was nonsensical and unprecedented.

If James replied to this outrageous decision – and he must have done, vociferously – it has not survived. But the churchwardens certainly did – they repeated their acceptance of Dr Barry's arrangement and that they were adhering to it. The Colonial Secretary informed them that they had no choice: the government would not support the scheme.[18] The churchwardens, outmanoeuvred and angry, sent the entire correspondence on the case to Lord Glenelg. Meanwhile, the Governor also made Mr Reed Health Officer of the port. All Dr Barry's schemes for improving public health came to an end. By this point, despite evidence of Reed's dishonesty, Middlemore was fixated on finding anything that would help him finally get rid of Barry. Unhappily for James, he found something.

*   *   *

Most of the records of what happened have not survived – not in the usual way with old documents, but because they appear to have been deliberately destroyed shortly after the event. But enough were preserved to piece together what occurred.[19]

It began on 8 October 1837, when Assistant Surgeon Eddie of the 91st Regiment was called to attend Captain John Thornhill, commander of the regiment's elite grenadier company, who was reported to be 'seriously ill'.[20] Eddie examined him, and found nothing physically wrong with him; next day he submitted a routine report to Lieutenant Colonel Robert Anderson, commanding officer of the 91st, advising that no officer in the regiment was currently sick (clearly implying that Captain Thornhill was malingering). There the matter might have rested, but Thornhill wasn't happy; he wrote to Colonel Anderson asking that a medical board be convened to review his case and determine whether he needed to be sent home to Britain for the sake of his health.

The commander consented; however, instituting a medical board put the matter beyond the regiment – the Principal Medical Officer would have to handle it, as repatriation was normally only permitted in cases of serious, chronic or preterminal illness or injury. Anderson wrote to Dr Barry, and Dr Barry duly headed out to the 91st's officers' quarters to examine the patient. On the way, he met Mr Eddie and they had a conversation that resulted in James turning about and going straight home in a fury, refusing to examine Captain Thornhill.

Precisely what Surgeon Eddie said to Dr Barry is not known, but the general drift of it emerged at the later inquiry. Clearly Eddie was unhappy about the case – he knew there was nothing wrong with the Captain, and it seems that the Colonel had taken it upon himself not only to order the examination of Thornhill but also to insist that his being returned home on health grounds be authorised. In fact, he had no such power.

This would be enough to put James Barry's back up and cause him to decline to visit the Captain. But it would not be enough to explain his extreme anger and disgust. The subsequent inquiry hedged and minced words for all it was worth, but the only inference to be drawn is that there had been an arrangement between Captain Thornhill and Colonel Anderson to have Thornhill sent home, and the 'illness' was a sham that they expected both Mr Eddie and Dr Barry to rubber-stamp. The rumblings that ensued might also indicate that there was more to it than this – not merely a commander doing a favour for one of his captains, but perhaps a stratagem to get rid of an unhappy, unwanted officer, or to avoid some scandal being revealed.

Whatever it was, the cordial relationship that James had previously enjoyed with Colonel Anderson and the whole officer corps of the 91st was torn apart. With typical lack of reserve and discretion, James let it be known publicly that there had been a disgraceful incident. In response, he was barred from the regimental officers' mess, where he had previously been welcomed. General Middlemore naturally supported the regiment.

Evidently hoping that this would be the lever that would prise Dr Barry out of St Helena once and for all, Middlemore ordered a court of inquiry, and wrote to Lord FitzRoy Somerset to report the matter.[21]

The proceedings – during which James apparently repeated all his calumnies against the regiment – did not run smoothly. The court found that the case against James was not clear, and it took five months of obscure deliberation before a conclusion was reached. When it came, on 21 March 1838, the decision – dictated by His Excellency the Governor himself – leaned heavily in one direction, fudging the details and ignoring the root cause of the matter (the apparent conspiracy between Thornhill and Anderson to rig a medical board and force the Principal Medical Officer to collude):

> The Major General entirely approves of the resolution entered into by the Lt Col Commanding and the Officers of the 91st Regiment, in removing from their Mess a person who, after having experienced their utmost hospitality and kindness, gratuitously brought forward unfounded accusations calculated to raise injurious reflections upon the Honor and Character of the Officers of H.M. 91st Regiment and Dr Barry moreover declared that these accusations have been transmitted by him to England.
>
> The harmony and high character of a Family Mess of Officers of the 91st Regiment have demanded this act of Justice to themselves and the Honor of their Corps. The Major General has perused with the deepest regret, the very gross and offensive expressions Dr Barry has made use of in his address to the Court of Inquiry.
>
> It is scarcely to be believed that Dr Barry could have been induced so far to forget his position as an Officer and a Gentleman, to make use of such expressions, not only highly insubordinate and insulting to a

Board of Officers assembled by General Orders – but also calculated to lower the character of a British Officer in the estimation of the world.

Dr James Barry is placed under arrest and is hereby ordered to return to England and upon his arrival will report himself to the Adjutant General of the Forces.[22]

'Lowering the character of a British Officer' forsooth; in a quarter-century's service, James Barry had seen every side of the British officer, and suffered no illusions about his character, about the dishonourable deeds that sometimes occurred under the rose, or about how precious an officer could be – sometimes hypocritically – about his public honour. But James had not, until now, realised the ability of a whole regiment to close ranks against him:

> Lieut Barnes 91st Regt, Town Major at St Helena will ascertain when a favourable opportunity may occur of which Dr Barry can avail himself for embarking on his passage from this command – upon the receipt of a Report from the Town Major that such an opportunity has offered, Dr Barry will be struck off the strength of this garrison.[23]

In sending copies of the documentation of the case to Lord Hill via Lord FitzRoy Somerset, Middlemore had the gall to add: 'I regret exceedingly that I have been compelled to order Dr J. Barry home under arrest, but it has become absolutely necessary that Dr J. Barry shall be removed from this command.'[24]

Undoubtedly the lives and health of the poor and sick of St Helena – especially the civilians – would be materially worse once Dr Barry left, and the life of Dr Hopkins significantly more hard-pressed. The population also suffered as a result of Middlemore's other self-serving decision – the ousting of James Barry and installation of Mr Reed the surgeon. Just two weeks after James Barry's dismissal and arrest, it emerged that Reed had been unable to cope with visiting the sick of the town *and* inspecting ships; this on top of the fact that he had been improperly charging seamen and passengers exorbitant fees for medical advice (10s 6d for ordinary seamen, 21 shillings for captains and passengers: astronomically high prices for an ordinary surgeon at that time).[25] In addition, shipping agents reported that Reed took bribes from ships, and when he ordered a Dutch merchant vessel into quarantine for no good reason, he blamed it on Dr Barry.[26] Middlemore chose to believe this preposterous claim, but it did little to ease his own embarrassment.

On Monday 2 April 1838, the very same day that Reed was reported to be charging his outrageous fees to credulous sailors, Dr James Barry was marched down to James Bay under arrest. Charles Dickens described the scene, based on an account from an eyewitness:

> On one of those still sultry mornings peculiar to the tropics, the meas-
> ured steps of the doctor's pony woke up the echoes of the valley. There
> came the P.M.O. looking faded and crestfallen. He was in plain clothes.
> He had shrunk away wonderfully. His blue jacket hung loosely about
> him, his white trousers were a world too wide, the veil garnishing his
> broad straw hat covered his face, and he carried the inevitable umbrella
> over his head so that it screened him from the general gaze. The street
> was deserted, but other eyes besides the writer's looked on the group
> through the Venetian blinds. No sentry presented arms at the gates,
> and the familiar quartet proceeded unnoticed along the lines to the
> ship's boat in waiting.[27]

James was rowed out to the Indiaman *London*.[28] He went aboard under arrest and in disgrace. As an officer he had no chains put on him, nor confinement on board. But it was unlikely he would be welcome among the ship's officers, with whom he would normally expect to socialise. It would be a weary and dismal voyage, with an ignominious homecoming to look forward to.

26

Friends in High Places

St James's Palace, London: Wednesday 18 July 1838

Three royal carriages escorted by the Household Cavalry rolled slowly off the Mall and into Marlborough Road. Since the new Queen's accession the previous year, St James's was no longer the main royal residence, and for this afternoon's levée Victoria had travelled the stone's throw from the newly remodelled Buckingham Palace.

Among the host of guests was an unusual abundance of European royalty and nobility – German, Dutch, French – and foreign ambassadors, here to pay their respects to the new monarch. There was the usual preponderance of generals, admirals, clerics and lords, sirs, honourables and plain misters, all waiting to be presented, and among them was Dr James Barry.[1]

Although Lord FitzRoy Somerset was present, on this occasion James's sponsor was Viscount St Vincent. Discretion was required; James's arrest, along with the preposterous charges against him, had been quashed as soon as he set foot in England, and in time all records of that unfortunate business would be expunged,[2] but it was known about in military circles, and some Irish newspapers had recently reported the court martial and acquittal.[3] It was best that Lord FitzRoy not be seen publicly sponsoring Dr Barry, whatever he might do for him privately.

Viscount St Vincent was a genial-looking old fellow, with flowing silver hair and gentle, fleshy features that concealed a ruthless side. He represented the Conservative cause in the House of Lords, and had a particular interest in Jamaica. In the wake of the slave uprising and the Abolition Act, the Jamaican Assembly had been sticking to its noxious principles and passing a series of measures that sustained slavery in all but name;[4] so now the Whig government at Westminster was planning to introduce a bill suspending the island's constitution and installing what the plantocracy called a 'dictator' to force them to change. There was opposition from all parties in the House of Lords, with St Vincent to the fore.[5] He had vested interests in Jamaica and was prominently involved with the association of absentee Jamaican planters and landowners.[6] At this point, the passage of the Jamaica Bill was still in the future, but St Vincent was keen for intelligence from any source, and James had been there for several years during the rebellion and aftermath. But unless James was uncharacteristically emollient – which he may have been, given his awkward situation – St Vincent would be unlikely to hear any facts or opinions to his liking.

Another person present at the levée was William King-Noel, who had just been made Earl of Lovelace. His wife, Ada, Countess of Lovelace, was of course not there; she might be one of the great mathematicians of the age, but women were not invited to events like this; their role at court was to look beautiful at parties and be steered towards good marriages.

James Barry was now the sixth most senior staff surgeon in the British Army; outside of combat and the purchase system – neither of which applied to doctors – promotion in the British armed forces was based largely on seniority, which was determined by time in-rank on full pay. With eleven years' seniority, James was now only a few retirements, deaths or promotions away from an assistant inspectorship.[7] As far as the Army was concerned, he was doing well for his age, since according to his record he was still under forty. But underneath, Margaret was now in her fiftieth year, and it would become harder in the future to sustain the focus and drive of a person ten years younger than herself.

After spending the summer and autumn in England, on 24 November 1838 James Barry took ship again for the Caribbean, cleansed of all dishonour. He had no notion whatsoever that he was heading into the most dangerous posting he had ever undertaken.

His new appointment was finely judged – the West Indies were in the swim of the British Empire (unlike poor St Helena), yet the Windward and Leeward Islands command was relatively out of the way. And he was not to hold a command position this time.

Before proceeding to his final destination – Antigua – James was obliged to call at the headquarters of the Windward and Leeward Islands command in Bridgetown, Barbados, a tiny inverted comma of land on the threshold of the Atlantic, as unlike St Helena as an island could be, and quite different from Jamaica too: thoroughly cultivated for sugar, with low hills almost bare of trees. Bridgetown was on the sheltered west of the island, and James landed there in early January 1839. It was a troubled place, where many of the black population were reduced to begging and outlawry.[8] This was undoubtedly the fallout from emancipation, which had begun the previous year and would be complete by 1840 – the liberated slaves might have their freedom, but their former masters were no longer obliged to feed, clothe or house them, and any whose labour was not required by the economy could be left to fend for themselves.

James was confined to Bridgetown for some days while he waited for a vessel to take him on to Antigua. Like Kingston it had something of a Mediterranean feel – the same low houses in buff or amber stucco with balconies and verandas; one visitor found it a down-at-heel place: 'the plaster falling off from alternate damp and sun, leaves dark ugly patches, which give a dilapidated look'.[9] Eventually James took passage on one of the myriad ships plying from island to island – cattle boats, American brigs, the colonial schooner, and the steamers that sailed regularly and cost the earth.[10]

The journey took James north past Martinique and Guadeloupe, where Private John Bulkley had suffered in the bloody campaign against the French thirty years earlier. Antigua, standing at the end of the chain, was one of Britain's oldest West Indian possessions, going back three centuries. It was larger and more interesting to look at than Barbados – a land 'fenced round by immense dusky-green headlands ... mountains, bold in outline and volcanic in their forms, their sides, serried into ravines by ancient streams of lava, give them all the grandeur of mountains of far greater height, a delusion assisted by their dark green vegetation.'[11] Between the hills, which sank away towards the northeast, were valleys cultivated for sugar.

The capital of Antigua was St John's, a pretty little port, but English Harbour, eleven miles away, was where the military strength was concentrated. There was a naval dockyard, and the garrison was housed on low hilltops overlooking the harbour entrance and separated by marshy ground. The total garrison was between five and six hundred men (mostly white), some of whom were stationed on Montserrat and Barbuda, both dependencies of Antigua.[12]

The hospital was on Shirley Heights: a building with two storeys and a basement, two wards for patients[13] and a commanding view over the harbour and the blue Atlantic. For all its greenery, Antigua lacked the coconut palms and forests of other islands; there was little rain, no rivers (other than small rivulets in the hills), and its climate was prone to drought. The mortality rate was generally below four per cent:[14] very good for a command in the West Indies. From now on, this would be Dr Barry's domain, as the island's medical officer.

The Governor of the Leeward Islands was his old friend and ally from the Cape, Major William Macbean Colebrooke, former Commissioner of Inquiry, who'd arrived in 1837 after a period as Lieutenant Governor of the Bahamas. One visitor found him 'affable and courteous', and he was a friend to emancipation, believing that Antigua had been 'greatly improved' by it, achieving it in a single swoop, without the long transitional period of 'apprenticeship' used in other colonies; he claimed that all the planters agreed.[15]

This was just as well, since of Antigua's population of thirty-seven thousand, only two and a half thousand were white.[16] The ethnic mix showed on market day in St John's, when people came from all over the island, forming a 'dense mass of all hues ... The ground was covered with wooden trays, filled with all kinds of fruits, grain, vegetables, fowls, fish and flesh':

> The whole street was a moving mass. There were broad Panama hats, and gaudy turbans, and uncovered heads, and heads laden with water pots and boxes, and baskets, and trays ... all moving and mingling in seemingly inextricable confusion. There can not have been less than fifteen hundred people congregated in that street – all, or nearly all, emancipated slaves ... At the other end of the market-place stood the Lock-up house ... The whipping post is hard by, but its occupation is gone.[17]

The lash might have a been a thing of the past for slaves, but not for British troops, for whom flogging was still a common punishment, particularly in hot countries where troops grew fractious and drunkenness and fights were common. The formula was well established and ritualised: the entire regiment formed up in a hollow square; two halberds were planted with their heads crossed, and the victim, stripped to the waist, was tied up by his wrists and ankles. The regimental drum major brought out the cat o' nine tails, made from knotted cords bound to the end of a drum stick. A drum rolled as each stroke was administered, and the victim's back was soon a bleeding mass of lacerations.[18] The regimental surgeons were required to be present – with the authority to stop the proceeding if they judged it dangerous: 'the instant a military culprit receives a lash,' stated an Army manual, 'the surgeon becomes responsible for his life – He is, in fact, paramount to the commanding officer.'[19] Invariably the surgeon was then left to deal with the results. One authority commented:

> Upon the number of lashes which a man may receive without endan-gering his life, it is extremely difficult to speak with precision. Five hundred lashes with the common army cats, was always considered a very full punishment; and although in former times I have seen many men receive more than this number, yet such punishments are generally to be considered as hazardous.[20]

Sometimes the injuries were so severe that the victim had to be hospital-ised. On these occasions James Barry – who as a staff man would generally have been spared the sight of the ritual – would see the worst cases, the men flogged to within inches of their lives. Margaret had once coolly told her brother that he must live with the consequences of choosing to take up the musket, and perhaps she still viewed such brutalities in the same way.

James worked away at the fruitless task of pestering the local Colonial Secretary for reimbursement of the pay he'd missed while under arrest at St Helena,[21] without success. On the brighter side, Antigua afforded plentiful opportunities for botany, the island abounding in plants with medicinal value: absinthe (wormwood), aloe, aniseed, rosemary, ginger, the hallucinogenic and anticholinergic jimson weed (*Datura stramonium*), which was useful in various afflictions from gastrointestinal to respiratory, lignum vitae (*Guaiacum officinale*), the tree *Quassia excelsa* whose bark was used as an appetiser and digestant, and castor oil. From this bounty, James could extend the personal pharmacopoeia on which he had been working since his days at the Cape. In July 1840 Major Colebrooke left Antigua to take up a new post, and in the autumn James was recalled to Barbados to serve as Acting Principal Medical Officer for the whole Windward and Leeward Islands command. The man in charge (Thomas Draper, James's old friend from Jamaica days) was retiring, and his replacement, Inspector General Dr Hugh Bone, had to travel from Corfu, which in the event took him over a year.[22]

The command was large, its constituent islands numerous, and the prevalence of disease sometimes calamitous. But for the first time in his career, James managed to get through an extended period in high authority without antagonising his superiors, getting himself arrested, court-martialled or threatened with imprisonment. His service earned him official thanks in General Orders.[23] James was now the Army's fifth most senior staff surgeon – slowly climbing towards command rank. When Dr Bone finally arrived, James sailed for Trinidad, where he was to take up a new post as Principal Medical Officer.

Trinidad was altogether different from the Windward Islands – far larger, with great tree-clad hills and camel-backed mountain ridges.

Sailing into the Gulf of Paria through the Bocas del Dragón, a bare three miles to starboard James could see the coast of South America – the fabled Spanish Main. That green band filling the view was Venezuela. At last James was in sight of the destination Margaret had intended to reach thirty years earlier. All of this – the disguise, the study, the terrible risk – had been originated in order to bring her to that land, where she had meant to discard 'James Barry' and be herself again, Dr Margaret Bulkley, living on her own terms under the protection of General Francisco de Miranda. Now Miranda was long dead on the far side of the ocean, and Venezuela was a different place – fully independent since 1831 but still torn by infighting and rebellion. Neither James Barry nor Margaret Bulkley would ever set foot on it. The ship turned towards Port of Spain, and the Venezuelan peninsula slipped slowly astern, never quite sinking below the horizon, a reminder of the changeability of life and the fallibility of plans.

Port of Spain – where Miranda had taken refuge after the failure of his first expedition – exuded warmth and colour. The bay had 'a very foreign air; feluccas, canoes and other odd-looking craft skim about', and the town was crowded with 'Indians, Spanish Americans, French, English, Bengal coolies, Scotch and negroes, from all sorts of places, speaking all sorts of tongues'.[24] Having been taken by the British as recently as 1797, it was still predominantly Latin.

James Barry's role here was slightly odd: officially the island was an outlier of the Windward and Leeward Islands command, staffed from Barbados, but in the coming year Dr Barry would make it so much his own that by 1843 it would be given to him as a fief within the command's medical staff.[25] His immediate superior was the Lieutenant Governor and Commander in Chief of Trinidad, Colonel Sir H. G. Macleod.[26]

Port of Spain, for all its attractions, occupied an unhealthy location near the great eastern marshes of the Gulf of Paria, with swampy ground between the city and the sea, but it was airy and set against a beautiful mountain backdrop. Only about forty to fifty soldiers were based in the town, with the rest dispersed around the island. James took a house not far from the barracks – where the hospital was also located, unhealthily near a swamp – and settled to his work. The hospital had four wards, and was on dry, elevated ground with clean running water from a rivulet. The annual mortality rates were about ten per cent for white, and four per cent for black troops,[27] the whites' worst afflictions being fevers and diarrhoeal disorders. (The Royal York Rangers had been stationed in Trinidad in Private John Bulkley's day, and suffered appallingly from fever; with war against the French and the hazards of disease, only the fortunate had survived that campaign unscathed – including John, his luck running good for once in his life.)

Smallpox and tuberculosis plagued the black soldiers, and James undertook a successful programme of vaccination. A large prevalence of leg ulcers was noted. Sir Everard Home of the Royal College of Surgeons had once stated that 'no surgical complaint incident to the soldier has deprived His Royal Majesty's service of so many men as that of ulcers in the legs'.[28] This chronic and disabling disorder usually occurred on the lower leg, developing from a trivial injury or an insect bite that became infected and produced a rapidly spreading and destructive ulcer. Those already debilitated – such as alcoholics – were particularly susceptible, and as there was no effective treatment the patient often faced amputation.

Chronic alcoholism was one of the most intractable problems faced by the Army in the Caribbean; mainly because drinking was not only tolerated but encouraged, with each soldier receiving his daily ration of a quarter-pint of rum. One senior doctor called the West Indian rum ration 'the most effectual means for destroying both the mind and the body – the moral sense and physical powers of the individual – the general discipline of the Army, and the national character of the country'.[29] All attempts to stop it invariably failed, usually due to the threat of mutiny. Alcoholism led to drunkenness, which led to disorderly behaviour and crime, which inevitably led to the hollow square, the crossed halberds and a chequered back. Attempts to substitute other drinks for rum (such as wine or porter) were quashed by local vested interests – sugar and rum being the Caribbean planters' staple products. James Barry opposed the rum ration, and repeatedly criticised it in his medical reports to London, apparently with little or no result.

Doctors had to cope with another side effect of this rampant alcoholism: delirium tremens (referred to as 'brain fever of drunkards'), which occurred when an addicted man was suddenly deprived of his drink – as happened if he was hospitalised (after a flogging, for instance). He experienced confusion, delirium and hallucinations. In one twenty-year period 'brain fever' was diagnosed in more than 1,500 men in both the Jamaica and the Windward and Leeward commands, of whom 217 died.[30] It was such a chronic problem that Sir James McGrigor, the Director General, sent out a circular to all Principal Medical Officers requesting detailed reports on delirium tremens from every surgeon.[31]

James set about the task with his only colleague then in Trinidad – Dr Henry Schooles, assistant surgeon with the 81st Regiment (the station was decidedly short on staff, with the regimental surgeon having gone home through ill health and James's assistant seconded to care of invalids).[32] Among Trinidad's 385 white soldiers, there had been three deaths from delirium tremens in the past ten months. Dr Barry's report stated: 'There can be no question but that the primary cause is the continued use & abuse of ardent Spirits.'[33] He went on:

> Delirium Tremens occasionally commences with ferocious Delirium but invariably where the paroxysm subsides it assumes the trembling nervous Delirium from which it derives its name; in many cases every species of Blue Devil torments the Sufferer inducing him, if not watched, often to commit suicide:– all stimuli cease to have effect:– the stomach rejects every thing & low mutterings are succeeded by stertorous breathing which precedes death.[34]

As for treatment, Dr Barry found that measured quantities of the standard range of 'stimulants' – brandy, champagne, opium, capsicum[35] – together with 'Keeping the Bowels open' and a 'light nourishing Diet' could be effective in the patient's first or second attacks. But the problem of addiction remained. As one patient put it, 'The weather is always so hot:– Rum always so cheap:– and man always so Dry.' Dr Barry suggested that 'perhaps the only chance would be to embark the subject in a Temperance Vessel* for a Cold climate, with plenty of nutritious Diet.'[36]

Endemic drunkenness notwithstanding, this was one of the quieter reaches of the Empire. Early in 1842, while James was still settling in at Trinidad, a piece of news came ricocheting through the Army that appalled everyone. The Empire had been more or less at peace for many years now – give or take the occasional colonial skirmish, there had been no wars, no real battles. Then India's Northwest Frontier blew up, and the British Army in Afghanistan was massacred. James's old comrade General Sir Willoughby Cotton had narrowly avoided the disaster; after leaving Jamaica he'd been sent to take command of the occupying force in Kabul, but had been replaced at the eleventh hour by the hopeless, worn-out General Elphinstone. After the murder of several British diplomats at a conference with the tribes, the Afghans had forced the British to retreat to India. En route the whole sixteen thousand-strong convoy was cut to pieces in the snowbound passes, entire regiments wiped out. The only person to make it through alive was William Brydon, a young assistant surgeon in the East India Company's 4th Light Cavalry, who rode into Jallalabad exhausted and – according to legend – with a broken sword trailing from his hand.[37] Britain and its armed forces were shaken to the core, even in the remotest, most peaceful outposts. Afghanistan was like an omen, the beginning of a period when war, not peace, would be the abiding state somewhere or other in the Empire.

For the time being, Trinidad at least was peaceful, and the only thing to ruffle Dr Barry's existence was the occasional affront to his sensitive pride. One of his old friends, Edward Bradford, who'd been an assistant surgeon with the 56th in Jamaica in 1832, was now in Trinidad with the 23rd Royal Welch Fusiliers. He recalled decades later: 'I had the misfortune to give him great offence by stating in an official report that he was probably 50 years of age.' It was a reasonable guess, and in fact below Margaret's true age. However:

---

* ship whose commander banned alcohol

He called the report a 'base attempt to blast his prospects'. Yet he for-
gave me afterwards. The same singular craving for authority and power
was here manifest in him as during his whole life. He was gifted with
much acuteness, and had a good memory. So long as he was treated
with deference he was good humoured, and would enjoy mirth at his
own expense; but if anything touched his importance, his anger knew
no bounds; there was no authority or station which he (secure in his
own importance) would not set at defiance.[38]

The higher James rose, the greater became the fear of falling. At the heart
of it was the fear of discovery – of absolute ruin. James's apparent age
had caught up with Margaret's actual age. In 1842 James was forty-three
years old, and Margaret fifty-three – and they had not been quiet or easy
years. Those around him believed that Dr Barry saw his own authority as
an entitlement. Combined with the volatility that came from the stresses
on Margaret's life and the constant risk she ran, this attitude was perceived
as overweening arrogance. A civilian physician, Dr R. T. McCowan, who
knew James intimately in Trinidad, recalled of him:

> He was a very bold person, and challenged one or two of our officials
> for naming him a diminutive creature. He had a favourite little dog,
> which he always carried about with him … He was highly respected,
> and was a frequent attendant at the Governor's levees. He was a strict
> vegetarian, and his regulation sword was as long as himself … I may
> state that Dr Barry was looked upon by some in this Island as the
> illegitimate offspring of some English nobleman, from the great influ-
> ence and haughty bearing which he used to possess.[39]

An officer who came to Trinidad to sit on a court martial was left with
a distinct impression:

> On the assembling of the court an individual appeared as spectator
> who at once attracted my attention. He was in the full dress of an
> army surgeon, but had all the appearance of being a woman. On
> making inquiries I was told that the individual was Dr Barry, the
> principal medical officer of the district. The impression and general
> belief were that he was a hermaphrodite, and as such he escaped much
> comment or observation in places where every one was used to him.

But I was under the belief that there had never existed a true human hermaphrodite so that I was convinced James Barry was a woman about sixty years of age, and being much interested in him I cultivated his acquaintance and we became very friendly. He frequently asked me to visit him, and I endeavoured to draw out his antecedents, but found him very reticent. The only thing that I discovered was that Lord Fitzroy Somerset … was a friend of his from which I inferred that it was to him Barry owed his high position. He was a vegetarian and drank only water.[40]

About 1842, after decades of exposure to exotic hazards and contagions, Dr Barry at last succumbed to a serious illness. The clinical features were not described precisely at the time, but it was a fever of some kind – some spoke of yellow fever, but it was more likely malaria.[41] It began with a visit from a female *Anopheles* mosquito, which would have existed in numbers in the watery, swampy land around the barracks. The *Plasmodium* parasite was introduced into the bloodstream via the anticoagulant injected into the victim through the feeding mosquito's proboscis. Following the bite, the disease would take from a week to a month to show. The victim experienced flu-like symptoms – joint pain, headache, shivering, vomiting, fever and jaundice (which could cause misdiagnosis as yellow fever). There would be long periods of delirium and unconsciousness.

Probably for the first time in her career as James Barry, Margaret faced two equally terrifying dangers: the possibility of a dreadful death, and the likelihood of her secret being discovered. Unable to look after himself, James was taken in by a female friend in Port of Spain; he made her promise that if he should die, his body must be wrapped in the sheet in which he expired, and then buried without examination. The persona of James Barry had become so habitual and so well known that Margaret now feared not only worldly ruin but also post-mortem shame. But ruin remained the first concern, and James gave out a strict order to all his medical subordinates not to visit him.[42]

One of them decided to ignore this instruction.

Dr Nicholas O'Connor was apparently not a particularly good practitioner. Despite seven years in the Army, he was still at the lowest surgical rank, and destined never to rise much higher. Quite possibly his lack of advancement was connected with his indiscretion and tactlessness. He was assistant surgeon in the 59th (2nd Nottinghamshire) Regiment, but was on the verge of quitting (or being ejected from) the regiment to join the medical staff, which he entered at the bottom rank – assistant surgeon (which was lower than its regimental namesake).* O'Connor would soon be heading back to England to take up his post at the depot hospital at Chatham, but for the time being he'd been placed with a regimental detachment in Trinidad.[43]

One day O'Connor happened to be out walking with a friend, Lieutenant Robert Lowry of the 47th (Lancashire) Regiment. It occurred to O'Connor that, in spite of the strict order against it, he ought to visit Dr Barry. 'I feel bound to call,' he said to Lowry, 'and see how he is.' True, it was worrying that a person with a severe febrile illness should refuse to see any medical attendant, but if O'Connor knew Barry at all well, he ought to know his probable reaction if he were disobeyed. O'Connor's urge perhaps sprang as much from curiosity as from professional concern. 'Will you come with me?' he asked, and Lowry agreed.[44]

The guest bedroom opened onto a veranda, and the two officers found the door unlocked; leaving Lowry outside, O'Connor went in. Approaching the bed, he found Dr Barry deeply asleep – a tiny, slight frame sweating feverishly beneath the sheets, the dyed red hair stuck to the pale forehead. O'Connor began a routine examination; after taking the pulse and the temperature, he drew back the sheets to listen to the chest.

Lieutenant Lowry, idling on the veranda, was startled by his friend calling excitedly from the bedroom. The doctor beckoned him frantically to the bed. 'See!' he exclaimed, raising the sheet and exposing the naked body. 'Barry is a woman!'

Margaret woke in a sick confusion, to find two men in her bedroom, staring down at her in amazement. Despite her bewilderment, she recognised them both, and realised immediately what had happened: the sheets were drawn back and her body exposed. The very thing she had most feared throughout the past thirty-six years had finally happened – discovery not by some busybody nurse or laundress, but by James's male peers – and *two* of them! Had she been less thoroughly, irrevocably exposed, these snooping interlopers might have received the full lash of the renowned Barry temper; instead, Margaret gathered her senses,

---

* The system had been revised: the rank of hospital assistant renamed 'assistant surgeon' and the old assistant surgeon's rank renamed 'staff surgeon second class'.

covered herself hastily, and pleaded with the two officers not to tell a soul so long as she lived.

Whatever their faults, they were both gentlemen, more or less, and they both swore.

A gentleman's oath ought to count for something, but it was a fragile thing to have as the only barrier between Margaret and disgrace, ruin and public humiliation. The riskiest of the two was Dr O'Connor; his discretion was in limited supply, and he did tell a fellow officer, Lieutenant Joseph de Montmorency of the 59th, on condition that he too swear to keep it a secret. So now there were three men who knew. By 1845 O'Connor was back in England, and the following year he took up a posting at the Cape of Good Hope, where he must have heard many tales about the peculiar Dr Barry and would be sorely tempted to tell what he knew. Margaret had no choice but to trust and hope.[45]

Among the victims of malaria, James Barry was one of the fortunate ones. He survived, recovered his health and returned to duty. He remained hard at work for another three years – by which time the three witnesses had all gone home with their regiments or to new postings, apparently thus far keeping the secret to themselves. Then, in the middle of 1845 James fell ill again with severe fever. This time the medical outcome was worse: it was the deadly yellow fever. The symptoms were similar to malaria, with headache, fever, muscle pains, fatigue, nausea and vomiting. After a few days the sufferer either recovered or entered the second, toxic, frequently fatal, phase. That was when jaundice appeared, accompanied by gastrointestinal bleeding and bloody vomit. A doctor with years of experience in the West Indies would recognise the disease immediately.[46]

Again James survived, but this time he was left debilitated, his constitution damaged and his body and mind too weak to continue in his demanding work. In late 1845 the assistant surgeon of the 19th Regiment, Thomas Longmore, was posted to Trinidad to take over Dr Barry's duties.[47] On 14 October James boarded a ship for England.[48]

Living in the small colonial community in Trinidad, Longmore became acquainted with the lady with whom Dr Barry had stayed during his first illness; he was told the story of the doctor's strange request not to be examined, but neither the lady nor Longmore had the slightest notion of the reason for it. The truth had left Trinidad, safe – for now – with the only four people who knew it.

PART IV

The Most Hardened Creature
1846–1856

The Navel of the Mediterranean

The news from India began its journey to England just as James arrived there, at Christmas 1845. Trouble had been brewing in the Punjab for months. The Sikh state with its vast, well-equipped, modern army threatened to invade British-ruled India. On Thursday 5 February 1846 *The Times* reported excitedly that the express overland mail from Bombay had brought the latest despatches; the Sikh army – horse, foot and guns in their tens upon tens of thousands – had crossed the River Sutlej on 12 December, and the British forces, scattered and outnumbered three to one, were fighting for their lives.[1] Britain went mad with anxiety and agitation, every newspaper full of speculation, with snippets of fact buried within, and it was the topic of discussion at every social gathering.

On Thursday 18 February Queen Victoria held a levée at St James's Palace, and James Barry, after months of recuperation, found himself well enough to attend. The Queen had married since James had last met her, and Prince Albert was there at her side. Lord FitzRoy Somerset was not present for once; the staff at Horse Guards were on an emergency war footing and had little time for socialising. The war was especially personal to Lord FitzRoy, as Arthur, the elder of his two sons, a major in the Grenadier Guards, was out in India as Military Secretary to the Governor-General.

So again James was presented to the Queen by a substitute: this time the politician William Lowther, 2nd Earl of Lonsdale, an old friend of Lord Charles Somerset.[2] Lonsdale, who was close to Margaret's age, had been a keen electioneer in his younger days, but had lost out to the Whigs. He now sat for the Tories in the Lords.[3] James took to him, and the feeling was mutual; this was surprising, because although Lonsdale had supported the abolition of slavery (as had most Tories), he'd spent much of the 1820s opposing the emancipation of Catholics. Margaret's family had suffered from the English repression, although James's necessary allegiance to the Anglican Church had forced him away from those roots.

Lonsdale was a lively character – an energetic, well set-up dandy with fine features (he bore a startling resemblance to Lord Charles), exquisite taste in clothes and a penchant for opera, and although he'd never married he was known to have fathered three children by three different opera singers. He had an intellectual streak, and was a Fellow of the Royal Society; Disraeli was said to have used him as the model for the erratic character of Lord Eskdale in his novel *Coningsby* (published in 1844), using him again in *Tancred* a few years later, where his attraction to talent and his tolerance of temper ('genius always found in him an indulgent arbiter'[4]) might explain his fondness for James Barry. He was soon added to James's small but priceless collection of sponsors.

In the few days following the levée news came that two dreadful but victorious battles had been fought against the Sikhs – including a two-day slaughter at Ferozeshah on 21–22 December, reckoned later to be the 'Indian Waterloo', the bloodiest battle ever fought by the British on Indian soil. *The Times* reported peevishly: 'We had hoped that the importance of the event … would have so stimulated the ordinary slothfulness of the persons to whom the publication of the *London Gazette*[*] is intrusted that we might have presented our readers this morning with a copy of the despatches.'[5] There followed a list of British officer casualties from the two battles; among the wounded of Ferozeshah was 'Major A. W. Fitzroy Somerset, Military Secretary to the Right Hon. the Governor-General, mortally – since dead'.

The following day, the *London Evening Standard* reported: 'We regret to hear that Lord and Lady Fitzroy Somerset are plunged into the deepest grief by the melancholy information received from India.'[6] Still, Lord FitzRoy knew the service, had helped his son into it, and must accept its dangers. Their second son – now their only child – was a civil servant. As for the war, it was over within weeks – one more extremely violent battle brought it to a close and British India was under control for the time being.

---

[*] paper responsible for military announcements

James Barry spent that spring and summer convalescing, and probably stayed for a time at Lowther Castle, the Earl of Lonsdale's spectacular estate near Penrith in Westmorland. By early November he was well enough to return to service, and travelled down to Southampton to take ship. For the first time in his career he was going not to the far corners of the earth but to the Mediterranean.

Valetta, Malta: Monday 16 November 1846

If the Mediterranean had a single pivot upon which military dominance of the region turned, it was Malta. Empires had fought over it for centuries, and since the 1814 Treaty of Paris it had been British. The key to Malta was the fortified capital of Valetta and its Grand Harbour – viewed from above, it resembled a gaping mouth: a vast expanse of harbourage with peninsulas projecting into it like fangs, divided lengthways by a long tongue of land whose tip lay in the harbour entrance. The teeth and the tongue – on which stood the city of Valetta itself – bristled with fortifications and around them lay the harbours and dockyards of the merchant fleets and the Royal Navy.

The P&O steamer *Achilles*, sails furled and paddle-wheels churning the blue water to foam, eased into the harbour.[7] On the Valetta quayside, companies of red-coated soldiers paraded, a military band was playing and a huge crowd had gathered. On deck, Dr James Barry, the station's new Principal Medical Officer, looked out at the parade, the crowds, the warships dressed in their best and firing guns in salute. The man they were honouring was his fellow passenger, Lieutenant General Sir Patrick Stuart, Governor of Malta, who was returning after a period of home leave. While Sir Patrick and his retinue went through the reception ceremony, James looked out from the ship's rail, out over the pale, warm stones of the city, the domes and arches, bastions and guns, all echoing to the drumming of the bands. When eventually he and John went down to the quayside, the troops were turning about with a crash of boots and marching off to the drums and pipes – 42nd Highlanders, the Black Watch, in swaying blue tartan, the 97th Earl of Ulster's with sky-blue facings on their scarlet coats, the West Norfolks, the Connaught Rangers, and the Royal Malta Fencibles, the local colonial regiment.[8]

It was a large, prestigious garrison for an island not much bigger than St Helena and a fraction of the size of Trinidad. Aside from its strategic importance, Malta was a popular posting – its pleasant climate and lively social scene attracted officers of both the Army and the Navy. For James Barry it was his first appointment as Principal Medical Officer in a major command, and his most responsible job since his time as Colonial Medical Inspector. Given his remarkable record for kicking over ants' nests and defying authority, a lot of trust was being placed in him by Lord FitzRoy and Sir James McGrigor; they could only hope he would repay it with good behaviour.

After settling into lodgings in Sliema, the peninsula forming the northern lip of Grand Harbour's mouth, James set about his work. Although he had only two men on his staff – a surgeon second class and an apothecary – there were eleven regimental surgeons and assistants, each regiment with its own hospital. In addition he had three hospitals under his direct control – Station Hospital, the small Chambray Hospital on Gozo and the great Sacra Infermeria* on the Valetta harbour front, built in the sixteenth century by the Knights of St John. Parts of it had been reused for purposes as various as a Royal Navy ropewalk† and Marsala blending, but it had considerable medical facilities, including an eighty-bed ophthalmology ward (trachoma‡ being endemic among soldiers in some stations).[9]

Less than a month into his posting, James managed to misbehave in a manner that earned him a severe reprimand – a record even for him. What motivated him to do what he did is a mystery. One Sunday he entered the Anglican Church of St Paul in Valetta during a service, went to the sedilia (the recessed seating in the chancel wall reserved for clergy during mass) and sat in it.[10] That alone was enough to cause grave offence to every person there, but rather than take action, the priest, the Reverend John Cleugh, Anglican Chaplain of Malta, seethed inwardly and carried on with the service, afterwards writing a letter of complaint to the Governor.

For a person who took religion very seriously, James's act seemed calculated to give offence – a specifically anti-Protestant offence. Given

---

* Holy Infirmary
† long space used for manufacturing rope
‡ contagious eye infection

Margaret's upbringing and the sacking of her father from the Weigh House, she would have had every reason to sympathise with the situation of Catholics under British rule (of whom there were thousands in Malta). And yet James had been more than thirty years in the British Army – which did not welcome Catholics – and had even made a good friend of the anti-Catholic Earl of Lonsdale. It may have been an anti-clerical protest by a devout but eccentric Christian or a personal spat with Reverend Cleugh. James Barry was, after all, beginning to acquire a record for antagonising clergymen.

His act in the church earned him an extremely stiff rebuke from Sir Patrick Stuart, who issued a garrison order barring such actions. The *Malta Mail* commented severely:

> We express our unqualified disapprobation that an officer and a gentleman presuming on his position should ... behave in so highly indecorous a manner, as Dr Barry is represented to us to have done. If a report has been done by the clergy to the Governor, they too are to blame for giving out of their hands the power delegated to them in things spiritual connected with the Church of St Paul. Had Dr Barry been properly punished, Mr Cleugh would have stopped the service till the Clerk or the Beadle had ordered the intruder out. We fancy that the little great man would have blushed turnips and cauliflowers, and the effects on his sensitive mind would have been even greater than that produced by the Governor.[11]

Fortunately, the incident proved to be a mere hiccup in Dr Barry's Maltese career. But he did act as arbiter in a case of officers causing offence. It originated in a really remarkable medical case. Lieutenant David Cahill, paymaster of the Connaught Rangers, had fifteen months earlier suffered an illness diagnosed as rheumatism, depriving him of his sight and the use of his legs. He suffered a number of relapses and was left with total paralysis of the left leg, partial paralysis of the right hand and arm, and permanent loss of sight in his right eye. His condition was probably multiple sclerosis, but this was unrecognised at that time,[12] and the case occasioned a good deal of discussion between James Barry and Cahill's doctor, James McGregor, regimental surgeon of the Black Watch (the patient had been left behind when his own regiment left Malta).[13]

Two regimental assistant surgeons upset Lieutenant Cahill badly by informing him of a private conversation about his case between Dr Barry and Dr McGregor: a conversation in which McGregor was alleged to have implied that Cahill was malingering, because he had opted for quack treatment by a civilian doctor rather than approved treatment from a military one. Cahill wrote a rude letter to McGregor accusing him of telling lies, but in fact McGregor hadn't said any such thing to Dr Barry. It was all very complicated, very nasty and very trivial, and James was forced to arbitrate. He was furious with the two assistant surgeons (whose names he didn't know). 'Here's a professional conversation between medical men which should be sacred and secret,' he wrote to the Governor; 'told to a patient, a poor, unfortunate sick man, and even the truth not told ... I do not wish to know who these two gentlemen were, as I should feel contempt for them and it would not be possible for me to have any confidence in them.'[14]

With his intimate knowledge of the disciplinary system (gained first hand), he recommended that Cahill be court-martialled for unbecoming conduct, since he knew he would be acquitted and that it was the only way to clear up the matter. His opinion of Cahill's letter was that 'no gentleman should write such a letter, and no gentleman should receive it', and added that 'I deeply regret being subjected to hold intercourse with tattling, gossiping individuals, who appear to me to have no regard for simple verity; but by their garbled statements endeavour to excite strife and discontent in the Garrison.'[15] Himself a maker of 'ungentlemanly' accusations and purveyor of gossip *par excellence*, James wrote these words without any appearance of irony. Of course his real concern was the breach of medical confidentiality. As expected, the patient was found not guilty and returned to duty.

Most of the parties involved soon left Malta as the garrison changed; the regiments were posted elsewhere and replaced by four battalions from the 44th East Sussex Regiment and the 69th South Lincolnshires. The 44th was a relatively fresh regiment; it had been one of those destroyed during the retreat from Kabul in 1842 – wiped out to the last man in a final stand at Gandamak – and had had to be rebuilt from scratch. The 69th had recently returned from service in Canada, and with it came James's old friend and colleague from Trinidad, Assistant Surgeon Henry Schooles, formerly of the 81st.[16] One man was left behind in the change-over; James had taken on a new orderly in addition to his manservant

John – Private Thomas Salter of the 42nd Highlanders, who was sufficiently content in his new position that when the regiment sailed for Bermuda in 1848, Private Salter stayed behind.[17]

The Malta garrison offered Dr Barry quite an array of unusual and fascinating medical conditions. There was one particularly odd case of rabies. As usual, it was fatal, yet the patient did not manifest the typical hydrophobia (fear of drowning in one's own saliva or any mouthful of fluid), neither did he become disoriented – according to James's report 'he was sensible to the last'.[18] This was probably an instance of the rare aparalytic ('non-furious' or 'dumb') form of rabies.[19] Tragic but very interesting. At around the same time, James was so fascinated by a case of bilateral testicular tumour that he described it in some detail in his annual report, even though he wasn't the surgeon involved. The patient had been seen the previous year with a right-sided scrotal swelling – thought on clinical examination to be a hydrocoele (a collection of fluid around the testis). However, during surgery a fleshy mass was found to be present having the appearance of what was believed at the time to be *fungus haematodes* – 'blood fungus' – a vascular growth, which was removed. It was in fact a malignant tumour. Following this first operation, the man was discharged from hospital after thirty-five days and returned to light duty. However, according to Dr Barry's report:

> After a lapse of four months, the left Testicle became diseased, a Medullary fungus protruded through the scrotum, rapidly increasing to about a quarter of an inch in 24 hours, great absorption of the scrotum taking place, the Testicle was removed by Surgeon Dr Dawson, aided by his assistant Dr Moorhead.[20]

The operation was as interesting as the condition; it was the first surgery in James Barry's career (as practitioner or superintendent) known to have been performed under anaesthetic: 'Surgeon Martin of the Naval Hospital administering Aether with a sponge which appeared to occasionally produce stupor interrupted by violent shouting.'[21] Ether had been first tried in 1842, and first publicly demonstrated in the United States in 1846. It was absolutely at the leading edge of surgical science, and still imperfect – leading to the bouts of 'violent shouting' when its effects failed. Unfortunately, there was a haemorrhage about three hours after the operation, necessitating further exploration and ligature of the

bleeding vessels. The patient remained 'in a delicate state of health' and
was invalided to Fort Pitt at Chatham. (Hardly surprising, as these highly
malignant tumours spread widely throughout the body, especially to the
lymph glands and the lungs.)

In 1847 news came from Margaret's homeland. The crisis in Ireland
known as the *Gorta Mór* – the Great Hunger – was out of control;
the potato crop had failed and people were dying in their thousands.
Charitable subscriptions were raised in England and throughout the
Empire, including the Mediterranean stations. Governor Sir Patrick Stuart
gave £20, the Archbishop of Malta £12, the Bishop of Gibraltar £5 and
Dr James Barry £5 – a sizeable sum, more than most individuals and one
of the most generous in proportion to James's wealth.[22]

However, as an Irishwoman who had lived on the fringe of the great
rebellion of 1798, Margaret must have been aware that the matter of
charity was a thorny one. The Irish nationalists saw the famine as a political issue; good food was flowing out of Ireland to the export market
while the people starved – yet another example of England bleeding
Ireland white. The 'universal sentiment', claimed one nationalist orator
to loud cheering, 'has been that we will accept no English charity ... The
resources of this country are still abundantly adequate to maintain our
population: and until those resources shall have been utterly exhausted, I
hope there is no man in Ireland who will so degrade himself as to ask the
aid of a subscription from England.'[23] Yet the subscriptions came; some
were saved, others died and thousands emigrated. And nothing changed.

28

A Question of Numbers

Casal Curmi, near Valetta: late September 1848

Two carriages rattled along the rough, holed road into the middle of the village and drew to a halt, sending squawking chickens fluttering among the pigs snuffling in the gutter. Several gentlemen descended, stepping gingerly between the pats of dung – five in Army and Navy uniforms and two civilians. One of them – a short, feminine-looking fellow in a red uniform coat – was seized by the arm and urged along the street by one of the civilians towards a ramshackle house where a policeman was waiting. The civilian conferred with the policeman, and his face lit up. 'Aha, Dr Barry!' he exclaimed. 'You cannot now crow over us – here are two cases of cholera!'

'I was shocked and disgusted,' wrote James later, 'at this unchristian burst of indecent joy:– these expressions need no explanation and on them I shall make no comment.'[1]

The odious civilian was Dr Collings, a physician attached to the colonial government; he, along with police physician Dr Chetcuti and several military surgeons, with Dr Barry in overall charge, had been ordered to visit Casal Curmi, a village three miles inland from Valetta to investigate a reported outbreak of cholera. The cause of Dr Collings's unholy delight was a debate that had been running for some weeks over a controversial outbreak of illness in the city.

It had begun on 6 September with the death of Benedetto Tonno, aged sixty-four, a citizen of Valetta; then in Casal Curmi there had been ten more cases, four fatal; then three more deaths among the washerwomen who worked for the Civil Hospital, 'in consequence of the excrementitious and filthy state' of the linen they had to wash.[2] All had been diagnosed as cholera. But not everyone agreed, and Dr Barry was one of the dissenters.

Unusually for him, he was being politically sensitive. In a place like Malta, special care had to be taken – the mere name of cholera spread terror, and if word got out that it was here in Malta – the navel of the Mediterranean – it could ruin trade, destroying the livelihoods of local people as well as harming the Empire's economy and security. Therefore doctors had to be absolutely sure before a diagnosis was given out.

It was particularly problematic because the diagnosis could be misunderstood, there being more than one affliction bearing the name cholera, not all of them serious; moreover, it could be difficult to diagnose, as several other diseases could cause similar signs and symptoms. The one to fear was Asiatic cholera – known also as epidemic cholera, which had first come out of India in the great pandemic of 1817–24, which James had witnessed in Mauritius. It didn't always oblige by presenting with the classical clinical picture: the dramatic onset, with unrelenting diarrhoea and vomiting, shortly compounded by profound shock due to the huge loss of fluids, followed – in the absence of sound treatment – by the rapid downhill course to circulatory failure and death.

Rumours had already escaped from Malta that there had been an outbreak on the island. The Governor, Richard More O'Ferrall (who had taken over the previous year), had been informed by Vice Admiral Sir William Parker, Commander of the Mediterranean Fleet, that the harbour authorities at Leghorn,* Naples and Civita Vecchia were quarantining all vessels arriving from Malta.[3] The Admiral had protested, and urgently implored the Governor to do likewise, but it was no good – the damage was already done. The outside world needed to be reassured that there was no cholera in Malta. O'Ferrall convened a Board of Health, made up of military and civilian doctors chosen and headed by Dr Barry. It was an eminent collection, including Dr Chetcuti (President of the Società Medica d'Incoraggiamento di Malta), two regimental men and a pair of Royal Navy surgeons, one of whom was Dr Andrew Millar of the Admiral's flagship, the 104-gun first rate HMS *Hibernia*.[4] They were required to answer the following questions:

1st Are you of the opinion that the Cholera of an Epidemic Character exists, or has existed, at Malta in the year 1848?

---

* Livorno

2nd What is the present state of the health of the island?

3rd Are you of opinion that clean Bills of Health may be given?[5]

It had been reported that there had been several cases of Asiatic cholera in Casal Curmi, and Dr Barry and his board – with the wider situation sharply in mind – had been sent to investigate.

The group entered the house guarded by the policeman. It was a wretched hovel, and the patient, a woman, lay on her bed without any covering, apparently unfed, sucking pathetically on a piece of orange. 'Nothing could exceed the misery and destitution of this poor woman,' James commented.[6] The local doctor said he had given her calomel (mercury chloride, often prescribed for syphilis, which was believed to have a purgative effect on the bowels) and opium. Dr Collings and Dr Chetcuti examined her, questioned her and 'in the most unqualified terms' declared it *not* to be cholera. Instead they concluded that it might be sporadic cholera, but not Asiatic – and therefore not properly 'cholera' at all, according to the awkward classification of the day.[7] All the doctors present 'fully agreed', according to James. The next case 'was a poor man, with a large family – his case was also unanimously declared not cholera' while 'the state of poverty and destitution was equal to that of the former'. The doctors managed to obtain him some food, which he needed more than medicine. (James happened to see him again some time later, and found him recovered.) Proceeding, the doctors found no cases of cholera among the reported victims, and James returned a report:

> That no case of Asiatic Epidemic Cholera has occurred on the island.
>   The island is Healthy.
>   Clean Bills of Health may be given, and we are happy to be able to add that all cases of bowel complaint with symptoms styled Cholera usual at this season are of a mild character and much diminished in number.[8]

Quite how the board reached that conclusion Dr Barry did not explain in his subsequent statement, but part of it would undoubtedly have been based on the number of people who were ill. Even if one found cholera-like clinical features, if there were only a few cases it was called 'sporadic cholera' or 'cholera morbus' and regarded as a different disease with a different prognosis.[9] The situation was further complicated by attitudes to medicine among the poorer Maltese people; they were often averse to taking internal medication at all, and when they did, it was often dangerous patent medicines. Dr Chetcuti reported that he had been 'consulted in two cases, in which the capsules of balsam of copaiba* produced acute gastro-enteritis, which in both was followed by the death of the patients'.[10]

The board resolved that military and civil medical officers must not use the word *cholera* to denote any recorded illness unless it could be firmly diagnosed as Asiatic cholera, and that terminal cases must be subject to post-mortem.

About a week after the visit to Casal Curmi, Lieutenant General Robert Ellice, Commander in Chief of the Malta forces, asked Dr Barry to visit the village again and review the situation. This time James took with him just Dr Montanaro of the Fencibles and fellow board member Daniel Armstrong, surgeon of the 44th (another old friend and comrade of James's, Armstrong had been an assistant surgeon at the Cape in the late 1820s).[11] The poor woman previously diagnosed with mere sporadic cholera was found to have died – of typhus, according to the local doctor. He reported two other new cases, and took Dr Barry and his colleagues to see them: a twelve-year-old boy lying on a patch of straw under some stairs in an open yard, and in a hovel adjoining the yard an old woman. Both showed signs of typhus. James commented:

These wretched beings were in the most deplorable plight, surrounded by filth and stench intolerable, without sustenance or support. In fact I feel inadequate to describe the scene and shrunk from it with horror. On speaking to the Civil Commissioner and the other persons present, we learned that every year the inhabitants of this village suffer much from Remittent and Typhus Fever owing to the locality as well as to their living miserably poor and crowded.

I shall only add the deleterious effluvia arising with which the atmosphere was impregnated from the many sources about Valetta, particularly about the residences of the swine, are sufficient in themselves to generate at this Season of the year manifold malignant diseases, severe and equally destructive if not more so than the so much dreaded Cholera.[12]

---

* preparation of sap from *Copaifera* trees, taken for lung, bowel and bladder complaints

James was angered by the rumours of cholera, which 'I regret to say, have filled the multitude with terror' and driven many to 'drunkenness, disease and not a few to death', and he took refuge in his religion, concluding that 'should it please the Almighty God to inflict this awful scourge on us, we have only to commit ourselves to the never-failing mercies of our Heavenly Father, and with deep humility and resignation bowing down to say "O Lord thy will be done."'[13] This fierce religiosity was extremely unusual for Dr Barry when referring to a professional matter, and perhaps an indicator of the uncertainty about whether the diagnoses of typhus and sporadic cholera really were correct, and the potential costs if they were wrong. For the disease had now spread to Fort St Elmo, the old star-shaped fort originally built by the Knights of St John at the tip of the Valetta peninsula, and was beginning to look awfully like Asiatic cholera.

Several men of the Royal Artillery had been taken ill and died within hours. Dr William Richardson of the Ordnance Medical Department had performed an autopsy on one man – Gunner Abraham Middleton, 'a fine, robust Soldier' – and was firmly of the opinion that it was Asiatic epidemic cholera.[14] On 6 October James himself autopsied another of the victims and concluded that the cause of death was 'a quantity of fruit in a marked stage of fermentation from bad wine and brandy'.[15] Yet Dr Richardson's autopsy and clinical report could not be rationally gainsaid – they showed the clear clinical features of Asiatic cholera. Of the eleven doctors who observed Richardson's autopsy, five shared his conclusions, two would not commit themselves and four disagreed. Among the dissenters were Dr Barry and Dr Armstrong, who would admit only to sporadic, non-epidemic cholera (and attributed some other cases to 'bilious mucous diarrhoea').[16]

In all, twenty-eight men in the St Elmo barracks showed similar symptoms, and only seven survived. Generally, medical officers were not prepared to diagnose epidemic cholera until an epidemic was clearly under way. By any reasonable metric, twenty-eight cases in an area as small as St Elmo's was an epidemic, but the doctors were not prepared to certify it based on a single autopsy. How many cases must there be before they would change their minds – hundreds? Thousands? Eventually the unhappy answer would emerge, and it appeared that the threshold was a rate of dozens of deaths per week.

Was James Barry being clinically rigorous in denying the presence of Asiatic cholera in Gunner Middleton, and thereby removing the foundation for declaring a potential epidemic? Or was he – again utterly unlike him – being politically expedient? For once in his life his nerve may have failed him, shrinking from making a diagnosis that would require the immediate quarantine of Malta, placing a halter on all its external trade, with all the vast economic consequences that would follow. James had tried to do the right thing many times before, and had often landed in severe trouble for his pains (memories of the Tronk and the Fiscal must have haunted him). Dr Richardson could afford to stick his neck out – if the quarantine proved unjustified it wouldn't come back to bite him; ultimate responsibility lay with the Principal Medical Officer.

Governor More O'Ferrall could make neither head nor tail of the doctors' conflicting opinions, and asked Dr Barry (via General Ellice) to explain to him the confusing terminology and the lack of agreement: 'It is very desirable that the Medical Officers should find some ground for agreement both as regards the credit of the Profession and the Safety of the Public.'[17]

With an obstructiveness that was more like his usual self, James replied: 'I regret that not being conscious of any expressions used by me requiring explanation, I am prevented from offering any, but I will most cheerfully undertake the task, if such expressions be pointed out.'[18] He produced an eleven-page letter explaining the differences between Asiatic cholera and other similar sicknesses. The key differentiating factor, so far as most contemporary doctors saw it, was whether or not a very large number of people became sick. When few cases occurred – even if exhibiting the classical symptoms of Asiatic cholera, or with similar clinical features – confusion arose. There were eight or more different names applied to these supposed non-Asiatic choleras: sporadic cholera, bilious diarrhoea or bilious cholera, spasmodic cholera, mucous diarrhoea, algid cholera, lienteric cholera, English cholera and so on – all of which Dr Barry meticulously itemised,[19] hiding the precariousness of his position behind semantics and the primitive state of contemporary medical knowledge.

In avoiding taking responsibility, James was taking an enormous risk. If Asiatic cholera *was* loose in Malta, with a constant, unfettered maritime traffic in and out, he was risking the spread of a deadly epidemic to Gibraltar, the Levant, Italy and beyond.

It was his extreme good fortune that this did not happen. The small epidemic of Valetta and Casal Curmi died out, and James Barry reaped the reward; the population, the civil government and the mercantile class – which had hung on anxiously throughout, torn between the fear of disease and of financial ruin – rejoiced, and attributed their economic salvation to Dr Barry. While the disease was still running its course, the *Malta Times* reported:

> A penny subscription is talked of to be got up in the island to purchase a suitable piece of Plate to be presented to Dr Barry for his having in his unremitted exertions and perseverance saved us from a calamity which by false assertions of some of the faculty might have tended to ruin many families.[20]

The very evening that story was published, Edward Doughty, a marine corporal aboard the Malta-based receiving ship HMS *Ceylon*, died. An autopsy was performed in the presence of nine Army and Navy medical officers. They agreed unanimously that Corporal Doughty had died of Asiatic cholera. He was one of the last of the few dozen fatalities. While it is unlikely in the extreme that any of them would have been saved if James had declared a cholera epidemic, it is certain that only the luck of the draw had prevented his inaction from causing thousands more deaths. He must have been acutely aware of this, and never again would he put political and economic considerations before medical ethics.

Two years went by in relative peace, and then cholera came back to Malta; this time it came like a whirlwind, and the island experienced its full, stark terror:

Medical Intelligence
THE CHOLERA ON THE CONTINENT

Vienna and Venice—This disease has recently made its appearance at Vienna and in Venice, and has occasioned numerous deaths.

Prague—... the cholera has been very severe in that city during the last three weeks. From the 16th to the 23rd June there were 57 cases, of which 28 proved fatal.

Algiers—The cholera has reappeared on the northern coast of Africa. It destroyed, in one day, at Tunis, 150 persons.

Malta—Letters from Malta of the 2nd inst. state that there is now no
doubt of the cholera being on the island.

London Medical Gazette, 12 July 1850

It could have come from anywhere – ships and people from every part
of Europe, the Levant and North Africa called at Malta, and traffic even
came from east of Suez via the land bridge from the Red Sea. The disease
first appeared in June aboard ships of the Mediterranean Fleet moored
in Grand Harbour, then made its way ashore and found a fertile ground
in which to multiply. It gained its first foothold among the soldiers of
the 44th Regiment in their barracks at Floriana, the inland part of the
Valetta peninsula, and then spread to the civilian population. Within a
couple of weeks there had been eighty-two cases and sixty people were
dead. Although not thought initially to be a particularly dangerous form
of cholera, it proved especially virulent among children.[21]

This time there was no debate and no prevarication; an epidemic was
declared, and quarantines were established at Naples, Leghorn, Corfu and
elsewhere on all traffic from Malta. By the second week of July there had
been 173 cases and 126 deaths. After that, it appeared that the epidemic
was in rapid decline,[22] but this soon proved to be an illusion; the worst
was yet to come. In late July the numbers steadied, and although the
infection rate went down for a while, the number of deaths stayed the
same; the men of the 44th and their families were badly hit. Not a single
infected person survived. In the Royal Navy the picture was quite the
reverse – the Mediterranean Fleet cruised off the coast, communicating
with the shore only by boat, and although there were hundreds of cases
of cholera among the seamen, they suffered only fourteen fatalities that
month.[23]

The doctors struggled to contain the epidemic, but they had no
certain knowledge of how cholera spread. The accepted view was the
miasma theory – that disease travelled in foul or 'vitiated' airs – but
most accepted that it was fundamentally a mystery. In England the previous year a physician called John Snow had published a pamphlet, *On
the Mode of Communication of Cholera*, in which he aimed to 'open up to
consideration a most important way in which the cholera may be widely
disseminated, viz., by the emptying of sewers into the drinking water
of the community'.[24] Snow adduced a good deal of epidemiological and
pathological evidence to support his hypothesis that infection entered

the alimentary canal from the water supply rather than infecting the blood through the air. But he had no notion of the exact means of transmission, which was a crucial problem, and his hypothesis hadn't been widely accepted. The *London Medical Gazette* felt that Snow had failed to prove his case, but 'deserves the thanks of the profession for endeavouring to solve the mystery. It is only by close analysis of facts, and the publication of new views, that we can hope to arrive at the truth.'[25] It would be some years before Dr Snow managed to prove that he was entirely correct.

What doctors did widely agree on was that the key to prevention was cleanliness. In that respect James Barry was ahead of most of his colleagues, but faced challenges in the confined, crowded spaces of Valetta and the deprivation and squalor of the rural populace. The vulnerable state of the city had not been improved by a recent redevelopment in and around the barrack complex of Floriana, where the ground sloped down steeply to the harbour shore. The old House of Industry had been converted into a new Civil Hospital, while a new House of Industry had been established by converting some buildings near the Lunatic Asylum, and a new prison had been built, all at a fairly parsimonious cost.[26] The result was a tightly packed, densely populated group of buildings hard against the curtain wall of the city fortifications on the harbour edge, with the Floriana Barracks in the middle, where the 44th Regiment was housed.

By the end of July the regiment had lost sixty-five men, ten women and nine children, while the units housed elsewhere, including the 69th and the Royal Artillery, had lost only a handful.[27] James was convinced that this was due to the layout and drainage of the new redevelopment, and wrote to Commander in Chief General Ellice's secretary:

> The Barracks are surrounded by a capacious (new) Civil Hospital facing S. East on the higher ground, an Infirmary below the Barracks on the opposite face immediately adjoining an extensive Cemetery, and the Quarantine Harbour. It is notorious that these Barracks and the suburb have been at various times visited by malignant diseases – Dysentery, Fevers, Ophthalmia and Cholera.[28]

James reminded the General that in 1837 there had been a ferocious cholera epidemic in Malta that had begun in this very spot. The drainage of the barracks was 'very defective from the absence of any flow of water'; there was one partly open sewer running through the middle of the barrack yard that carried the effluent from the suburb of Floriana and was regularly sluiced with water from a storage tank. The barracks had gun casemates instead of proper windows, so ventilation was poor, and the windows of the Civil Hospital overlooked the yard with the open sewer, which went through the curtain wall and emptied onto the rocks below, where the quarantine harbour was situated. According to the beliefs of the time, shared by Dr Barry, 'blowing upon these channels, blocks up the drain throwing back the vitiated air on to the contiguous buildings, which being inhaled must necessarily be followed by increase of disease with intense malignancy'.[29] He was incorrect about the vitiated air, but almost certainly right that the open sewer and the crowding of the buildings played a part. He concluded:

> I have no hesitation in averring that, at no very distant period, either the Barracks or the Hospital must be abandoned. The former have been temporarily vacated in consequence of the late mortality from Cholera among the 44th Regiment, even the Sentry's post has been shifted owing to the intolerable stench in the vicinity emitted from 7 or 8 (often more) dead bodies awaiting interment in the Dead House of this Civil Hospital.

General Ellice preferred leaving the sewer where it was and keeping it open 'as its cleanliness can be ensured by constant slushing', but otherwise he agreed with Dr Barry that the barracks had been harmed by the alterations to the surrounding buildings.[30] He particularly disliked having the punishment yard overlooked by the hospital, causing a 'total want of privacy' during punishment parades, which he considered 'most objectionable and an inconvenience to which the Troops ought not to be subjected'.[31]

By late August the *London Medical Gazette* was reporting Asiatic cholera in Alexandria and Cairo, Cuba, Schleswig, Brunswick and a few cases in London, while in Malta:

> The cholera still pursues its deadly course. Many hope it is on the decline, but it is to be feared that it is only subsiding in places where its ravages have been most severe, to commence in places hitherto free ... The progress of the disease is dreadfully rapid. On Thursday afternoon

Captain McQueen, of the Royal Artillery, who has but recently joined
the garrison, was attacked. At half-past 2 am on the following morning
he breathed his last, at the early age of 27 years.[32]

In September a man-of-war, HMS *Bellerophon* (a later namesake of the
vessel that had brought Napoleon to Plymouth), came in from the Fleet
to fill up with water and provisions; twenty seamen aboard came down
with cholera, several of them dying within hours.[33] There was little the
doctors could do even to alleviate the patients' suffering, death being so
swift, and nothing could cure them. All they could do was try to enforce
cleanliness and plead for changes in the city to assist it.

In October General Ellice sent copies of James Barry's report to
Governor More O'Ferrall and to the Quartermaster General at Horse
Guards, while James sent a copy to Sir James McGrigor in London. The
Governor was mortified – this was, he claimed, the first he had heard of
any objections to the building alterations. He drafted a lengthy rebuttal
of Dr Barry's report, 'to correct its manifold inaccuracies and exaggeration, for, if unaccompanied by the explanation and contradiction which
I am about to offer it would tend to mislead the department to which it
may be sent'.[34] First and foremost (and not very relevant in the current
circumstances) he pointed out that the building project had taken two
years, and that the plans had been available for scrutiny by all, yet there
had been no objections that he had heard of. He denied at length that the
arrangement of the buildings was problematic, and concluded that 'The
Poor House has always been remarkable for being Healthy, while the
Barracks have been for years equally remarkable for being unhealthy', as
if this proved his point, when in fact it confirmed Dr Barry's statement
that the area of the Floriana Barracks had a history of cholera and other
epidemic diseases. Two days later, the Governor sent his rebuttal to Earl
Grey, Secretary of State for War and the Colonies.

By early October the epidemic was in decline, and by the end of the
month it was over. The total number of notified cases throughout Malta
and Gozo ran to 4029, and 1736 people had died.

In November, worn out by his duties in overseeing the management of
the epidemic – for at sixty-one, weakened by illness, Margaret no longer
had the energy of youth – James embarked on a cruise to the Levant and
the Black Sea 'for the recovery of my health'.[35] On his return he received a
copy of the Governor's rebuttal of his report. As requested, James studied

His Excellency's letter and 'most carefully reperused and reconsidered my own Report' in the light of his comments, with the conclusion that 'I deeply regret and most respectfully decline to alter one single assertion in the Report alluded to, the correctness and truthfulness of which I still maintain.'[36] Restraining his habitual indignation, he added:

> His Excellency is pleased to call in question my zeal and foresight. I would simply respond that after a very long service in many parts of the World (and often under very trying circumstances) this is the first time either has been impugned, having endeavoured through life fearlessly and conscientiously, to perform my duty to my Country, my Sovereign and my God.

It appeared that for once higher authority agreed with him. The correspondence generated by the case passed not only through the hands of Earl Grey, but also Lord FitzRoy Somerset and the Duke of Wellington (eighty-one years old and back in place as Commander in Chief of the Forces). Wellington officially thanked Dr Barry for his services – one of the proudest moments of his military life.[37]

This was a good note on which to end a tragic period in Malta's history and James Barry's part in it. On 1 April 1851, accompanied by John and Private Thomas Salter, he boarded the iron paddle-sloop HMS *Triton*, bound for his next posting.[38] He had served Malta for four years and five months, and on his departure the *Malta Times* noted that 'the soldiers and the poor particularly, as well as numerous acquaintances amongst the first circles in the island will regret their loss'.[39]

29

The Most Kind and Humane Gentleman

When the god Poseidon wrecked Odysseus's raft, stranding him on the shores of Corfu, he set in train one of the great unfulfilled love stories of legend: Odysseus's lifelong adoration of his saviour, Nausicaa, never consummated, never openly spoken of. If Margaret recalled that story from her classical studies with Dr Fryer she might have thought of it now, watching the rocky green coast rising above the noon horizon, its shallow bluffs slipping past *Triton*'s port bow, and might have remembered a similar love of her own, a long time ago, thousands of miles away on another foreign shore.

Standing like a sentry at the threshold of the Ionian Sea and the Adriatic, the island of Corfu — a dagger blade of land forty miles long — had variously belonged to Greece and Venice, then to France under Napoleon, and had become a British protectorate under the 1815 Treaty of Paris, as part of the independent United States of the Ionian Islands. Ahead of *Triton*'s prow lay Corfu town, its bay dominated by the old round-topped fortress on the headland, with the Venetian citadel in its own huge fortifications of beetling square bastions of grey stone looming over all. Offshore, guarding the roadstead, lay the small island of Vido, and further west Lazaretto, named after its leper colony. Closing off the sea to the east, turning the roadstead into a vast anchorage, was the mainland coast of Greece and Albania.

Above the quays stood the palace of the British Lord High Commissioner, Sir Henry George Ward — a fine classical edifice in white Maltese stone fronted by the open Spianada* (currently used

---

* esplanade (Greek)

as a parade ground) and overshadowed by the massive citadel. The views over the town were spectacular – the battlements, the terraces overhanging the sea.

This was James Barry's new home. For over twenty years he had lived almost exclusively on small islands – Mauritius, Jamaica, St Helena, Antigua, Barbados, Trinidad, Malta and now Corfu – as if fate were trying to maroon him. In fact, he had been gaining valuable experience; hitherto, only islands had been small enough to allow a mere staff surgeon to hold command postings (which were normally given to deputy inspectors). That period had now ended; he was the most senior first-class staff surgeon on the Army List, and within two months of his arrival at Corfu, his promotion came through. As of 16 May 1851 he became Deputy Inspector General of Hospitals James Barry MD, his rank equivalent to a lieutenant colonel.[1]

Some room had been created at the top by retirements, including that of Sir James McGrigor, replaced as Director General by Dr Andrew Smith. Only six years earlier Smith had been a staff surgeon and actually junior to James, then leapt to his deputy inspectorship the following year and this year bounded to the very top.[2] (Smith was a brilliant man – a distinguished naturalist and an old acquaintance of James's from the Cape, where he'd served seventeen years; he had been given charge of Cape Town's Museum of Natural History by Lord Charles Somerset and subsequently became a friend of Darwin.) He wasn't the only one overtaking James Barry – John Kinnis, who'd been a lowly but gifted hospital assistant when James worked with him during the cholera out-break at Mauritius in 1819, had leapfrogged to a deputy inspectorship in 1844 while serving in China.

James had been held back by his period on half-pay at the Cape and by his reputation for waywardness, but his talent, his long service and the influence of his friends had kept him moving steadily upwards. Now, although Corfu might be only an island, as Principal Medical Officer his authority covered the Ionian Islands, from Corfu and Cephalonia to Cerigo* and all islands in between. It was a major command, right on the brink of a region of Europe where political friction was about to build to a white heat.

*   *   *

---

* Kythira

Directly under him James had a staff of three surgeons, three assistant surgeons and an apothecary. One of the surgeons, George Reade, was an aged veteran with medals from the Peninsular War and the War of 1812,[3] while another was James's long-time friend from Malta and the Cape, Daniel Armstrong, who had supported him through both cholera outbreaks. Armstrong had left regimental service and transferred to the staff,[4] his move to the Ionian Islands command was apparently arranged at James's request.

There was a large British force at Corfu, with seven infantry regiments in all, plus artillery.[5] There were several hospitals to be inspected, including two within the citadel itself, where the commanding officer, Major General Charles Conyers (another Peninsular veteran), had his headquarters. James inspected both, along with the barracks, and rode across the island to look at the convalescent hospital in the old monastery on the peninsula at Palaiokastritsa, the very bay in which Odysseus was said to have landed and been found by Nausicaa; it was a beautiful spot in which to convalesce – a wooded promontory with views over the blue bay and the white stone bluffs and cliffs. To inspect the rest of his domain, James had to travel by sea.

As in Malta the general health of troops in the command was good for an overseas station. Even so, on average the entire garrison strength would be seen by the hospital staff at some point each year, with over 1100 admissions per 1000 troops, with every affliction from fevers to ulcers, venereal disease, and injuries from accidents, fights and punishment. This better-than-average record was partly due to improvements in the barracks, but also the age of the troops; in 1837 the Army had introduced a regular system of rotation whereby most regiments, having had a period of recruitment and build-up in Britain, served three or four years in the Mediterranean, then a similar period in the West Indies, followed by another in Canada, with the result that the average age of troops in the Mediterranean was lower than elsewhere.[6]

The classes of disease were different in the Ionian Islands from those in Malta, with a worrying number of 'paroxysmal fevers' (malaria and yellow fever) that were virtually unknown in the other Mediterranean commands. Notably, health was best on Corfu and Paxos, close to the centre of the command, and worst on Zante, an outlier. For the Principal Medical Officer it was a tricky command to supervise, especially an officer as meticulous and active as Dr Barry, and it required a lot of sea travel.

James's health and fitness were not what they had been. The artificial distinction between his and Margaret's ages was becoming meaningless. Margaret was in her sixties, and James looked it, and nowadays Dr Barry was more a figure of humorous remark than of curious gossip; an elderly eccentric, irascible but kindly, with his odd diet and teetotalism, followed everywhere by his growing menagerie of dog, cat and parrot, and given a leeway not generally granted to the young.

At about this time an anonymous artist (said to be Edward Lear, who toured the Ionian Islands in the 1850s) drew a pen-and-ink caricature of the doctor in the full dress uniform of a deputy inspector general – the coatee with huge epaulettes, the high-crowned bicorne hat, rank insignia on his cuffs, trousers with stripe, boots and spurs, a gleaming sword, and his ever-present fly-whisk riding crop.[7] Although he was a little stooped, he maintained the classic officer's posture: knee bent, hand resting on the hilt of the sword, which was slung fashionably low so that it would serve like a dandy's cane and had to be carried to prevent it dragging on the ground. The years had brought out the Bulkley-Barry features to the full – the Ciceronian nose accentuated and the underlip protruding in the permanent semblance of a scowl.

Age blurs the distinctions of sex, and his servant Thomas Salter, despite years in his company, never guessed that Dr Barry was female; he thought him delicate but not suspiciously so, and regarded him as a sort of kindly martinet – a tyrant to his subordinates but tirelessly caring for the health and welfare of the men in his charge. He was obsessed with cleanliness, and when the troops were lined up in ranks for medical inspections, he would pass among them, muttering in his squeaky voice, 'Dirty beasts! Dirty beasts! Go and clean yourselves!'[8]

He was unpopular among some of the senior officers for his 'interfering ways', but one man of the Royal Engineers at Corfu who was treated by him during a life-threatening illness recalled that there must be 'many officers and a great many of the ex rank and file who remember [him] with gratitude'.[9] One of James's junior assistants in Corfu – a compounder or medicine mixer – told a friend what it was like to follow him on his ward rounds, loaded with the day book and patients' medical records, which he was required to consult on the doctor's orders:

He was punctuality itself and he insisted on the medical officers being at the hospital in uniform, to meet him on his approach. To the sick,

however, Dr Barry was the most kind and humane gentleman he ever
met; but patients who contracted disease through their own folly – and
there were not a few – he would not look at.[10]

On one occasion Dr Barry found this same assistant sitting by the bed of
a dying soldier, an old schoolfriend, writing a letter to his parents. James
was touched, and 'The doctor complimented him on his good, and as he
termed it, humane conduct, sent his servant for him in the evening, and
presented him with a few dollars, and a dozen blood oranges for the sick
patient. He, poor young man, was past all earthly help, and died a few
days later.'[11] James received regular deliveries of fruit by the mail steamer
from Naples and Sicily, and often called the assistant to his quarters to
give him 'a few choice oranges for some poor sufferer' and a dollar for
himself. James took a liking to this young man and offered to use his
influence to help him get into the medical profession. But 'carried away
by the unreasoning silliness of youth' and not liking the idea of being
shot at, the young man declined, 'much to the doctor's surprise, if not
disgust'.[12]

On Wednesday 5 April 1852, after a year in Corfu and a total of nearly six
years in the Mediterranean, James departed for ten months' home leave.[13]
    He took his time getting home, arriving in England in mid-May.
In London he took the finest lodgings he could afford; he was now
on a decent Army salary (over £540 a year), and with no dependants
his expenditure was modest. Moreover, now that he was off-duty he
was able to take private patients – specifically his friend the Earl of
Lonsdale, becoming his personal physician.[14] He took rooms in Down
Street, between Piccadilly and Park Lane,[15] a choice probably determined by associations with Lord Charles Somerset (Lady Mary, now
in her sixties, lived nearby). As a keen equestrian, James would have
been attracted by the nearness of Hyde Park and the Row, where
gentlemen and ladies went to ride and drive on the tree-lined avenue
and be seen by the *beau monde*. As everywhere, he made an impression
in society. One little girl who became acquainted with him about this
time recalled years later:

He was very short and spare, and a smooth, not very prepossessing face,
scanty and carroty locks and a high, thin voice which might be termed

squeaky, but he was considered very clever and a skilful surgeon and
much respected. He seemed to seek the society of nice young girls and
I have heard my eldest sister joke about his intentions to her.[16]

Margaret, of course, had never experienced life as a mature woman; all she
had to draw upon was her girlhood, so may have been attracted to these
girls for that reason – perhaps, indeed, she was striving for a long-lost past.

James spent the summer between leisure, socialising and occasional
work, looking forward to spending the harvest season at the Earl's
Westmorland estate, Lowther Castle. Then, on Wednesday 15 September,
the whole of England was shaken; a black-bordered panel appeared in *The
Times*: 'Death of the Duke of Wellington'; the previous day, he had been
'seized with illness' while staying at his official country residence, Walmer
Castle near Dover, and died the same afternoon.[17] He was eighty-three
years old. The nation was shocked; the Iron Duke was invulnerable, with
no signs of illness and still working hard as Commander in Chief of the
Forces. The following day, more details emerged:

> A sudden death, caused by fits of an epileptic nature, at a very advanced
> age, left no opportunity for final adieus or parting words. The usual
> interval of sickness and suffering was spared to an exhausted frame,
> bowed down by the weight of years ... the Duke ... was permitted to
> pass from the present scene so silently that the exact moment of his
> departure could not be detected by those who watched his deathbed.[18]

James Barry would always treasure the memory of the thanks he had
received from Wellington after the cholera at Malta, but never spoke of
the earlier impingement on Margaret's life when, as Sir Arthur Wellesley,
he had planned and plotted with Francisco de Miranda to bring about a
military expedition to Venezuela – the liberation that never was – before
being diverted to the Peninsula and immortal fame.

The funeral – expected to be the public event of the year, if not the
decade – would take two months to plan. In the meantime, James and
Lord Lonsdale travelled north to Lowther Castle. A railway now ran
all the way from London to the northwest, with stations at Penrith and
Carlisle. England was a brave new world indeed, full of progress, smoke
and industry – and grinding poverty – all starkly visible from the train
windows.

Lowther was a magnificent spread – a fine turreted stately home with sweeping wings, huge walled formal gardens, and hundreds of acres of rolling, wooded parkland on the fringe of the Lake District, a couple of miles from Ullswater. Later that month they travelled on to Lonsdale's estate on the coast, Whitehaven Castle, where he was to host the West Cumberland Agricultural Society's show in his grounds. James became a well-known figure in Whitehaven, going for morning rides with Lonsdale's cousin, Eleanor Lowther, the unmarried thirty-three-year-old daughter of the Rector of nearby Distington, so often that a local paper later remarked that he must be 'that lady's *beau ideal* of a *perfect man*'.[19]

The Agricultural Society show got thoroughly rained on, and wasn't well attended.[20] James was guest of honour at the gala dinner that evening. When the toasts were made, the Earl rose to his feet and proposed the Army and Navy. (Cheering.) He spoke about the death of the Duke of Wellington – 'I believe that his name will live among men as long as the history of the country is known on the earth.' (More cheering.) The *Carlisle Journal* reported: 'The noble Earl concluded by coupling the toast with the name of Dr James Barry, army physician.'[21] Brimming with pride, James rose and replied on behalf of the Army.

That October, amidst the flood of grief and adulation towards Wellington and all those closely associated with him, Lord FitzRoy Somerset was raised to a barony, becoming the 1st Baron Raglan, of Raglan, in the County of Monmouth,[22] and James was included in the quiet family celebration of the event. There had been some doubt as to whether Lord FitzRoy could afford to be ennobled in this way (it carried quite significant fees, and he wasn't a rich man), but Prince Albert, on behalf of the Queen, offered to pay on his behalf. Shortly afterwards Lord Raglan moved from his post as Military Secretary to the Commander in Chief and became Master-General of the Board of Ordnance, a cabinet-level post that Wellington had once held.

At last, on Thursday 18 November, the great funeral took place – a vast affair that was reckoned to cost £80,000.[23] The weather was appropriately grim, after a night of heavy rain and with a slate sky threatening more. The immense procession, beginning at Horse Guards, went along Piccadilly, where James would have been among the thousands of spectators. The decorated hearse – made from eighteen tons of bronze from French cannon captured at Waterloo – was so large and lofty that the Duke's coffin, with his hat and sword laid on it, had had to be lifted aboard with a crane. It was accompanied by a fleet of coaches; every great military man of the day was there (including Lord Raglan), along with a host of coroneted heads (Queen Victoria came out onto the balcony of Buckingham Palace to pay her distant respects while the procession paused for her). The cortège was escorted by companies and squadrons of soldiers – all the regiments of Horse and Foot Guards and most of the infantry and cavalry regiments whose names were associated with the Duke and his victories: the Rifle Brigade, Scots Greys, Life Guards, and more. The succession of columns kept on coming, horse, foot and guns, and only spectators perched on the rooftops could see its whole extent at once. The pavements and park railings were jammed with people, many of whom had camped overnight, and on Piccadilly, *The Times* reported, 'the windows and balconies were completely occupied by the families who inhabit them and their friends'.[24] In fact, many of the people were neither – householders all along the route had been advertising for weeks, offering to let windows, rooms and even whole floors for the day, with prices ranging from a guinea to £20.[25] James Barry would not have had a view from his rooms in Down Street, but would have found space with one of his friends. If he was rash enough to go into the streets, he must have been swamped; every open space was thronged, the ends of the streets opening onto Piccadilly 'completely built up with living masses of men and women, forming, to all appearances, a mound or rampart of heads, which were all duly and respectfully uncovered'.[26] It was the same along the whole route to the City and St Paul's Cathedral, where the service took place.

For once a vast state funeral was entirely justified; the Duke of Wellington was sincerely mourned, having been a legend during his lifetime. And he was one of those rare figures whose fame would continue through the lapse of centuries.

By March 1853 James's period of leave was drawing to an end, and on the 2nd he began his journey back to Corfu. On this occasion, for the first time in his career, he journeyed by land. Lord Raglan had suggested to him that he visit Vienna, where Raglan's brother-in-law Lord Westmorland was British Ambassador. (Raglan and Westmorland were old comrades from their time as aides to Wellington, and had both married daughters of the Earl of Mornington. Westmorland's family also had connections with the earls of Lonsdale.) Raglan provided James with a letter of introduction and off he went.

Well-travelled as he was, James had never visited Continental Europe. It could be a primitive place to travel; while the railways had already snaked their way across much of Britain, in France most journeys were still by road. James, used to waterborne transport and reasonable comfort, would more likely have chosen to go up the Rhine by steamboat, taking the railway across Germany and a final steamer down the Danube to Vienna. Accommodation in southern Germany would not be at all to James's taste: unclean inns in which man and beast lived in offensive proximity. As one contemporary guide expressed it, 'The extreme disregard for cleanliness and sweetness, which is most annoying and disgusting to Englishmen, merits the utmost reprobation. The Germans themselves do not seem to be aware of it: let it be hoped that their increased intercourse with the English will introduce a taste for cleanliness.'[27] Crossing from the German to the Austro-Hungarian Empire was a polite but officious business; the list of contraband included all cigars, tobacco and snuff (tobacco being an imperial monopoly in Austria) as well as playing cards, almanacs and sealed letters.[28]

Austria was an interesting as well as a beautiful country, with a progressive public health system − very much to James Barry's taste − in which each district had medical officers who were paid by the state for attending the poor; the vending of food was also regulated to prevent the sale of unwholesome stuff, and selling medicines was prohibited without a licensed physician's prescription.[29]

Vienna was gorgeous but expensive, and the authorities even more draconian than in Germany; James's passport was taken from him on entering the city and his details recorded; as a British subject, he was treated politely, while people of other nations were subjected to an inquisition. Eventually he was issued his *passierschein* − a ticket without which he would be unable to leave Vienna (it was impossible even to obtain post horses without written permission from the Office of Foreign Affairs).[30] As a guest of the British Embassy, he was in a slightly more privileged position, but still had to observe the rules.

The Embassy itself was worth travelling a distance to see − it occupied the Coburg Palace in the Seilerstätte (between the imperial Hofburg Palace and the Stadtpark), a magnificent confection of Viennese Palladian in white marble fronted by tiers of pillars, high windows and statuary.

Lord Raglan's letter having gone ahead of him, James was invited to dinner with Lord Westmorland and his family. They had been warned to expect a person of peculiar appearance, but assured that he was a man of great ability. As it happened, Lord Raglan had done James few favours in directing him here; although Lord and Lady Westmorland were polite and respectful (a rather soulful-looking couple, he with drooping, sleepy eyes, she with a pretty, dreamy stare), the youngsters were not. Their eldest daughter, Lady Rose, recalled of Dr Barry:

> When he arrived we saw a small man with small features, a very smooth, though wizened face, very fair (not red) hair and a most peculiar squeaky voice and mincing manner, the whole effect of which was so irresistibly comic that it kept all the youngest members of the party in agonies of suppressed laughter all through the dinner (which is probably the reason why my recollection is so vivid). My mother, whom he sat next to, however, said that in spite of his ludicrous appearance his conversation was most interesting, though his manner was that of a mincing old maid![31]

(When in later life she heard the truth about James Barry, Lady Rose altered her view, perceiving instead an 'adventurous, strong-willed girl, consumed with a passion for surgery and medicine' who 'could find in those days no possible training in what was her ruling passion, and so adopted this extreme course' and 'earned the respect and esteem of her colleagues and superiors'.)[32]

From Vienna James travelled on to Trieste, where a ship took him down the Adriatic to Corfu, where he resumed the reins on April Fool's Day 1853 – just in time for the build-up to war.

30

Prodigality and All Wickedness

It was conceived as a war of religion – Islam in collision with two opposed brands of Christianity – but, as usual, beneath the surface lurked the vying of nations for power and strategic influence. Strange alliances had been formed to serve the needs of the moment, and the whole thing got wildly out of hand.

There had been rumblings east of the Ionian since the very beginning of James Barry's time there. As was so often the case that century, the trouble began in France. In late 1851 Louis-Napoleon, President of the Second Republic, yearning for the greatness of his uncle Napoleon Bonaparte, staged a coup and had himself proclaimed Emperor Napoleon III. He then embarked on a plan to make France powerful again. To do this he needed Catholic support, and decided that the best way to achieve it was to gain ascendancy for the Catholic Church in the Holy Land of Palestine, which was in the possession of the declining Ottoman Empire. The Eastern Orthodox Church was currently the representative of Christianity there, and supplanting it would put France one-up against its old enemy, Russia. It was a plan with no apparent flaws, from Emperor Napoleon's viewpoint. The French Ambassador forced Sultan Abdülmecid I to recognise French Catholic protection of Christian sites in Palestine, but Tsar Nicholas I countered with diplomatic pressure of his own, and forced the Sultan to tear up France's treaty and continue his existing agreements with Russia.

In response, Napoleon despatched the new eighty-gun ship of the line *Charlemagne* to the Black Sea – a show of force that was in violation of international law. The Sultan caved in and agreed a new treaty with the French. Tsar Nicholas I, unable to match France's naval power, sent two armies to occupy Wallachia* north of the Danube, threatening Ottoman territories to the south. At this point, the Russians saw the faithless Ottomans as the greater enemy, and in early 1853, just as James Barry was on his way back to the Mediterranean, the Tsar began using diplomatic channels to try to ensure that neither France nor Britain would intervene if Russia went to war with the Ottoman Empire. His diplomacy with the Sultan was aggressive, and with Britain charming.

But the British weren't having it. Although they'd allied with Russia against Napoleon I, they now saw the Russians as a threat to British possessions in Asia; indeed, this had been at the root of the recent crises in Afghanistan and the Punjab – tensions brought about by Britain's attempt to secure the northwest door of India against the Russian Bear. The prospect of the Tsar gaining further power in the Black Sea and greater influence in the Levant was profoundly worrying. Accordingly, Britain and France combined to send a naval task force to the Black Sea to protect Constantinople, while Russia prepared to seize Ottoman territories in Moldavia and Wallachia.[1]

The British government, under the Earl of Aberdeen and the hawkish Foreign Secretary Lord Palmerston, pushed hard against Russia; Benjamin Disraeli, for the Opposition, accused the government of careless aggression that would make war inevitable. But the public were all for it, whipped into a jingoistic fervour by the conviction that defending against Russia was essential for the preservation of freedom from tyranny.[2] In the House of Lords, the Marquess of Clanricarde, a former ambassador to Russia, spoke out against Russian aggression, and with the wilfully short memory of the politician, added that he could not speak highly enough of 'the loyalty, good faith, and honour of the Emperor of the French'.[3] The House cheered him to the rafters. Soon the country, in alliance with both France and the Ottoman Empire, was fully at war with Russia. The conflict centred on the Danubian territories and the Russian Black Sea port of Sevastopol in the Crimea. Eventually the Danube would be abandoned, and the Crimea would be the exclusive focus of fighting.

In February 1854 Lord Raglan was released from his dull duties at the Board of Ordnance and given overall command of the Eastern Army, and

---

* historic nation bordering the Black Sea, comprising parts of Bulgaria, Hungary and Moldavia

shortly afterwards sailed off to join the huge Anglo-French force in the Black Sea.[4] Suddenly Britain's strategic footholds in the Mediterranean assumed an importance they hadn't had since 1815; and of them all, the closest to the scene of the action was the Ionian Islands command.

When James returned in spring 1853, he found Corfu all but overrun with British troops. There'd been just four regiments in the garrison when he left; now there were ten.[5] Most were here temporarily, as part of the military build-up occasioned by the growing crisis. Barracks crammed to bursting, officers' messes springing up everywhere, the shops and parks teeming with subalterns and the streets and taverns with rankers, while officers and seamen from the fleet of transports and warships took up what little space was left.

There was also an unsettling shock for James. Among the new arrivals stationed on the island of Vido were his acquaintances from Trinidad, the 47th Lancashires, including Captain Robert Lowry, one of the three officers who knew James's secret. Lowry was married in Corfu in June,[6] and within a few months the 47th transferred to Malta. Lowry continued to keep James's secret to himself.

This was just as well, since the last thing James needed was more stress. With war looming, there was heightened tension everywhere, more drinking than ever, more whoring and more fights; a Presbyterian missionary deplored 'this scene of prodigality and all wickedness' and was dismayed that so many soldiers rejected his 'bread of life'.[7] Regardless of questions of morality, such behaviour caused more injuries, more venereal disease, more floggings and more strain on the medical services. Each regiment had its own surgeons, but it all had to come under the authority of the Principal Medical Officer.

As if this wasn't bad enough, certain regimental commanders insisted on tyrannical regimes of parade-ground drill for their men. In the hottest weather, on the baking Spianada, troops marched and sweated in their heavy serge, pipeclayed crossbelts and packs, the fortress walls echoing ceaselessly to the crash and stamp of their boots and the screams of the sergeants. Inevitably the number of admissions for heatstroke increased. One of the worst was Lieutenant Colonel William Denny, the commanding officer of the 71st Highland Light Infantry, which had previously been stationed at Cork, and so were hardly acclimatised to the Mediterranean heat;[8] he marched his men constantly, even in the full glare of the sun. James would see them in their flat-topped kepis and thick tartan trews (unlike their fellow Highlanders the 92nd Gordons, also at Corfu, the 71st were not a kilted regiment), weighed down with heavy packs and muskets, their faces as red as their jackets, and it made him furious.[9] One afternoon in early November – with the weather still unseasonably hot – James saw them being marched out of the barrack yard of the citadel, heading for the Spianada, and his temper snapped. He hurried after them and caught up with Denny on the bridge over the moat, blocking his path and remonstrating angrily. A furious argument exploded – James, gesticulating wildly and underlining his points with his riding crop, caught Denny a violent swipe across the face (possibly accidental, but James did have form for this kind of violence). A vigorous scuffle broke out, the Colonel trying to wrest the whip from the doctor's hands. Fearing that it would be used against him if he lost hold, James flung it over the railings into the moat. It was said that Denny would have heaved James into the moat after it if he hadn't been restrained by a friend. Instead the Colonel placed Dr Barry under arrest and had one of his ensigns escort him to his quarters.

As Denny and Barry were of equal rank there was no insubordination to answer for, and the matter blew over, seen as part of the high emotions inevitable under the circumstances (although they must have been roasted in private by General Conyers). Shortly afterwards both were back on duty. But the incident hadn't gone unnoticed – there had been plenty of witnesses, and the *United Service Gazette* carried a short report on the 'military quarrel' that had 'caused a little sensation from the rank of the parties'; it was reproduced in newspapers across Britain and Ireland, and remembered in the Army for decades.[10] Some claimed that Dr Barry had taken sweet revenge on Colonel Denny, but in fact that would come two years later in sad and unexpected circumstances.

In the meantime they had to get on with one another, for when the regiments were marched one by one down to the harbour to board transports for the Crimea, the 71st was not among them; with three others it was held back as part of the permanent garrison. And when General Conyers retired from his position, Colonel Denny became acting garrison commander.

The war rumbled on hundreds of miles away. In October 1854, when news came of Lord Raglan's victory at the Battle of the Alma – the first great engagement of the war – Denny held a parade of the whole garrison on the Spianada, where they fired a *feu de joie** in celebration; it was reported that 'The officers and soldiers of the 71st Regiment expressed unceasing anxiety to follow their brave comrades' to war.[11] It took another three months, but they finally got their wish, and on 20 January 1854 they took their places in the transports and went off to battle,[12] Denny taking his wife with him, oblivious to the hell they were heading into and the effect it would have on him. James saw them go, unaware that they would meet again before long.

Corfu had suddenly grown deathly quiet. Not only had the bulk of the troops gone to the war, the remaining garrison had been dispersed to ease the overcrowding – the 1st Royal Scots to Cephalonia and the 31st Huntingdons to Zante – leaving only the 48th Northamptonshires in Corfu, occupying barracks intended for four regiments. The 71st shouldn't have been needed, but the war wasn't going well. The high water mark had been reached on 25 October 1854 with the Battle of Balaclava, when the pride of the British Army, the Light Brigade, was thrown against the Russian cannon by the arrogance and rashness of its commanders and the vacillating folly of Lord Raglan himself. The Russian army was badly mauled at the Battle of Inkerman the following month, Sevastopol was laid under siege and the war settled into a slow, horrible attrition.

The casualties were dreadful – not only from battle but from the cholera brought by the French; cholera cases outnumbered the killed and wounded five to one. In charge of the overstretched medical services for the Eastern Army was Inspector General Dr John Hall, who had been saddled with it unwittingly. Director General Andrew Smith had originally appointed Deputy Inspector William Burrell as Principal Medical Officer for the expedition, but the Eastern Army rapidly grew, so Smith – thinking to assist Burrell – recalled the very experienced Hall from Bombay to handle the medical services in Constantinople. Deeply offended, Burrell resigned, leaving the entire operation to Hall.[13] Hall, badly overworked, felt uneasy about his position in relation to Lord Raglan, confiding to his diary: 'I am conscious of having exerted myself to my utmost ability'; but 'It is possible that His Lordship wants to get rid of me and make room for his protégé Barry.'[14] In fact James had applied for a posting to the Crimea as soon as the war started, but no role was

* celebratory salute, with a rapid sequence of shots

given to him[15] and the gentlemanly Raglan had no intention of depriving any man of his post.

James did what he could for the war effort. In about October he received an urgent message from Lieutenant Colonel Lockyer of the 97th (Earl of Ulster's) Regiment, which had been temporarily stationed at Piraeus in Greece ahead of a posting to the Crimea; there'd been an outbreak of cholera, ninety-two men had already been taken ill, and a supply failure had left the surgeons with no medicines or medical facilities. Within two hours of receiving the letter, James had embarked the necessary supplies and arranged to send weekly deliveries. He provided similar emergency supplies to two other stranded regiments – the 3rd East Kent (the Buffs) and the 91st Argyllshires. He later received official thanks from Director General Andrew Smith and the commanding officers of all three regiments. Presumably this action made good his awful breach with the officers of the 91st in St Helena sixteen years earlier (there were probably none in the regiment now who remembered it; Colonel Anderson at least had gone).[16] James also earned the thanks of Admiral Lord Lyons of the Mediterranean Fleet for his 'zeal and services' in discovering 'the cause of the Malignant fever' on board the eighteen-gun corvette HMS *Modeste*, stationed at Corfu, and for his 'successful treatment of the sick and the purification of the Ship'.[17]

Although most of the regiments were gone, Corfu didn't stay quiet for long. In late 1854 James suggested to Raglan and Hall that his facilities be used for convalescents. During that terrible winter Corfu received about five hundred men, casualties of Alma, Inkerman and Balaclava, of whom eighty per cent were later deemed well enough to return to active service.[18] A constant stream of convalescents came from the hospital established at Scutari Barracks in Constantinople; some went to Malta, some to Corfu, while the less fortunate were placed in hulks moored off Scutari.[19] Recovery rates under James Barry's regime were excellent; one of the batches, arriving from Scutari in February, comprised 462 sick and wounded men; after only two weeks, fifty-three were fit for duty, sixty-three for slight duty and sixty-nine not yet ambulant. There were 260 men, although up and about, still under in-patient treatment, while only seventeen had died.[20] The convalescents were quartered on the islet of Vido, a short distance from Corfu town. Mr Charteris, a Presbyterian missionary, visited them from time to time during the first month:

They are located in almost all the wards of the forts; and if comforts of every kind, and good fresh healthy air, can restore them, we may hope to see many of them soon fit for service. Some died on the passage, six have died since they came here, and, I rejoice to believe that almost all the others are convalescent. Some have received severe wounds, one of whom has brought from Inkermann ... a grape-shot of about a quarter of an inch in diameter, which passed through his limb ... He is rapidly recovering, but I fear may be somewhat of a cripple for life.[21]

On his first visit, when they had only just arrived from Scutari, Charteris found the men in a terrible state – ragged and unclean:

Many of them were very indifferently clothed, and wore an expression of wretchedness corresponding to their tattered habiliments. But on my second visit ... their countenances were quite changed – every one seemed improved, and was clad in the blue hospital-dress ... They were moving over the island in knots of four and five together, with the air of 'monarchs of all they surveyed'. When accosted, they expressed themselves generally perfectly satisfied with their lot.[22]

Only three days had passed between those two visits. This was outstanding, a testament to James Barry's management, commitment to hygiene and welfare, and excellence as a doctor. Unfortunately, the pattern was not followed elsewhere – including at Scutari, whence the men had come. Florence Nightingale had recently taken up her post there, but had evidently not applied her reputed standards of care to these men. (Mr Charteris did note, however, that Miss Nightingale had provided some of them with prayer books.)

The sheer number of patients put enormous pressure on Corfu's Commissariat and stores; their uniforms were in rags, infested with lice, and had to be incinerated; there were no replacements, and the men had been obliged by the administrators to pay for their own hospital uniforms, fatigues and coats, which were made locally until supplies could be obtained from Scutari. Major General Alexander Fisher Macintosh, who had just arrived to take over command of the garrison, was determined to get the men returned to duty and out from under his feet. He was also under pressure to provide reinforcements to the war. He and Lord High Commissioner Sir Henry Ward had already sent off the

34th Regiment from the depleted Corfu garrison; they went singing and cheering.[23] With so much strain on the Army, which was being driven hard against Sevastopol and suffering appallingly in the freezing conditions, the more convalescents who could be returned to active service, the better.

Dr Barry complied as far as he could. In April he approved 213 men for service. However, instead of embarking them on the civilian steamer as expected, Macintosh (perhaps trying to save money) tried to have them transported by two Royal Navy steam-frigates en route to Turkey. But they already had regiments aboard, and more than half the former convalescents were left stranded on Corfu.[24] The British Army could not abide having men idle, so Macintosh decided to put them to work, doing routine fatigue duties. Dr Barry objected vehemently to this treatment;[25] one can only suppose that he had bowed to pressure from above and had rated men fit who were not sufficiently recovered. If they were not going to be used for vital service, he preferred that they be allowed to continue their convalescence in peace. This interference with Macintosh's orders had predictable results.

The point of impact was Lord Methuen, commander of the Royal Wiltshire Militia, a regiment mobilised especially for the war. Some of Methuen's men were among the disputed ex-patients, and Dr Barry had a heated altercation with His Lordship, in the course of which he threatened to report the whole matter to Lord Raglan, boasting that he enjoyed special favour with the Commander in Chief. Profoundly offended, Methuen spoke to Macintosh, who wrote to Lord Raglan himself in an attempt to both forestall and blacken Dr Barry:

> Apparently with a view to impress Lord Methuen with a belief that he possessed more than usual influence with your Lordship, [Dr Barry claimed] that he was a private friend of yours, and had resided 13 years in the house of your Lordship's brother. This avowal, coupled with his injudicious interference with the management of these men, [came] after he had pronounced them fairly recovered, and therefore properly speaking, beyond his immediate control.[26]

Macintosh hoped 'that your Lordship's mind will in no manner be biased by any statement' from Dr Barry. In fact, Macintosh's anxiety was unnecessary. Lord Raglan replied genially:

I am sorry to learn that Dr Barry, of whose zeal for the service I entertain no doubt, should have thought fit to interfere in a matter … which rested with you alone. You will be glad to learn that he has not written to me, and I should hope that he may upon reflection feel that such a course would not only be highly improper, but would be utterly disapproved by me.[27]

Raglan had been promoted to field marshal with effect from 5 November 1854, the day of the Battle of Inkerman; it was the culmination of half a century's service, but he didn't have long to enjoy it. He had proven himself a poor commander in chief – he was old and unwell, too genial to make harsh decisions, and couldn't cope with the complicated management of a major war. His staff and subordinates knew him as a kind commander – far kinder than a commander ought to be. By 1855 the Eastern Army was little short of a shambles, clinging on in the trenches around Sevastopol – which they had failed to capture – and protecting the port and headquarters at Balaclava, the whole operation brought low by cholera and inadequate systems of supply and medical care.

On 21 June Raglan fell ill with a diarrhoeal illness, believed to be either cholera or dysentery, compounded by depression. He held on for over a week, rallying a little from time to time, under constant care from his physician, Dr Joseph Prendergast, but on the 29th he died. James's last link with the Somerset brothers expired with him. The entire Eastern Army mourned him ('We did not know until he was taken from us how dearly we loved him,' said one private, while an officer said, 'I see no one to replace him … Everyone who knew him loved and respected him and rightly so … he was gifted with the most sensitive feelings and kind heart.'),[28] but few can have grieved for him as deeply and sincerely as James Barry, hundreds of miles away in Corfu.

The soldiers – who had their own immediate problems to cope with – recovered quickly enough under the command of Sir James Simpson, Raglan's chief of staff, until he was replaced by Sir William Codrington. But conditions did not improve. In October, James Barry set out for the front to have a look for himself.

31

The Land of Mornise

Üsküdar, Turkey: October 1855

On the eastern shore of the Bosphorus where it met the Sea of Marmara, on the edge of Constantinople, stood a remarkable building. From a distance it resembled a palace – a long, noble frontage in pale stone and roofed in red tiles, stretching back at both wings to form a vast square, with a slender tower at each corner. The Turks called it Selimiye Barracks, after Sultan Selim III who founded it. Part of it had been handed over to the British for the duration of the war, and they called it by the name of the district – Üsküdar, or Scutari. Despite its grand façades, within it was a thoroughly functional building, in which the British had created a hospital from part of the barracks. Scutari was the principal way-station for British troops going to and from the Crimea and the main base hospital.

As James approached, he rode past hundreds of tents, laundry draped on their ropes, the smoke of campfires everywhere, and people, animals and vehicles teeming, the whole lot giving off the ripe stench of an army encamped – woodsmoke, musty canvas, serge, sweat, dirt and horse dung. Companies marched in full parade order or loafed about in fatigues and slouch caps. The atmosphere of the East was represented in a mosque's dome and minarets beyond the building and the robed and turbaned figures mingling with the troops.

So this was Scutari, notorious for its nightmare conditions and famous for the miracles reportedly worked by Florence Nightingale and her nurses. Hardly a week went by without some town, city or guild in England raising a subscription to support her work. She was a heroine in Britain, used as an adviser and exemplar by people planning new charitable hospitals (which alarmed some doctors, who feared that the novelty

might cause funding for existing hospitals to decline).[1] Miss Nightingale
supported the proposals, and insisted that her system of unpaid voluntary
nursing should be adhered to, which was all very fine and commendable,
but rather restricted the pool of talent to those who came from wealthy
families, as did she.

James Barry had not come to Scutari on duty; he was curious to see
the war at first hand, and had obtained leave of absence to travel up to the
front. He'd arranged a locum for Corfu – Dr James Henderson, surgeon of
the 82nd Regiment, who'd worked at Balaclava and Scutari; Henderson
was close to Miss Nightingale, having treated her when she was seriously
ill with the 'Crimean fever' (diarrhoea and dysentery) in May.[2] Older than
James, with his daughter in tow, Henderson was now free to spend time
in the gentler environment of Corfu. 'I was glad to find that you escaped
at last from the tender mercy of the "Sanità",' James wrote to him.[3] His
view of Florence Nightingale was somewhat jaundiced.

With both his servants, his horse (a beautiful grey Arab), his dog
and a pet goat[4] (which provided him with milk), James Barry entered
Scutari through the archway in the front façade, arriving in an enormous quadrangle – part parade ground, part store yard, busy with
wagons, horses, nurses and men, and scattered with hutments and
stores. Although it was autumn, the sun was blazing and the space
was drenched in heat. A small crowd had gathered – soldiers, servants
of the Commissariat and a variety of camp followers. James noticed
a young woman, severely dressed with white cuffs – clearly a nurse –
walking across the courtyard.

She was fine-featured and serious-looking, with a broad forehead,
cold eyes and a pointed nose; despite the heat of the sun she wore only
a simple cap, which in James's opinion was quite inadequate; he had
developed quite a crotchet about the ill effects of exposure to full sun,
and he was quite unreasonably angered by this young woman's careless-
ness. He addressed her sharply and called her to him. She knew right
away who he was – Dr Barry was expected, and his peculiar appearance
was known throughout the Army. James was rather more surprised
to discover that this woman was the great 'Sanità' herself, Florence
Nightingale. They disliked each other on sight. Dr Barry scolded her
harshly for her negligence in being out in the sun with only a cap,
subjecting her to a long and demeaning lecture in front of the crowd
of spectators, who all stood silent, pretending not to notice. 'I never

had such a blackguard rating* in all my life,' Miss Nightingale recalled, '– I who have had more than any woman – than from this Barry sitting on his horse … he behaved like a brute.' She thought James Barry 'the most hardened creature I ever met'.[5]

Decades later, when Dr Barry's secret was known, Florence Nightingale showed no sign of understanding, no indication of fellow feeling or comprehension of the forces that might have made 'James' the way he was. He was merely an uncivil brute who happened to be a woman in disguise. From James's – or rather Margaret's – point of view, Nightingale was a woman who had been born into a wonderfully wealthy, progressive middle-class family with a good education and excellent social connections, who had never had to fret about money; having been seized with a drive (revealed to her by God, she claimed) to devote herself to caring for the poor and sick, Miss Nightingale had been able to use her connections and influence to pursue her vocation openly. While working at a clinic for gentlewomen in Harley Street, she'd been moved by the awful news coming out of the Crimea, and embarked on the great project of her life; she managed to get both the Secretary at War and Director General Dr Andrew Smith on her side, and in October 1854 they'd sent her to Scutari with her train of thirty-eight volunteer nurses, supported by a fund from *The Times*. And thence flowed all the fame and worship that an enthusiastic nation could heap on her. She hadn't had to struggle against debt, hadn't needed to spend years studying medicine and surgery or work her way up the ranks of the profession, and she had not been forced to do all this in disguise. And the reforms for which she received such acclaim – and would in time be credited with by history – were identical to the improvements James and the more enlightened of his colleagues had been instituting for decades in hospitals throughout the Empire – hygiene, clean water, and properly ventilated, rigorously organised wards with soundly built beds and skilled nursing staff – all with tangible results. It was quite simply unfair.

But at the same time Margaret apparently didn't take into account that Miss Nightingale would never be able to treat the sick as a surgeon or physician could, would never enjoy the life and freedom of a man, and in spite of her connections had had to fight against resistance to follow her vocation, especially in establishing herself at Scutari. The medical

---

* *rating*: in this context, an angry rebuke; thus, a telling-off fit for a blackguard

staff here, overwhelmed by the influx of thousands of sick and wounded
from the Crimea, and sometimes afflicted themselves by sickness, had
failed to give her the warm welcome that she felt was her due; instead
she sensed insolence and frank hostility. She'd had to struggle to improve
conditions and reduce the suffering and mortality to the extent that she
had. When the manager of the *Times* fund arrived at Scutari he found
that the Army medical officers had 'made no facilities for the proper
distribution' of the fund, and seemed indifferent to it; he also found that
no accurate records of patients were being kept, and 'small provision had
been made for converting the barrack hospital into an hospital at all'.[6]
It was a disgrace to the Army Medical Department and the inspector
generals who were in charge of it.

Perhaps Margaret and Miss Nightingale might have perceived one
another as sisters in spirit if they hadn't met under such fraught circumstances. But even that is improbable. They were entirely different in
temperament – Margaret high-spirited, gregarious, fond of the luxuries
of life, and furious of temper, Florence as chilly and austere as a nun.

That first day, having thoroughly upset a national heroine, James
went and introduced himself to the Principal Medical Officer, Inspector
General Dr Alexander Cumming, one of the men who had been unsym-
pathetic to the Nightingale mission. He wasn't very receptive to Dr Barry
either. After James had gone, he wrote to John Hall, Principal Medical
Officer of the Eastern Army in the Crimea:

> I may as well warn you that you are to have a visit from the renowned
> Dr Barry. He called on me yesterday, and as I never met him before, his
> appearance and conversation rather surprised me. He appears to me to
> be in his dotage and is an intolerable bore, so would recommend you
> to be prepared for him as he seems to have the intention of Quartering
> himself on you ... He will expect you to listen to every quarrel he has
> had since coming into the Service. You probably know that they are
> not a few.[7]

If Dr Hall was still jealous of Dr Barry, this portrait of him might have
quelled it. Making just the briefest stay at Scutari, James sailed on for
the Crimea. Fascinating as the hospital was, it was Sevastopol he really
wanted to see – the front line. As an Army surgeon who had never seen a
real war, he felt an absence, and believed that the world was on the brink

of perpetual conflict; he approached it with some trepidation, and 'please God shall return as soon as I shall have lionized or rather vagabondised,' he wrote to Henderson; 'I must confess I am more than anxious to have a look at this Land of Mornise* … For my own part I think War has but just commenced & it is problematical if the 40 years will end it – I'll give you a line from thence if it please God that I am spared.'[8]

Balaclava was a nightmare, a nondescript village by the sea, altered by a year of military traffic into a mess of mud, hovels, disease and despair, spilling out onto the plain and the hills, where the troops had constructed underground dugouts and mud cabins that were sounder and more salubrious than their tents. Great mountains of stores – chiefly food, powder and shot – were piled up ready to go to the front, while stretchers of sick and wounded queued to go out to Scutari. Soldiers and camp followers wandered through the village, where the shops were kept by 'small-souled Maltese' who 'dealt largely in animated cheese, mouldy tobacco, cracked pipes, sour beer';[9] better goods were sold by traders outside the village, and few people lingered in the streets for long.

From Balaclava it was about eight miles up to the main siege camps around Sevastopol. Even though the siege had ended with the fall of the city and the Russian retreat in September, the Army was still up there, holding the line. A railway had been built to carry supplies up to the line, and as Major Alexander of the 14th Buckinghamshires put it, 'Guns and mortars could not have had their insatiable appetites satisfied' without it.[10] Most of the traffic, however, had to go by mule cart, on foot or on horseback by rough roads over the crags and valleys. With his servants in tow, Dr Barry steered his horse carefully up to the front line.

Sevastopol was Russia's great Black Sea port, positioned on the south shore of a broad estuary and surrounded by fortifications. The allied encampments fronted by trenches surrounded it from Inkerman at the head of the estuary to the coast. Major Alexander described how, even after the siege:

The British divisions were pitched in white rows of tents to the south of the city, and the French occupied ground to the right and left …

* possibly from French *morne*: dreary, dismal, bleak; or misspelling of French *morniste*: mockery, satire

ravines intersecting the encampments, and becoming deeper as they approached the ramparts of Sevastopol, which were thickened with well-rammed earth, and bristled with thousands of cannon.[11]

The landscape had been torn by continual artillery fire and, every evening during the siege, detachments of soldiers would make their way from the encampments to the trenches to relieve the previous lot: twenty-four hours of trench duty for each detachment:

> The men were in forage caps, red coatees, cross-belts, and dark trousers; they carried, with the light and handy Enfield rifle and bayonet, sixty rounds of ball-cartridge, their great-coats and water barrels; following them was a keg of rum, and last of all the stretchers – blood-stained – to carry the slain warrior to a hastily-prepared grave in the trenches, or the wounded soldier back to his hospital in camp.[12]

Although the battle was ended, the routines continued; the Russian army still lurked to the north, the investment of the city was still under way, the war still on, and preparations were in train to utterly destroy Sevastopol's port facilities. When James Barry arrived he joined the camp of the British 4th Infantry Division.[13] It was greatly expanded from its usual size of two brigades, and among the regiments temporarily attached to it James found two regiments from Corfu. Compared with the smart soldiers who had left on the transports, the men James met were frayed, grubby phantoms, hollow-cheeked and bearded to the eyes. The 48th Northamptonshires were his particular friends, having spent two years at Corfu and only this spring come out to the war. On first arriving they had shown the benefits of their time in the Ionian Islands; one military visitor noticed their 'quiet and steady demeanour' and 'found that their better conduct and superior condition were generally known and recognized', and explained thus:

> 'Why,' it was said, 'the 48th has lately been a lucky regiment: they have been regularly nursed. A regiment never gets into a first-rate condition when it is knocking about … [The 48th] has been at a Mediterranean station for the last two years, and came directly out to the Crimea. They have been carefully handled and treated, and are certainly a very superior set of men.'[14]

They were a credit to their officers, and also to the medical care given by James Barry and his subordinates. Their commander, Lieutenant Colonel Benjamin Riky, who had purchased his way up the ranks ('and was a little sore on that point'), was 'as proud of his regiment, as a father of his son' and felt that he could have no better death than with them 'on any Crimean path of glory'.[15] Since arriving here they had been hurled against the Russian fortifications, battered by the daily bombardments and wearied by the mud, sickness, and now the increasing cold of this, their first Crimean winter.

Given what he had seen and heard at Scutari and in Corfu, it was no surprise to James to see the condition of the camp hospitals, which were undersupplied and overstretched. Staff Surgeon Frederic Roberts, Principal Medical Officer of the 4th Division, reported later that 'there was no sanitary discipline observed in our army in the Crimea ... nor had the duties of departments suffered a reduction into anything approaching to science.' He clarified: 'It was not so much the want of means we suffered from as the want of arrangement. Every regimental surgeon had to work on his own account, from building huts to curing frost bites.'[16]

James Barry pitched in to help the 4th Division, and in particular the 48th Regiment; he spent three months there 'and made myself useful as opportunities offered', earning the gratitude of both Colonel Riky and Inspector General Hall, with whom he became good friends in spite of Cumming's snide letter.[17] During this time the depleted regiments were pulling themselves together, salvaging equipment from the frozen battlefield, and making themselves ready for more conflict.

Meanwhile, the loose ends of a two-year-old incident came together. Also in the Crimea about this time was James's old foe Colonel William Denny of the 71st Highlanders, whom he had last seen sailing away to war. In the event, Denny hadn't gone into action with his men; he'd been struck down ill, and was kept behind. A medical board declared him unfit and sent him back to England.[18] A rumour ran through the Army that Denny's illness was mental rather than physical, and later it was even alleged that Dr Barry had wangled the medical board (this was impossible, as the board occurred in the Crimea in May 1855 while James was in Corfu). Denny had since returned and was briefly reunited with the 71st during the siege, but in late October another medical board was convened for him; this might well have included Dr Barry, since he was present and senior. Denny was again declared unfit and given two months' leave; at Christmas the certification was renewed until April and he was sent home again, very possibly with James's involvement.[19] According to gossip, Denny repeatedly begged the Commander in Chief to allow him to return to his regiment but was refused – thus, James was at last revenged for the scuffle on the citadel bridge and his embarrassing arrest.[20]

By the time James left the Crimea in January 1856 the war was coming to an end; in February hostilities ceased and in March a peace treaty was signed in Paris. From a force that numbered about fifty-six thousand at any one time, the British Eastern Army had suffered over twenty thousand dead – more than sixteen thousand of them from disease. In the French army, sixty thousand had been killed by disease. The Russians, having lost about four hundred thousand men from all causes and seen Sevastopol's port destroyed, were forced to agree not to establish any naval force in the Black Sea.

In Britain, jingoism had been replaced by anger at the conduct of the war and the failure of British arms to produce glorious victories. The officers and men of Alma, Inkerman, the Charge of the Light Brigade and the Thin Red Line were welcomed as heroes, but their leaders were castigated. Inquiries were held; blame was apportioned, contested, redirected and argued over for years afterwards, and a good deal of it settled on the deceased shoulders of FitzRoy Somerset, 1st Baron Raglan. By contrast, one of the few names to emerge from the fiasco with laurels undimmed was Miss Florence Nightingale, her fame all the brighter against the dark background of a shameful war.

James resumed his post in Corfu in mid-January 1856; the garrison was back to its normal strength, and aside from the regular run of floggings and drunken fights it was now thoroughly peaceful.[21] Colonel Denny turned up again in mid-November, having had his medical leave repeatedly renewed.[22] This time he was apparently allowed to rejoin the regiment, which was then en route to Malta from the Black Sea. But it was the end of the line for Denny: he retired from the service the following year.[23]

For James, life was brightened by an event about a year after his return from the Crimea, when a launch from the Austrian naval forces arrived in Corfu harbour carrying a seaman who had been seriously injured during the firing of a salute. He was admitted to the Military Hospital, and Dr

Barry took him into his particular care. The injury was unspecified, but would have been one of two kinds that could occur when firing a heavy cannon: contusions and fractures caused by failing to keep out of the way of a recoiling gun carriage weighing over a ton; or (less commonly) lacerations and other wounds caused by getting in the way of a premature discharge. The patient did very well, and James was delighted to be rewarded with a beautiful diamond ring by the young Archduke Maximilian, brother of the Emperor and Commander in Chief of the Austrian naval forces, 'for his attention and humanity' to the sailor.[24]

On 23 June 1857 James Barry handed over his office and departed Corfu for the last time. He left it in a better state than he had found it, and the improvements he had begun would be continued by his successors – with such effect that six years later, when the British were winding down their occupation of the Ionian Islands in advance of handing them over to Greece, the command was singled out for its remarkably low rate of admissions to hospital.[25] By that time, James Barry would be on the other side of the Atlantic.

PART V

A Useful and Faithful Career
1857–1865

32

'This Vorld of Voe, this Wale of Tears'

Whitehaven Castle: Thursday 24 September 1857

James Barry loved a party. He'd been noted for it in his youth – dancing and playing the gallant with the ladies.[1] And tonight's ball, given by the Earl of Lonsdale as part of a small season of public events, would be one of the grandest he'd ever known. The Earl had spent a fortune on preparations, and was expecting over two hundred guests. Every window was ablaze with light, and specially installed gas jets lit up the driveway and the great gate, beyond which Lowther Street ran straight down to the harbour, where the ship lights and the lighthouse twinkled as if in answer.[2]

That morning the local agricultural show had taken place in the castle grounds – again marred by violent rain. The weather had cleared up now. The carriages began to arrive about nine o'clock in an endless line, 'to set down their freights of beauty' as the local paper put it,[3] and didn't stop until half past ten. The guests included local aristocracy, industrialists, clergy, squires, military men, professionals and tradesmen and their wives and daughters. The dancing began with a quadrille at half past nine, followed by a succession of polkas and waltzes, with music from Golightly's quadrille band, and the ballroom lit up in 'a scene to be lastingly impressed on the minds of the beholders'.[4] How different from the balls of Margaret's youth, with their courtly sets, cotillions and reels – now ladies and gentlemen danced promiscuously in each other's arms, like lovers – how different, and how much more exhilarating. At midnight a supper of the finest dishes, 'which the most refined taste could suggest or wealth command', was served in two dining rooms overlooking the illuminated forecourt, where the band of the Royal Cumberland Militia played popular airs. After supper the dancing went on until half past four.

For James it was a fitting way to bring his summer's leave in England to a close. The following month he'd be departing for his next posting. He was bound for Canada – 'to cool myself after such a long residence in the Tropics & *Hot* Countries'.[5]

England was a lonelier place now that Lord Raglan was dead – not James's last link with the Somerset family, but the most significant. Of Margaret's family there was no trace. Her mother, Mrs Bulkley, who astonishingly had still been alive as recently as 1851 at the age of eighty-six, had been living with her daughter-in-law Elizabeth in a tiny terraced house in Albion Street,* Bethnal Green.[6] John had died, and Elizabeth supported her teenage daughter Esther and her mother-in-law by dress-making. If Mary Anne Bulkley, as a young mother sixty years earlier, had been able to see the end she would come to, it would have mortified her and perhaps driven her into the early grave she had always threatened to occupy. The little household had been tragically broken up when Esther fell ill and died in May 1851,[7] after which they disappeared from the records.[8] They had long since become strangers to Margaret, leaving no trace whatsoever in the life of James Barry – except perhaps one. Two letters were written by James in 1857 on black-bordered mourning sta-tionery sealed with black wax; possibly Mrs Bulkley, who would now have been in her nineties, had at last succumbed. Certainly James acquired one of the mourning rings Mrs Bulkley had had made back in 1809, with 'Sacred to the memory of Mary Anne' engraved on it.[†]

There was a lot going on in James's life. Professionally he was con-cerned about the report of the special Sanitary Commission on the Crimea; it thoroughly damned the condition of the hospitals, and was energetically supported by Florence Nightingale. Inspector General Sir John Hall, despite having been knighted for his services during the war, felt profoundly slighted by the report, on behalf of himself and the Army Medical Department. Like James (with whom he was now on friendly terms, having got over his jealousy about Raglan), Sir John was frustrated by the credit being given to Miss Nightingale and the Commission, and had published his *Observations*, in which he remarked that the Sanitary Commissioners 'were more likely to borrow hints from the Army Medical Officers' than the officers were to require advice from the Commissioners.

* now Hemming Street
† see Chapter 33

He added that although the report's practical conclusions were sound, they were 'unexceptionable' and 'so common place, so well known, and so generally admitted that it is amusing to see them paraded as the result of so many months' deliberation on the part of functionaries invested with almost unlimited power to correct bad smells'.[9]

The day after the Whitehaven ball, James wrote (on his black-bordered notepaper) to Sir John. He'd read his *Observations* with keen interest: 'Our Dept has been treated in a most extraordinary manner,' he wrote,[10] puzzled that Sir John himself was not appointed to the Royal Commission on the Crimean War rather than Dr John Sutherland, the civilian who had headed the Sanitary Commission.

In time the Royal Commission would expose the dreadful state of the Scutari hospitals and the improvements made by Florence Nightingale and the Sanitary Commission. The facts were incontrovertible; the war hospitals had been execrable, and ultimately Sir John Hall was responsible. The whole military operation had been arranged in haste, with insufficient decision by Lord Raglan and Director General Andrew Smith, and inadequate support from the government (as in almost every other war in history), but Hall's responsibility it inescapably was.

With hindsight, the Army Medical Department's biggest mistake was not putting James Barry in charge of Scutari and giving him the resources that were allocated by popular acclaim to Miss Nightingale. He might have truly transformed the whole situation rather than merely improving it.

Sutherland, indignant at being accused by Hall of lying and of stealing other men's credit, replied to the *Observations* disclaiming any intention of blaming the Army Medical Department for the catastrophe, for it was 'a medical and not a sanitary department' (from the doctors' point of view, this disclaimer was as insulting as a direct accusation); Sutherland praised the hospital organisation and the 'single-minded devotion of the medical officers'.[11] Hall published a rejoinder decrying Sutherland's 'paltry subterfuge to throw discredit on the medical department of the army', which had been 'written with a species of special pleading cunning, which is intended to damn by implication, rather than by direct open manly accusation'.[12] By the standards of the day, one couldn't have had plainer allegations of incompetence on the one hand and cowardly dishonesty on the other, and had this been a half-century earlier it might have ended in pistols at dawn on Calais Sands.

Meanwhile, James was at leisure. On the Tuesday after the castle ball it was the Whitehaven Races,[13] where for the less equine among the crowds there was a wrestling tournament – a rare opportunity for an outsider to see the spectacle of Cumberland's martial art, with its unique garb of socks, long underwear and skin-tight shorts, the whole outfit elaborately embroidered in colourful patterns; a comical appearance belied by the sober gravity of the wrestlers' deportment and the spectacular violence of their matches. The holiday season was busy, and the whole area was alive with visitors – particularly the Lakes. The local paper reported that Charles Dickens and his friend Wilkie Collins were on a walking tour, the latter severely spraining his ankle.[14]

A few days after the races, James Barry and Lord Lonsdale travelled down to London,[15] James to prepare for his Canadian posting. When he returned to his lodgings at 29 South Street, just off Park Lane, he found an envelope waiting, bearing the stamp of the War Office. He opened it to find a sheet of thick parchment, written in the familiar copperplate:

> VICTORIA by the Grace of God of the United Kingdom … To Our Trusty and well beloved James Barry Esquire, MD. Greeting. We do by these Presents Constitute and Appoint you to be Inspector General of Hospitals.[16]

There were the wafer seals and stamps, and at the top left the Queen's signature.

At last – the penultimate rung on the ladder. His new rank was effective only in Canada for the time being, but it was still a powerful moment. Not only was this the very peak towards which he had been working all his career (the only person above him now was the Director General), it was also a historic milestone. Inspector general was equivalent to brigadier general – the first level above field rank. For the first time in history, a woman had achieved general rank in the British Army. It had never happened before, and more than a century and a half would go by before it happened again.[17]

There was a good deal of business to be done – new boots, clothing, uniforms (now in dark blue rather than scarlet) and gear to buy for the cold climate. 'On each change of station,' he later commented, 'I was put to an immense personal outlay, the Climates of each being of such different temperatures.'[18] This required a visit to his Army agent, the distinguished firm of Sir Charles McGrigor & Co at 17 Charles Street,* St James's Square, where he dealt with the manager, Mr W. B. Barrie (no relation). Army agents were inseparable from the lives of officers – known as the 'bankers of the British Army' they managed (among other things) the collection of each officer's pay and emoluments, and acted as personal banker, accountant and adviser. James also booked passage from Liverpool for Montreal for 21 October aboard the fast mail steamer.[19]

Although he had his orders for Canada, it wasn't certain that James would ever get there. There was a crisis in India again – a crisis to beat all others. News had first reached England in May 1857 of a mutiny among the East India Company's native regiments; it was unprecedented in its savage, pitiless violence, and had spread like a plague, developing into an all-out Indian rebellion, a conflict far greater and more urgent than the Sikh wars. It would overshadow the Crimea for bloodiness and terror, and troops and transports were being hurriedly diverted from all over the Empire to fight the flames. James had heard that a large number of medical officers would be sent out (and commented sourly that the Sanitary Commissioners and their civilian friends should be sent out too – 'they shd all go in the same Boat').[20]

James had spent the summer keeping his ear to the ground, gathering every bit of intelligence about where his colleagues were being posted. He wasn't exactly happy about Canada – his comment about being sent to cool himself after years in hot countries referred as much to his tempestuous reputation as to climate. The man he would be replacing, Inspector General Thomas Alexander, was expected to be transferred to Malta,[21] but in fact was destined for other things; he had served in the Crimea and impressed Florence Nightingale, who was acquiring a lot of political influence and moving for reform of the Army Medical Department – Andrew Smith would retire soon, and Nightingale would ensure that Alexander would serve on the Royal Commission on the Crimea and be his replacement as Director General.[22] Sir John Hall, who had been next in line, suffered a stroke and had to abandon his plans to write a medical history of the Crimean War.[23]

---

* now Charles II Street

Everything could have turned out so much worse for James Barry; as it was, there was no sign of him being redirected to India, so Canada it was – 'thus much for Changes and Chances in this "Vorld of Voe, this Wale of Tears" – as schollars say,' he wrote, bemused by the official claim that older officers' postings were being 'decided for our Wellfare'.[24] He still considered himself fit for any duty.

The British had worked hard to keep Canada. First they'd fought the French for it in the previous century, then during the War of 1812 they'd fended off American attempts to seize it; latterly, in 1837 there had been two major anti-colonial rebellions. And still there was tension, largely between the old provinces of Upper Canada (the area north of the Great Lakes, which was wholly British in character) and Lower Canada (Quebec and Labrador, which was culturally French), while hundreds of thousands of new British and Irish settlers were colonising the vast open lands westward as far as the Pacific.

James's posting was to Montreal, in Lower Canada. He arrived there on 3 November 1857, just as winter was beginning to bite.[25] He hadn't experienced cold like this in decades – not since his days as a student in Edinburgh when Europe was still in its 'little ice age'. It would get much, much worse with the passing months, as the mercury sank far below freezing and the world turned white and crisp.

The territory for which James was responsible was enormous and militarily unusual. For the whole of Canada there were only two British regular regiments – the 17th Leicestershire (veterans of the Crimea) and 39th Dorsetshire[26] – together with the Royal Canadian Rifles and a large body of militia. The country yearned for independence, and was already slowly moving towards it; therefore the situation of the British colonial government was complicated and delicate, with civil territories that didn't match up with the military regions. Canada and New Brunswick (but not Nova Scotia) came directly under James Barry's purview, and within Canada there were Army stations at Quebec, Montreal, Kingston and Isle-aux-Noix.[27] It was a tangled mess spread over a vast area that would be virtually impossible for James to superintend in the hands-on manner to which he was accustomed. But, once in Montreal, he took charge and busied himself with settling in.

There was little enough to concern him professionally – in health and medical terms, Canada was a fairly well-run station. But for a reformer there was always room for improvement. He thought the men's diet could be varied a bit, and lobbied for a 'cheering change ... from eternal boiled beef and soup' as 'nothing contributes more to general health than a change of Diet'.[28] He requested improvements to the water supply (which depended on wells in summer and carts in winter) and the barracks' drainage and sewerage. He also recommended proper mattresses instead of straw palliasses, and barracks heating: 'I have invariably found Wood as fuel for the use of Troops much more healthy than Coals', because coal gave off a gas that was 'exceedingly deleterious in generating fevers of the typhoid type and diseases of the respiratory organs' and could 'render exceedingly unhealthy the surrounding atmosphere'.[29]

There were further suggestions, but by Dr Barry's standards it was routine stuff. He had a good staff of four surgeons and three assistants, plus all the regimental men,[30] and on the whole Canada was as healthy as could be expected given the extremes of climate – from summers as hot as any in England to winters beyond anything a Briton was accustomed to. During that first winter the temperature fell to a barbarous low of −28°C. For a person approaching seventy years old, accustomed to heat and sunshine, his survival was a wonder.

One thing James was deeply concerned about was alcoholism among soldiers' wives – a problem throughout the Army. The regimental commanders had made efforts to curb the soldiers' excessive drinking, but their wives were another matter. The root cause was the distress these women suffered due to a complete lack of privacy; James asked his superiors to consider 'a woman, humbly born, but modestly and religiously educated', who suddenly found herself in her husband's barrack room with ten to twenty other men behaving as soldiers will. Subjected to the coarseness, the foul language, the aggressive and obscene conversations, 'she becomes frightened and disgusted', he wrote, and if she failed to get used to it she was likely to take to drink, which in turn tended to encourage the husband, who inevitably 'becomes the occupant of a cell in a Military prison'.[31] Here, for the first and only time in one of his official reports, James Barry gave the briefest accidental glimpse into Margaret's own early experience in a masculine world. She'd had the fortitude to adapt to it in spite of the added stress of her disguise. For the wives' benefit, Dr Barry recommended that separate accommodation be provided for married couples as a matter of policy.

*   *   *

Montreal was unlike any place he'd been accustomed to. Built on an island at the confluence of the St Lawrence and Ottawa rivers between Quebec and the Great Lakes, it was Canada's largest and most prosperous city, with a population of about sixty-five thousand – a mere village compared with London, but a metropolis next to any colonial town he'd lived in for the last thirty years. It was dominated by the round green hill that gave the city its name, which the locals were pleased to call a 'mountain'. The lower slopes were covered in orchards and pleasant villas and criss-crossed by popular carriage drives. Between the foot and the water stood the city itself, a grid of long, straight thoroughfares lined with large houses and good shops.

James rented a handsome new-built house with a pillared front at the corner of Durocher Street and Sherbrooke Street* near the edge of town, equipped himself with a very fine sleigh and horses, and began his usual process of becoming known – not to say notorious – about the town, a familiar sight to the locals, speeding along in his sleigh, wrapped up in furs.[32] He quickly made friends in the top drawer of Montreal society, and joined the newly established St James's Club, modelled on a London gentlemen's club, with all the exclusivity that implied.[33]

James became particularly friendly with Sydney Bellingham, an Irishman who'd come to Canada as a penniless teenager; thirty-five years on, he had a fine estate on the slopes of Mount Royal and tens of thousands of acres on the Ottawa River. Bellingham was an odd figure who lived on the boundary between the eminent and the disreputable. He had recently gained a seat in the Canadian Legislative Assembly and been accused (and acquitted) of electoral fraud.[34] 'I knew Dr Barry very well,' he recalled, 'and was a frequent visitor at his house.'[35] He later heard that Barry was 'the child of one of the doctors of George III', and was inclined to believe it, since he seemed 'abundantly supplied with money' and 'maintained the establishment of a gentleman of fortune, keeping a handsome carriage and a retinue of servants'. Unlike some others, Bellingham was impressed rather than disgusted by Dr Barry's eccentricities. The menagerie had increased, and he now had 'half a dozen small tan terriers for whose use he imported from London a special kind of biscuit'. As a vegetarian who didn't normally like root vegetables, James discovered a delight in Quebec turnips. But he only liked them

---

* now Avenue McGill College and rue Sherbrooke

boiled, and one young society hostess – the daughter of an artillery colonel – who was encouraged by Bellingham to befriend him, committed the error of serving him a dish of *mashed* turnip and cream, 'which he rejected as indigestible'.[36]

Where James came by his new affluence is a puzzle. His Army pay had jumped up a level on his promotion, but officers of general rank were by no means rich. He may have inherited something from one of his wealthy connections, or been given an honorarium by Lord Lonsdale (as his occasional personal physician). More likely he was living beyond his means, as Margaret's mother had done, complacent about his situation now that he was at the top of the professional tree, and trying to emulate his rich friends.

Montreal regarded Dr Barry with interest, amusement and occasionally dislike. The first year passed and a second winter set in, and on 7 December 1858 – the forty-third anniversary of his appointment as an assistant staff surgeon – he was confirmed in his rank as full Inspector General (no longer confined to the locality).[37] His eccentricity stepped up a level also; indeed, a few in Montreal were beginning to wonder whether the old doctor was straying into the realm of insanity.

Durocher Street, Montreal: Sunday 23 January 1859

With a thumping of hoofs on the packed snow and a shiver of silver bells, Dr Barry's sleigh came rushing out of the driveway and swept along the frozen road. Everyone knew it by sight; it was the best sleigh in town, driven by a coachman and attended by a footman, both in bearskin caps and cloaks. In the back, wrapped in musk-ox furs, sat Dr James Barry himself, looking out on the world with a scowl and shrieking at the coachman to go slower. The sleigh hit an icy rut and swerved violently, pitching Dr Barry off his seat. As he struggled among the tangle of furs, squeaking indignantly and trying to climb back up, the sleigh hit another rut and tumbled him down again.[38]

It wasn't the first time this had happened; local gossips believed the coachman did it deliberately in revenge for the doctor's allegedly cruel treatment[39] (a highly improbable belief, given James Barry's history of cordial, even fond, relationships with his servants). More likely he'd made the mistake of hiring a coachman who couldn't handle the large sleigh and mettlesome horses. The sight of the little doctor, scowling and cursing as he was tossed about in the speeding, lurching vehicle, was said to be commonplace around Montreal.

This particular morning, James was especially cross, and not just because of the erratic ride. He'd recently made a request to the Reverend John Bethune, Rector of Christ Church and Dean of Montreal, that the regular church service, which normally took place at two o'clock in the afternoon, be moved to nine in the morning. His reason was given vaguely as 'on Sanitary grounds' (presumably the afternoon slot conflicted with some plans he had for the men).[40] Now he'd received a reply from the Dean – verbally, via Army Chaplain Reverend Rogers – which not only denied the request but 'chafed' him rudely about it. Well, he'd see about that.

Sunday morning service in St John's Chapel had just concluded, and the Reverend Bethune, along with the Bishop and Archdeacon of Montreal and other members of the clergy, were gathered in the vestry. Suddenly the door banged open and in stormed Dr Barry in a fur cloak and a tumult of rage. Oblivious to the presence of the Bishop, he tongue-lashed the startled Dean and Archdeacon, accusing them of refusing his perfectly reasonable request, and of being 'callous to the Spiritual welfare of Her Majesty's Soldiers'[41] – he assailed them at length with 'violence and insulting conduct' laced with the kind of language that vicars ought never to hear, and concluded by threatening to publish their actions in *The Times*. Then he turned on his heel, returned to his sleigh and departed, leaving the reverend gentlemen white-faced and stunned.

The following day, the Dean had recovered his wits sufficiently to write a letter of complaint to Lieutenant General Sir William Eyre, Commander of British Forces in North America. Bethune denied ever sending any message at all to Dr Barry, let alone any that would 'chafe' him, admitted that he'd had a conversation with him on the subject but received no official application, suggested that Colonel Cole of the 17th Regiment was the proper person to make any such application, and reminded Eyre that the Army had always been happy with the afternoon service.[42] (In other words, he hadn't exactly made himself very receptive to Dr Barry's request, and was now perhaps being a little disingenuous.) Strangely, the part played by the Chaplain, Mr Rogers, who ought to have had some explaining to do, was overlooked by all parties.

Having cooled down, James apologised for the scene; he admitted that 'I was both warm and excited' and wrote that 'if in so doing I used the words attributed to me by the Dean of Montreal, I beg to withdraw them, and to express my great regret, that I should have been led to use such expressions to him.'[43]

The Dean accepted the apology, and apparently forgot the matter. General Eyre did not; it was allowed to pass in silence for the moment, but fermented during the two weeks that passed before the next outburst.

Durocher Street: Monday 14 February 1859

The Canadian winter was at its nadir in the first two months of the year, when temperatures fell through the floor. A rider turned his horse in through a familiar gateway and trotted up the drive. Colonel the Hon. Robert Rollo, General Eyre's Assistant Adjutant General, was a veteran of the Crimea (like almost every officer in the North American command), an old warhorse furnished with an imposing set of regimental whiskers and walrus moustache. He'd formerly been a captain in the 42nd Black Watch and had known James Barry in Malta thirteen years earlier (at the time of the doctor's last major insult to the Anglican Church).[44] It wasn't normal for Rollo to dance attendance upon Inspector General Barry, but the old fellow was needed for a medical board and had fallen too ill to leave the house.

Colonel Rollo was admitted by the doctor's manservant, and found the gentleman himself in the drawing room, reclining on a sofa before a well-stoked fire. Sitting with him was his medical attendant, Surgeon William Ward of the 17th Regiment. Another toughened veteran, Ward had served through all the major engagements from the Alma to the fall of Sevastopol and been awarded medals by all three allies.[45] James must have found him a comfortable and trustworthy doctor, and the risk of discovery evidently didn't worry him, since his illness – probably the chronic bronchitis or bronchopneumonia from which he had begun to suffer – wasn't serious enough to be life-threatening or involve loss of consciousness.

Nonetheless, James looked thoroughly unwell, and Rollo hesitated to bring up the subject of his errand. (He may have guessed the effect it would have, since he'd known both the persons it concerned for a long time.)

They chatted for a while, but eventually Rollo asked Dr Ward quietly 'if I might enter upon official business with Dr Barry'.[46] 'Certainly,' said Ward. 'Indeed I think it would do him good.' Colonel Rollo told James that he'd had a memorandum from General Eyre ordering a medical board to be convened on Major Thomas Ormsby Ruttledge of the 17th Regiment, on the request of his commanding officer, Lieutenant Colonel Arthur Lowry Cole.

James was instantly galvanised, bursting out of the languor of illness. 'Cole wants to get rid of Major Ruttledge!' he exclaimed. 'I know what he's after!' In James's mind it was a familiar story – a commander exploiting the medical system to purge his regiment, and James supposed that General Eyre must be complicit. He immediately began plotting out loud: 'I shall order a medical board to assemble, and I shall be the president of it!'[47] He would fill the board with his own staff to ensure that it couldn't be rigged. The nightmare that had ensued from the case of Captain Thornhill in St Helena still rankled, but this time he would outmanoeuvre the Lieutenant Colonel and the General rather than defy them. Or so he thought. Unable to contain his righteous glee, he went on to Rollo: 'I know more of this case of Major Ruttledge than anybody – Colonel Cole wants to get rid of him; I know what he's up to, he tried the same thing at Malta, but I got the better of him in that instance.'

Colonel Rollo could hardly believe his ears. It was a remarkable outburst, and while it was true that Cole and Barry had been in Malta together when Cole was with the 69th Regiment, he'd been a mere captain then, and not in a position to order or request a medical board, let alone rig one.[48] Dr Barry must be wandering in his mind.

The doctor went on plotting aloud; if Eyre tried to forestall him by insisting on a board the very next day, James would still fox him in spite of his illness: 'I shall have it in this room, and I shall be the president.' Gesticulating with Eyre's memorandum and looking alarmingly unwell, he declaimed: 'I have a duty to perform between my conscience and my God, and I shall not allow anything of the sort!'

Rollo watched the performance with growing alarm. 'Dr Barry repeated these observations three or four times,' he reported later, 'and became so much excited that I was afraid he would do himself harm.'[49]

'There is no great hurry about the board,' he said, prising the memorandum from James's fingers. 'I shall write to you in a week or ten days.'

With that, he tactfully withdrew. After sitting on the problem for a couple of weeks, Rollo spoke to Colonel Cole and informed him of Dr Barry's allegations. Cole claimed to be mystified; he and Barry had always been on good terms. He informed Rollo 'that there was no truth whatever in the assertions' and that 'the old man could not have been aware of what he had been saying'.[50] He preferred to let the matter drop and not press any charges against the doctor.

Quite why James was so suspicious is unclear. Major Ruttledge, the subject of the board, was a seasoned soldier; besides the Crimea (where he and Cole had both been majors) he was a veteran of the First Afghan War, decorated for his part in the capture of Ghazni and Khelat, and by 1859 may well have been worn out. Although he wasn't boarded, that summer he was persuaded to give up his place in the 17th, exchanging with a major from the 32nd, and at the end of July he was placed on half-pay.[51]

By then, however, James Barry was no longer involved. Three days after receiving Rollo's report on Dr Barry's outburst, General Eyre (without any investigation beyond asking Cole whether the allegations were true) wrote to Major General Sir Charles Yorke, Lord Raglan's successor as Military Secretary to the Commander in Chief of the Forces:

> It is with unfeigned regret that I feel it necessary to bring under the consideration of His Royal Highness the General Commanding in Chief the conduct of Doctor Barry, Inspector General of Hospitals in this command. The conduct of this officer has been very extraordinary and repeated complaints have been made to me of him since his arrival. It is only a few weeks ago that he publicly insulted & without any provocation whatever the Dean and Rector of Montreal in presence of the Bishop & Clergy of this place.
>
> More recently he has made a gross, & I believe most unfounded charge against Colonel Cole ... Altho' these affairs have been brought officially to my notice I have endeavoured out of consideration for the age & infirmities of this Officer to settle them privately, & having done so I have no desire to revive them unless required to do so. I mention them merely as instances of the uncontrollable temperament of this officer which with his other infirmities really renders him unfit for his high position. I must add that the utmost allowance has been made by every one for Doctor Barry's peculiar constitution & eccentricities of

character but it is clear that there must be a limit to such consideration & it is most desirable that some arrangement should be made by which this officer may retire from the active duties of his Profession, for which, from age & natural infirmities, he is now *totally unfit*.[52]

A slightly disingenuous letter; one might even say duplicitous, Eyre belying his own stated intention of having 'no desire to revive' the matter. But it had its intended effect. James no longer had friends at Horse Guards; he didn't know General Yorke, and the Commander in Chief these days was Prince George, Duke of Cambridge, a royal blockhead who'd bungled the command of the infantry in the Crimea (crucially failing to support the cavalry at Balaclava when the Light Brigade was launched to its destruction); Cambridge had since dedicated himself to obstructing every effort to modernise the Army, and was, in short, a man with sins on his military conscience that would make any decent soldier die of shame.

The British Army could bear all that, but it would not tolerate officers making crazed, indecent allegations against other officers. Without help and influence, it was nearly the end of the line for James Barry. Besides, he was now seriously ill with bronchitis (or influenza – he stated both in different documents)[53] and took to his bed. No longer wishing to be seen by a military colleague, he called in a Canadian civilian friend, Dr G. W. Campbell. Whenever Campbell called, he would find the bedroom in near total darkness, and being young and 'in some awe of Inspector General Barry's rank and medical attainments', did not examine him thoroughly and never discovered his secret.[54]

In April James applied to be relieved of his duties – but only temporarily. However, he resigned his membership of the St James's Club – a sign that he guessed his days here might be numbered.[55] On 14 May 1859 he boarded a ship for home.

33

This Life and No Other

So all that great foul city of London there,—rattling, growling, smoking, stinking,—a ghastly heap of fermenting brickwork, pouring out poison at every pore,—you fancy it is a city of work? Not a street of it! It is a great city of play; very nasty play ... a huge billiard-table without the cloth, and with pockets as deep as the bottomless pit.

John Ruskin, *The Crown of Wild Olive*

The place had changed in fifty-odd years, and James had missed most of it – just glimpses at intervals, with great stretches of years in between. The streets were busier than ever with carts, coaches, carriages, gigs and omnibuses heaving through every thoroughfare. The city now seemed limitless, sprawling out into places that had been farms when Margaret was a girl, and whole districts had been demolished to lay railway lines, which added their smoke and smuts to the city's unbreathable air.

James Barry reached London on 1 June 1859, still unwell and exhausted by the sea voyage, having suffered terrible seasickness during the rough crossing, followed by another bout of illness at Liverpool.[1] He was accompanied by the ever-faithful John, his surviving pets and a diminished set of luggage. Only his most essential belongings had been brought with him from Canada – he'd convinced himself that he'd be returning there once his health was restored, and had left a lot behind in Montreal.

He'd scarcely had a chance to settle down when a letter arrived from the Army Medical Department, notifying him to appear before a medical board. The implication was clear and depressing; as James knew very well, when an officer of advanced years who was chronically ill was called to a board, it signalled the end of the line. James was indignant, convinced that he didn't need to be boarded; all he needed was to recover and get back to Canada. When he arrived at the department – which had moved to 6 Whitehall Yard, a narrow court opposite Horse Guards into which the government shovelled most of its small ancillary departments – he had another shock. Given his rank, he was entitled to a board chaired by Director General Thomas Alexander himself, or at least by one of the deputy inspectors based in England. Instead, his board consisted of three quite junior surgeons who were 'perfect strangers to me and to my peculiar habits'.[2] He didn't doubt their impartiality or their honesty, but they knew nothing of him and gave him only the most cursory interview. He admitted that as a result of his recent illness and rough voyage he 'looked unusually delicate and meagre', with the result that the board 'not unnaturally somewhat hastily jumped to the conclusion that [I] was in a bad state of health'.[3]

They reported accordingly, and Dr Barry was officially relieved of his position in the North American command.

On record James Barry was sixty years old, and in reality seventy – the three score years and ten regarded as one's lot. Yet he felt he had more to give, and it was unjust to deactivate him, disconnect him, reduce him to a state of powerlessness. Of more immediate concern, they had impoverished him, reducing him at a stroke to half-pay. Indeed, it was worse than that – under the rules of the Army, in order to receive the half-rate for an inspector general, he needed to have completed the full standard period of three years in that rank. Accordingly, he would receive only a deputy's half-pay.

Angry and indignant, James appealed, but got nowhere. Later that year, once his health had improved, he drafted an account of his career for submission to the Secretary of State for War, pointing out his achievements and dedication to duty, and applying to be returned to service. Writing his 'memorial' in the formal third person (as required when addressing a person of such exalted rank), he insisted that the board was wrong in its conclusion 'that your Memorialist was in a bad state of health':

> Whereas the fact is that he feels and believes himself to be stronger & in better health than he has been for the last two or three years and fully capable of effectively performing the duties of his rank.

Your Mem'st therefore prays that he may be restored to full pay and ordered back to Canada until he has completed his full period of Service, of which he requires nearly twenty months, by which means your Mem'st will be saved from great pecuniary loss.[4]

It had no effect; Canada was out of the question. In January he wrote a similar – but slightly less impassioned – memorandum to the Army Medical Department:

I am now prepared to serve Her Majesty in any quarter of the Globe to which I may be sent and am loath to close a career which impartially may be deemed to have been a useful and faithful one without some special mark of Her Majesty's gracious favor.[5]

He received neither a posting nor any mark of favour.

James Barry was already a relic of an old system. The Army Medical Department was changing character again – just a few weeks after this memorandum, the reformer Thomas Alexander died and was replaced as Director General by Dr James Brown Gibson, a man who'd been born in the same year James Barry performed his pioneering caesarean. Gibson had been the Duke of Cambridge's personal surgeon and was his protégé.[6] James Barry had no influence now.

For some reason – availability, courtesy, or possibly bureaucratic incompetence – nobody was posted to take Dr Barry's place in Canada for two years, and the work had to be managed by his former senior surgeon major (the ranks had been changed again – staff surgeon first class replaced by surgeon major).[7] But he would never go back. The full official summary of James Barry's army career had begun 'At Home' on 5 July 1813 when he took up his post at Chelsea; it then ran in a long list spanning the Cape of Good Hope, Mauritius, St Helena, the West Indies, Malta and beyond, and ended with a final simple entry: 'Half Pay, 19 July 59'.[8]

James was cut off from the source of his life and sense of identity. And there was more. Later that year the steamer *John Bull*, on which his trunks and boxes had been loaded at Montreal, had sailed down the St Lawrence as far as Quebec, and there, a dozen miles from the city, she was wrecked near the eastern tip of a river island, the Île d'Orléans. Everything on board was lost. As well as his general belongings, in those trunks had been James's books, documents, letters and paraphernalia stretching back throughout his life and career. At a stroke he was cut off from all but a sliver of his past.[9]

James was without purpose and all but without a past, his identity merely a shell. What could he do, what kind of life could he have now? His circle of friends shrunk still more when in June 1860 Lady Mary Somerset died, severing the final contact with his time at the Cape with Lord Charles.

In a bid to recapture some of his past, that year James took to the sea again, for only the second time of his own volition, on holiday. He went to the West Indies, and with him, as always, went his manservant, John; it was a journey into the past for John too, seeing his homeland for the first time in nearly thirty years.

They went to Jamaica first. It was a true revisiting; rather than stay in a Kingston hotel, James took advantage of his rank to secure free quarters at one of the Army camps – probably Stoney Hill, where he'd lived in the 1830s and which had the better accommodation. He made the acquaintance of the officers, including the Principal Medical Officer, a newly promoted deputy inspector called O'Flaherty, and grew particularly friendly with one of his assistant surgeons (a rank now equivalent to a hospital assistant in James's early days), a young Irishman from County Kildare, Charles Benjamin Mosse.[10]

Coming to the West Indies was a substantial physical risk for James; his career in Trinidad had ended with malaria and yellow fever, and he surely couldn't hope to survive a tropical fever now. But then, what had he to lose? He stayed for many months and settled into the community.

While he was in Kingston, he decided – or was persuaded – to have his likeness captured on camera. For the only time in his long life, James Barry emerges from obscurity, his image in life captured and impressed on paper, in a tiny, sepia-toned *carte-de-visite* print, four inches by two, not much larger than the miniature painted nearly half a century earlier. James is standing outdoors, drenched in sunlight. In the fashion of the day, he wears a dark broadcloth coat and loose grey trousers, the strand of a watch chain and a snow-white shirt with a high collar and a dark cravat secured with a small brooch. His right hand rests on the head of his dog, a little smooth-coated white terrier who sits blinking on a cushion in a cane chair; James's left hand hovers uncertainly – about to be raised in a gesture or reach out to the dog, or be placed on his hip, or perhaps reaching for the non-existent hilt of the sword he'd been accustomed to lean on for the past forty-odd years. He seems to have been caught before he has properly posed himself – an accidentally candid image at a time when photographs had to be staged. He looks uncertain – eyes narrowed at something beyond our field of view, the sullen lips pursed as if about to speak. His face is dominated by the nose, which in age is larger than ever, and his dyed hair is receding high on his forehead, swept across in a wavy lick. At James's elbow is the ever-present John; also dressed in dark broadcloth and white shirt with a watch chain across his front, he stands stolidly, hands at his sides with the thumbs forward like the soldier he once was. He is only slightly taller than James, but much broader; his dark face is handsome and gentle, also gazing curiously towards whatever or whoever James is looking at off-camera – sharing the experience with him as he had shared so much else. James gave the photograph to Mosse, who kept it all his life and passed it on to his descendants.[11]

James also made friends with a Scottish expatriate called M'Crindle, a chemist and druggist in Kingston. He and his wife were often invited to dine with James at his camp quarters. 'He had a well-set table for them,' their son recalled, 'but he ate only vegetables and fruit. When he wanted a haircut, he drove to their house, sent for the barber, and got his hair cut in the drawing room.'[12]

Eventually the inevitable happened, and James fell seriously ill. He sent for M'Crindle, whom he apparently regarded as his most trusted friend in Jamaica, and showed him 'a small black box'. If he were to die, he wanted M'Crindle to come and fetch the box and then keep it until it was sent for. Mystified, M'Crindle agreed, and, as if sealing the pact, James gave him a gold ring with the inscription, 'Sacred to the memory of Mary Anne', offering no explanation as to who Mary Anne might be.[13] With nobody else to reach out to, Margaret was securing a resting place for her mother's only legacy.

Despite his age, James Barry was still tough; amazingly, he weathered his illness and was soon back in society. Perhaps moved by his brush with mortality, he made the M'Crindle family a strange offer that was both touching and unsettling. James – and before him Margaret – had always been strongly drawn to little girls; there was a mothering urge whose origin can easily be guessed and which, despite never being afforded an outlet, had never gone away. Now James developed a deep attachment to the M'Crindle's baby daughter, and expressed a wish to adopt her.

He pressed his case, promising her an excellent life; she would be sent to a 'cousin' of his in Scotland, whose name they later recalled as 'Lady Jane Gordon' (conceivably a connection of the Earl of Buchan or the Earl of Lonsdale). He gave gifts to the infant, including a silver cup and knife, fork and spoon, engraved 'Presented by Dr James Barry', which he ordered specially from a jeweller's in Glasgow, the M'Crindle family's native town. Financially, he could not have given the girl a much better life than her parents, but he might have seen to her education and nurtured her ambitions. Like every other 'feminine' urge in James's long life, this one inevitably came to nothing – put down as yet another odd act of an eccentric character.

It was time to move on from Jamaica and dig deeper into the past. James set off for the Windward Islands; there was a friend there he wanted to see, an echo from the good old days.

Ebenezer Rogers, a lieutenant in the 3rd West India Regiment, en route to Barbados, found himself sharing his steamer cabin with a most peculiar fellow passenger. Rogers occupied the top bunk and the elderly gentleman had the lower, and they got to know each other, as cabin mates will. Rogers was intrigued by Dr James Barry, but how he'd been reduced to sharing a cabin, Rogers didn't speculate. Dr Barry had become a figure of remark during the few days' Caribbean voyage, with his pet goat and little white terrier. At dinner each evening he would dominate the table talk with amazing, unbelievable stories, portraying himself as a lady-killer who could win the best-looking woman at any party or ball. Each morning when he woke, he would demand the cabin to himself: 'Now then, youngster,' he would say 'in a harsh and peevish voice', 'clear out of my cabin while I dress.'[14] The young lieutenant never guessed the reason for it.

On reaching Bridgetown, at the earliest opportunity James took a carriage to the local commander's residence to call on the man he'd come all this way to see, one of his oldest acquaintances from the Cape of Good Hope – Captain Cloete, as was, his old duelling adversary. Like James, he'd risen in the service, and was now Major General Sir Abraham Josias Cloete, CB KH, Officer Commanding the Windward and Leeward Islands command. They'd kept distantly in touch, but had little contact with one another since those days at the Cape with Lord Charles Somerset. General Cloete had been in Barbados for some years now, and only three years earlier had got married.[15] He was also on his way out – his command was coming to an end and in June he'd be sailing back to England (which was nominally his home these days). His replacement, Major General E. Basil Brooke, would soon be arriving to take over.[16] Meanwhile, James and his friend got on with catching up and reliving the past. In James's case the reliving would become a little too real.

He met two other old acquaintances in Barbados – General Cloete's aide-de-camp, Captain Shadwell Clerke, and Surgeon David Reid McKinnon; both were in the 21st Royal North British Fusiliers and had been in the Crimea with the 4th Division (Clerke was another whose health had been permanently marred by his time in the trenches).[17] McKinnon was in the process of transferring out of the regiment to the staff and would shortly be returning to Britain;[18] he and James were close, and would remain friends for the rest of James's life.

Not so Captain Clerke. Quite how or why he and James fell out is unknown, but it may well be that Dr Barry's and General Cloete's duel came up in conversation – James did like to boast. One way or another, he had a conversation with Clerke; remarks were exchanged, and the remarks escalated into a dispute. Before anyone could stop it, Captain Clerke had grossly offended Dr Barry, and Dr Barry had challenged him to a duel.[19] Clerke, bound on his honour as an officer and a gentleman, accepted. The commonest cause for a duel was being 'given the lie' – called a liar. It may be that Clerke had openly doubted Dr Barry's claim that he had shot off the peak of Cloete's cap. If that was the case, then Dr Barry was hardly a person to shrink from attempting to prove himself right by the empirical method. Fortunately for the elderly doctor, General Cloete heard of the affair and called them both together, branded them 'a couple of dam' fools' and forced them to shake hands.

With that, James Barry's stay in the West Indies drew to a close. General and Lady Cloete sailed for England on 11 June aboard the screw steamer *Avon*, along with several other military families. James probably sailed with them. The ship reached Spithead on 1 July,[20] and as on countless previous occasions, James Barry stepped from a vessel onto British soil. He never left again.

Margaret's life was closing in. James no longer had a purpose. He had few friends left – few from the old times, anyway. He settled in London, in far more modest accommodation than he'd been accustomed to. He still socialised with the friends who remained, particularly the Earl of Lonsdale, and continued to be an occasional guest at Lowther and Whitehaven, going there for what would turn out to be the last time in October 1864.[21]

London was a miserable, oppressive place for a person with little income, as Margaret had learned the hard way in her youth. And now she was racked by age and bronchial illness; the toxic, choking London smokes were torment, and the constant presence of disease – especially cholera – was a perennial fear. Through James she had grown accustomed to the pleasant, wealthy side of London – the London of Mayfair mansions and aristocratic households – and all but forgotten the London of deprivation and dirt and debt. They welcomed her back. As if tracing her life backwards, Margaret took James to live in the district she had known when she was a girl. James took rooms in a house at 14 Margaret Street, near Oxford Market in Marylebone.

The house was owned by a Mr James Anderson, a middle-aged Scottish surgeon and dentist; he and his wife, Elizabeth, let out several sets of rooms, and as lodging houses went it was of the respectable but not affluent sort – moderately well-off gentlefolk who were styled as 'visitors' rather than lodgers. Some had servants of their own, although the young maid of all work, Sophia Bishop, could also be called upon.[22]

This was precisely the kind of accommodation in which Margaret and her mother had stayed during their early visits to London, when they were trying to prise some assistance out of the tight fists of James Barry RA. Indeed, exactly sixty years earlier Margaret had walked past this very street on her way from their lodgings to her uncle's rotting old house in Little Castle Street. She had come full circle, back to the origin of James Barry, having grown into the same irascible, eccentric old man her uncle had been.

While revisiting the scenes of her past, it isn't known whether Margaret went looking for any of her acquaintances from that time. Her namesake, Margaret Reardon, Daniel's daughter, who'd been born and named while the persona of James Barry was being conceived, was still in London; in her fifties now, she had never married, and lived in Islington with her sister – James's 'sweet Ellen', also unmarried – on an income from shares left them by their father.[23] They had both been infants when James came into existence and probably knew nothing of him.

Looking back on her life, had it been worthwhile? Fifty-six years she had spent deceiving the world, to the extent that she had effectively ceased to exist; James Barry had become more real – as such things are measured, in stature and presence in the world – than Margaret had ever been. The last dress she had worn, packed away in a trunk in anticipation of wearing it again in a few years, would be fit only for a museum now. Only after death would it be discovered how she had pined for it.*

What would her life have been otherwise? It was 1865, little more than a generation away from a new century, yet the situation of women had barely changed. In some ways it was more straitened than ever, the rebellious ghost of the Blue Stockings thoroughly laid by Victorian womanly virtue. Margaret would have been a governess at best, little more than an above-stairs servant, treated with contempt by families, cramming French irregular verbs and the use of the globes into generations of reluctant children, growing old and crotchety and lonely … Or perhaps married to a well-off man, rescued from penury and drudgery but with no personal freedom, and no identity – just a 'Mrs' tacked on to her husband's name. She might as well be 'Dr James Barry' – because even if the name wasn't the one she'd been born with, he was nonetheless her creation, and his achievements were all her own.

She had chosen this life and no other, and had lived it to the full, as few men or women did in this or any other age. In that respect at least, it had surely been worth it.

14 Margaret Street, London: Monday 24 July 1865

James was ill again. The oppressive summer heat magnified the suffering, but he was too sick to notice it, or be aware of the fact that the heat had exacerbated the infection seething in his innards.

He was unwell more often than not these days; his lungs had been bad for years, and the previous winter had done a lot of damage. It had been especially cold,[24] and the black ranks of chimney pots across the skyline churned out smoke, producing the thick dirty fog known as a London Particular, a damp, choking air that caused the equally distinctive London

---

* see Chapter 34

Blacks, the layer of soot dusting the snow, turning the sparrows black
and even marring the coats of livestock miles outside the metropolis; it
got into houses, grimed the skin, and caused a chronic affliction to the
lungs. Dr Barry had no longer been able to treat himself, and had had
to call in his old friend David McKinnon, now a surgeon major at the
Army Recruiting Office in nearby Duke Street. Throughout that winter,
McKinnon had examined and treated his elderly colleague without ever
discovering his secret (perhaps for the same reason as Dr Campbell in
Montreal). Spring and summer had eased the air pollution, but other
threats had arisen; James had succumbed to a new illness and it was now
bringing him to the edge of death.

Outside the window, London was sweltering under an unaccustomed burst of heat, driving the mercury up to 29°C.[25] Inside, the
room was foetid. McKinnon had seen several such cases in the past few
months, as had every other doctor; classified as epidemic diarrhoea,
it was a perennial problem in the city, but the unusually hot summer
had worsened it, and the disease had been carrying off Londoners at
the rate of up to three hundred a week.[26] It was causing a profound
concern in the medical profession, seen as a harbinger of the cholera
that was running rampant through the Mediterranean again. Twelve
years had passed since the last cholera epidemic in Britain, and as always
the very name elicited terror; for this reason, doctors were now reluctant to diagnose it officially – just as James Barry and his colleagues
had been in Malta.

The confusing classification of diseases labelled 'cholera' persisted,
but at least the epidemiology was understood. Medical authorities were
in agreement: it was conveyed through water contaminated with the
efflux of infected patients. Its exact pathology was not understood, and
would not be for a few years yet – the miasma theory of disease was still
influential, even though Louis Pasteur had demonstrated the existence of
pathogenic microscopic organisms and the new germ theory was gaining
ground. Either way, the authorities knew what had to be done to prevent these lethal gastrointestinal infections. For centuries city dwellers
had drawn their water from street pumps, a supply that was extremely
vulnerable to contamination; at the same time, the London sewers were
in an appalling state, crumbling, choked, discharging their slurry into the
rivers – some of which (such as the Fleet) had long ago been covered over
and turned into sewers themselves. The great new engineering project

overseen by Joseph Bazalgette, with its thousands of miles of new sewers and powerful pumping stations, had been completed this year, but it was too late for James Barry.

All week the temperature outside had been rising and James's condition worsening. Mr McKinnon faced a seemingly impossible challenge – as did all practitioners. One eminent physician wrote at this time: 'There is no remedy which has the slightest pretensions to be considered a cure for cholera; no drug or agent which, so far as we know, will neutralise the poison or lessen its virulence.' Portentously he added: 'I have not the faintest hope ... that a specific remedy for such a disease as cholera will ever be discovered.'[27] Meanwhile, doctors did what they could, decade by decade refining their notions of what worked and what did not. The old calomel and opium treatment was of indeterminate value, while inoculation with an extract of the plant *Quassia amara* (also used against malaria) was popularly thought infallible, though doctors had come to regard it as ineffectual but harmless.[28] Purgatives such as castor oil or Epsom salts to clean out the bowel were thought useful, and saline treatment – which was based on a theory known to be false (that cholera was caused by a deficiency of salt in the blood) – nonetheless had strong evidence to support its effectiveness; it was administered through well-salted beef tea or salt water after purging of the bowel.[29] But in the absence of a proper understanding of the pathology, a really effective treatment was as unattainable as ever.

All there was for James Barry to do was suffer, in a manner he had witnessed and treated in others but never experienced for himself. The diarrhoea was terrible – not copious but watery and producing a hideous stench. And what was worse, his secret made it impossible to permit any assistance with passing the diarrhoea or with personal cleanliness. Once he was past a certain point of weakness – and he had reached that point today – he could only lie in his soiled sheets and wander feverishly in his wits while McKinnon and John (who was accustomed to his master's quirks and knew better than to try to breach the boundary Dr Barry had built around himself) looked on helplessly.

Outside, London sweltered and racketed intolerably. James lay in a near stupor, his state so distracted, he had forgotten his longstanding wish that if he should die his remains must be buried as they were, in this nightshirt and this sheet, without examination. John mysteriously absented himself at this time, and James lay alone through much of the day and evening, although Sophia the housemaid sat with him at times. He was weakening by the hour.

The mind, in its mortal extremity, brings out all its deepest memories, and Margaret's would be no different. Her life had been rich: the voyages, the mountains and seas, the cities and coasts, the rank hospitals and sick soldiers, the glittering balls and country rides, and the red-coated ranks marching in the tropical heat … a baby brought out from the belly of its living mother … a message of thanks from the greatest general who ever lived … the regard of the man who knew Margaret more intimately than any other, who loved and supported her and suffered himself in part because of her … the sharp-featured, irresistible revolutionary luring her into an audacious adventure … the mother who had sacrificed her own health and well-being to help her to a life of her own … and the little girl with red-gold curls and blue-green eyes watching the ships come in at the Cork quays, seeing the troops march by, and wishing the impossible – that she might be a soldier with a sword and pair of colours …

She had made her fancy real, but now it was all over. Around four hours after midnight, in the darkened, stifling room, by the guttering candlelight, the last glow of Margaret Anne Bulkley's formidable spirit flickered and went out.

34

A Perfect Female

Nature with Barry Vy'd; She lost the Day
Then in revenge she snatch'd his life away

Margaret Anne Bulkley on James Barry RA, 1807[1]

London: Tuesday 25 July 1865

David McKinnon was disturbed at his breakfast table by Sophia, the
maid from Margaret Street. The news she brought was sad but
fully expected. As he'd done frequently in the past several months, Mr
McKinnon put on his hat, picked up his bag and set off with a heavy
heart to see his patient.

The room was as oppressive as ever, but silent now that the laboured
breathing had stopped. James's eyes were closed, his features greyed and
sunken in death. Only the most cursory examination was required.

Leaving Sophia to arrange the laying out, Mr McKinnon went off
to his office, where he wrote a brief note to Director General Sir James
Brown Gibson ('I have the honor to report that the Officer named in the
margin, died at 4 o'clock AM this morning.')[2] That done, he began seeing
to James Barry's personal affairs. As far as he knew, he'd had neither next
of kin nor friends in a position to take responsibility for him.

As the layer-out pulled the bedroom door to, she glanced back. The
corpse was wrapped in its winding-sheet, small, white and neat. She
could hardly credit what she had seen. She closed the door with a snap,

went below stairs to the kitchen, and without saying anything of the shocking discovery she had made, she told Sophia to go up and retrieve the copper of water. The mistress of the house wasn't at home, so the layer-out would have to come back for her tip; gathering her few things together, she went out of the door and up the steps to the street. It was not until some time later that it occurred to her that she might make more from this business than just her fee.

Later that day, the undertaker's men came to take the body away. The coffin was vastly oversized – made for a man six and a half feet tall.[3] With the mortality rate running so high at present, one had to take whatever was in stock, but in this case it almost seemed like a tasteless jest. Sophia stripped the bed, bundled up the soiled linen, and began airing the room. The next day, with Sophia in tow, Mr McKinnon took a cab to the Marylebone register office and entered the death. Name: James Barry; Sex: male; Age … McKinnon guessed at about seventy (a near estimate – Margaret had been seventy-six, James officially sixty-six). Cause of death: 'Diarrhoea: certified' (caused by 'errors in diet', although he didn't put that ambiguous opinion on the certificate).[4] Sophia, who was illiterate, placed her mark as informant, 'present at the death'.

During the days following Dr Barry's death, other visitors came to the house. One, who was remembered or heard about but whom nobody could explain, was a footman (or possibly two) in full livery, who arrived and took away the mysterious black box that Dr Barry had shown to Mr M'Crindle in Jamaica. This footman was apparently the agent of the secret owner. He also took away Dr Barry's little dog and gave John (who had returned after his unexplained absence) the passage money back to Jamaica.[5]

What was in that black box was never discovered, let alone why it was so important to the footman's unknown master. A 'black box' would probably be a cash box or a document case; the former is improbable, but the latter quite likely. One possibility is that it contained personal letters from Lord Charles Somerset. If such letters were of an intimate nature, Margaret would have wanted to keep possession of them until her last breath. He had been 'more than a father' to her, the most important and beloved person in her life. But if the Somersets knew of such letters, Margaret might in honour have agreed to have them discreetly returned to the family after her death to prevent a scandal if they were discovered.

Dr Barry's other effects were taken into the care of Sir Charles McGrigor & Co, his agents, for disposal. Like James Barry RA, James Barry MD had passed away intestate, but a few pieces went to persons he had named verbally. McGrigor's manager, Mr Barrie, received the doctor's gold watch chain, as well as a few valueless items – the Inspector General's commission, a visiting card and a battered old travelling trunk. The diamond ring from Archduke Maximilian disappeared; it passed through Mr Barrie's hands (he showed it to his daughter and told her how the doctor had earned it) but then fell into obscurity.[6] There wasn't much money to disburse (some said later that John was given £100)[7] and many of his belongings had been lost in the St Lawrence River five years earlier.

There was little left behind to mark the passage of James Barry's life. It was almost as if he'd never existed, and like countless millions of other old men he would fade into obscurity and oblivion. With no family to remember him, the fading would be more rapid than for most.

Or so it seemed in those first few weeks.

Kensal Green Cemetery, Chelsea: Saturday 29 July 1865

The funeral was a small one: a simple hearse and a handful of mourners took the path up to the open plot. The cemetery, a long band of green in the countryside just beyond Kensal New Town – bordered by the London and North Western Railway on one side and the Great Junction Canal and Great Western on the other – was large and only three decades old, so there was still a fair amount of open space still unused. Compared with the metropolitan burying grounds, which were swollen to bursting with packed corpses, Kensal was quite a pleasant place to be laid to rest.

At plot number 19301, purchased two days earlier for the sum of 3 guineas,[8] the oversize coffin was taken off the hearse and lowered into the enormous grave. There was no military ceremony, as the Queen's Regulations only allowed such honours for officers still serving. A great pity, as Dr Barry's rank would have entitled him to a brigadier general's funeral, with a battalion of infantry, two squadrons of cavalry and nine cannon.[9] No record survives of who was present – David McKinnon undoubtedly, perhaps Mr Barrie and Mr and Mrs Anderson, possibly Sophia the maid. Certainly John would have been there. Eventually a plain gravestone would be erected, inscribed simply:

DR JAMES BARRY
INSPECTOR GENERAL OF HOSPITALS
DIED 25 JULY 1865
AGED 70 YEARS

The age was based on McKinnon's estimate. Yet age was the least of the mysteries; nobody knew the truth about Dr James Barry, other than a handful of individuals who had faithfully kept it to themselves, and even they didn't know the half of it. It seemed that Margaret had succeeded in maintaining her secret intact beyond death, as she had always wished.

London: August 1865

David McKinnon took a hansom cab from the Recruiting Office in Duke Street to the offices of Sir Charles McGrigor & Co in Charles Street. Nearly two weeks had passed since the funeral, and he'd been summoned to attend to some unspecified business connected with Dr Barry's estate.

When he arrived and was shown into a side room, McKinnon was surprised to find the charwoman from the lodging house who'd laid out the body.[10] She informed him that the landlady, Mrs Anderson, had refused to pay her the perquisites to which she was entitled for performing the laying out, which was above and beyond her daily work. *Somebody* would have to pay her, she insisted, and it might as well come from Dr Barry's estate or from the Army. The woman was abrasive and in an ill humour, and among her imprecations she mentioned, in the manner of an insinuation, that she was aware that Dr Barry was really female.

McKinnon was taken aback; he'd known James Barry for ten years and been his medical attendant for many months, and knew nothing of the kind. The woman was surprised; she had assumed that she'd unearthed a conspiracy of secrecy. 'Well, a pretty doctor you must be not to know that!' she said. 'I wouldn't like to be attended by you.'[11]

Like most people acquainted with Dr Barry, McKinnon found the claim entirely credible. But he wasn't about to let this woman crow. 'It is none of my business whether Dr Barry was a male or a female,' he said. 'It is likely he might be neither – he might be an imperfectly developed man. Or a hermaphrodite.'

The woman poured scorn on this; she had examined the body and there was no question that it was that of 'a perfect female'. Not only that, she'd seen unmistakable signs of the deceased having borne a child 'when very young'. McKinnon inquired how she had formed this conclusion, and the woman pointed to her own lower abdomen. 'From marks here,' she said. 'I'm a married woman and the mother of nine children. I ought to know.'

It was becoming clear to the layer-out that this doctor genuinely hadn't had a clue that his patient was a woman, and that she truly had stumbled alone on a great secret. This might be even better than she'd imagined. She made it plain to Mr McKinnon that she would be willing to keep the secret if she were compensated sufficiently for it.

McKinnon was unmoved. 'All Dr Barry's relatives are dead, and it's no secret of mine.' And he bade the woman good day.

In the days after her conversation with David McKinnon, realising with considerable disappointment that there was nobody to blackmail, the layer-out began telling her story. She apparently began with the Army authorities, possibly attempting with them what she had tried with Mr McKinnon, for it was in the Army that the revelation first spread, passing rapidly from person to person. Inspector General Dr James Barry had been well known in the service and the constant subject of rumour and remark, and the news was readily believed and greedily consumed.

On Monday 14 August it broke publicly, appearing in Ireland first. 'An incident is just now being discussed in military circles,' reported *Saunders's News-Letter and Daily Advertiser*, 'so extraordinary that, were not its truth capable of being vouched for by official authority, the narration would certainly be deemed absolutely incredible.'[12] In an article packed with factual errors (including the claim that the doctor – as yet unnamed – had died in Corfu after resigning from the Army), the paper summarised a life of amazing deception: 'Our officers quartered at the Cape between fifteen and twenty years ago [sic] may remember a certain doctor … enjoying a reputation for considerable skill in his profession, especially for firmness, decision, and rapidity in difficult operations.' At least that part was true, as was the report that the doctor had been found to be not just a woman but a mother.

The story was repeated in newspapers across Ireland, and by Saturday 19 August it had crossed the Irish Sea and appeared in the London

Morning Post under the title 'A Strange Story'. It spread to Birmingham, Shropshire, Manchester, Sheffield, Liverpool, Newcastle, Aberdeen, Selkirk, then beyond Britain and around the Empire – everywhere that had a newspaper reproduced the same report, word for word (a typical practice at the time), and every officers' mess and governor's levée discussed it, particularly in stations where James Barry had served and where tales about his oddity were a part of local folklore. Initially the newspapers elided the late doctor's name, but within days he was being identified as Dr Barry. This did little to enlighten the public; the *Cork Examiner* printed the story, with no awareness that Dr Barry had any connection with that city (his being a nephew of the historical painter had been forgotten decades ago, quietly dropped from his own account of himself).[13] The author of the original piece in *Saunders's* had 'no doubt whatever' about the facts of the case but doubted whether even the novelist Mary Elizabeth Braddon (author of the sensational *Lady Audley's Secret*, a tale of a husband-murdering heroine) would have dared use it as a plot. Only one paper disdained to print the story; *The Times*, using the same title, 'A Strange Story', covered a tale from Suffolk about a vanished British soldier who'd married the daughter of Tipu Sultan after the siege of Seringapatam in 1799 then went missing leaving a huge estate that was now awaiting a claimant. The nineteenth century really did throw up all manner of remarkable characters.

One or two papers added their own commentaries to the story of Dr Barry. In Cumberland, the *Whitehaven News* – which detested the powerful Lowther dynasty – seized gleefully on the Earl of Lonsdale's embarrassment, and speculated on whether he knew Dr Barry's secret: 'we are not inclined to libel the noble Lord by supposing that his powers of discrimination are now so defective that he is unable to discern the difference between a man and a woman, after having employed them, day and night, with the same result, for upwards of half-a-century.'[14]

That paper also posed the question that was on everyone's mind, once they'd got over their glee and outrage at the scandal – *who was this woman?* Nobody could answer. Her identity was an absolute blank. And so they invented tales out of the clues James had left behind. Lord Albemarle (formerly George Keppel, who as a young lieutenant had met James at the Cape and been fascinated by him) was told by an officer's daughter that 'she believed the Doctor to have been the legitimate grand-daughter of a Scotch Earl, whose name I do not now give' (presumably Buchan);[15] Albemarle heard that this girl had studied medicine, disguised herself as a man, and joined the Army because she was in love with an Army surgeon. (As a woman, naturally, she could not have done it of her own volition.)

The medical profession tugged its whiskers thoughtfully and wondered how it was possible for a woman to live out a career as a surgeon and physician. After all, it was a given that women simply did not possess either the aptitude or the fortitude. The editor of the *Medical Times and Gazette* concluded that she could not have been a very good doctor; he suggested that there were doubts about the 'firmness', 'skill in operating' and 'decision of character' that had been attributed to Dr James Barry; but of course 'the querulousness, irritability, and quarrelsomeness' were all perfectly believable. The editor also reminded his readers that standards for entry into the Army's medical service hadn't been very high in 1813.[16] As far as the profession was concerned, that was the problem receipted and filed. Those who had actually *known* Dr Barry, of course, knew better.

Meanwhile, all that concerned officialdom was whether the body they had buried and recorded really was that of Inspector General Dr James Barry. The General Registrar wrote to David McKinnon asking if he could confirm it ('not for publication but for my own information'); in reply the doctor confirmed it and described his conversation with the layer-out.[17] However, as he could not claim to have ascertained Barry's sex personally, the records remained unaltered and the case was closed.

Île d'Orléans, Quebec: late 1860

The St Lawrence was nearly five miles wide just below Quebec, more like an inland sea than a river. The wreck of the steamer *John Bull* lay in the choppy grey-brown water, and a good deal of cargo had washed ashore on Orleans. The owners had arranged for salvagers to pick up what they could from the beach. They found not only items of cargo but a large quantity of books and papers strewn about. One of the men, idly curious, picked up a book; it was a Bible, and written in the flyleaf was a name: 'Dr James Barry'. He found the same name on a document lying nearby; this was a remarkable item – a sheet of vellum with a wafer seal, printed with florid letters:

In the Name and on the Behalf of His Majesty

> GEORGE the Third ... To Our Trusty and Welbeloved James Barry
> MD. Greetings: We do by these Presents Constitute and Appoint you
> to be Assistant Surgeon to the Forces ...
>
>   ... Given at Our Court at Carlton House the Seventh day of
> December 1815 in the Fifty Sixth Year of Our Reign.[18]

The salvager didn't know what to make of it, and had no idea who James Barry might be, but thought it an interesting document. He pocketed it, along with the Bible, and took it home. The Bible vanished at some point, but the document remained in his family's keeping for many years.

James Barry's first commission was one of a handful of curios of his life scattered in various parts of the world – a few letters here, a document there, the miniature portrait at the Cape. In London, Mr Barrie treasured the gold watch chain, but he also kept the old travelling trunk – one of the few items of dunnage that had sailed with James and been spared the fate of the *John Bull*. To his surprise, on opening it, Mr Barrie had found that the interior of the lid had been covered with a collage of fashion plates clipped from ladies' magazines – a parade of gowns, crinolines, bonnets, hats and coiffures pasted to the musty leather: a catalogue of loss and longing.[19]

The other traces of James Barry's life and Margaret's before him were scattered or destroyed, flotsam drifting down the current to the cold, wide ocean.

Epilogue

A garden in Constantia: summer 1932

The lady of the house was very proud of her family's history, and was surprised to find that her luncheon guest, despite being a military medical man, hadn't heard of its most noted connection, nor of the event that had occurred on this very spot over a hundred years earlier.

Colonel Nathaniel John Crawford Rutherford was in his late fifties, and had retired some four years earlier after three decades as a doctor in the Royal Army Medical Corps.[1] Despite serving for years on the South African station, he'd never heard of Dr James Barry.[2] Yet folk tales about him persisted even now, 104 years after his departure – particularly here, at the old homestead of Alphen. After lunch, Colonel Rutherford was led down to the gardens, where his hostess, Mrs Nicolette Bairnsfather,* showed him the very spot where Dr Barry had fought his duel with her kinsman, Captain Josias Cloete.

His imagination fired, Colonel Rutherford began researching the life of James Barry, and some years later produced a short series of articles in the Royal Army Medical Corps' journal telling his story. Rutherford had evidently been profoundly frustrated by the gaps and mysteries, and invented details quite liberally to fill the empty spaces and solve the puzzles. He couldn't conceive how a woman could be a medical student – 'One cannot possibly picture one of Barry's sex carrying it off in the constant company' of boisterous medical students, he wrote,[3] apparently forgetting momentarily that Barry had 'carried it off' in the company of soldiers for fifty years. Rutherford repeated the myth that this anonymous girl had joined the Army in pursuit of an unrequited

_____

* *née* Cloete

love who had fathered a child on her and abandoned her, and drew a portrait of an embittered man-hating female who quarrelled with men at every opportunity.

And so the myth of Dr James Barry went through another evolution. Colonel Rutherford was by no means the first to mythologise him, but like all the others he failed to find any clue to the identity of the girl who had hoodwinked the world.

Charles Dickens had begun it in 1867, piecing together a short narrative of 'Doctor James' for his magazine *All the Year Round*, based on the testimony of an anonymous informant who had known Barry in St Helena. Lieutenant (later Colonel) Ebenezer Rogers, who had met him en route to Barbados, researched his life not long afterward, preserving some details for posterity and using them in a novel, *The Modern Sphinx*. The story remained alive decade after decade, and was eventually dramatised. In summer 1919, eight months after the end of the Great War, St James's Theatre, London, announced:

MATINEE
In Aid of the EDITH CAVELL HOMES OF REST
FOR NURSES and ST GEORGE'S ORPHANAGE,
Cape Town.

Tuesday, July 22nd, at 2.30

FIRST PERFORMANCE of a Romantic Play founded
on South African history a hundred years ago,

Dr JAMES BARRY

By Olga Racster and Jessica Grove

Miss Sybil Thorndike
will create the part of Dr James Barry[4]

The play added new fancies to the known story – in addition to the duel (following which Dr Barry breaks down in tears), there was a plotline in which a young lady in love with Dr Barry is manoeuvred by him into loving another, more worthy, man. The reviews were mixed. *The*

Times thought Sybil Thorndike's performance in the title role 'unusually good', particularly impressed by the death scene, staged simply against black curtains lit by a single candle: 'One can hardly imagine a more trying ordeal for a young actress than the death scene of a woman of 60 or more masquerading as a man.'[5] *The Observer* was also impressed by the leading actress, but less so by the play – 'Dr Barry's existence ... was comparatively uneventful, and there were really no outstanding incidents on which to base a play.'[6] The *Manchester Guardian* thought that 'the skill of the authoresses ... was chiefly needed to clothe the incidents with credibility' and that the play was 'fairly exciting as a piece of melodrama'.[7] In 1932 – the year in which Colonel Rutherford visited Alphen and first learned of the duel – the playwrights turned their drama into a novel, *The Journal of Dr James Barry*, which stacked the fiction still higher and thicker.

It would be the 1950s before anyone got around to attempting a serious biography. By that time even more of the evidence had disappeared and all of the witnesses were long dead. And still nobody could discover precisely who the woman who pretended to be James Barry really was; the first true biographer, writing in 1958, had discovered the connection with the historical painter and his sister Mrs Bulkley, who had an unnamed daughter and looked after 'James' at Edinburgh, but still the true identities and connections remained out of reach ... until now.[8]

Over the same course of decades, another truth – a far more important truth, which had been there all the time in the story of Dr James Barry if only people had chosen to look beyond the scandal and romance – was playing out. Namely, the fact that had so disturbed the editor of the *Medical Times and Gazette* – that a woman, a seemingly delicate one, could be fully capable not only of studying medicine and training as a surgeon but also becoming an exemplary practitioner, as able to master the knowledge, wield the blade and stomach the horror as any man. Now other women were setting out to prove it.

In 1865, the year of James Barry's death, Elizabeth Garrett, a young woman who, like Margaret Bulkley, came from an aspiring lower middle-class family, overcame the obstructions placed in her way by the medical establishment and gained a licence to practise medicine. She'd had to obtain her education piecemeal through private avenues, having been refused entry by all the medical schools in Britain, and had been inspired by the example of the British-born Elizabeth Blackwell, who in

1849 had become the first woman in the United States of America to gain a medical degree. Blackwell had been forced to abandon her ambition to be a surgeon after losing an eye to an infection, and her bids to practise as a physician were frustrated by prejudice. But she began a private practice in New York and went on to eminence; in 1874, along with several other female practitioners, including Elizabeth Garrett Anderson (who had married in 1871 and who'd also had to begin with a private practice), she helped establish the pioneering London School of Medicine for Women.

The profession remained hostile. In 1873 the British Medical Association accepted Garrett Anderson as a member, then promptly regretted it and voted not to accept any more women. Other societies also kept their doors closed. Slowly the women wore the men down through sheer persistence, courage and ability. In 1906 the Royal College of Surgeons of England relaxed its policy, and for the first time since James Barry mounted the stairs to face the examiners, permitted women to take the College's now formidable examinations. In 1911 Eleanor Davies-Colley, who had studied at the London School of Medicine for Women (having been born in the year it was founded), was the first woman to pass and become a Fellow of the RCS.

Throughout the twentieth century, the male old guard renewed itself generation after generation, continuing to resist, block and hinder the female incursion; but there was no stopping it, and the resistance slowly weakened. In April 2014, more than two hundred years after James Barry's examination, the Royal College of Surgeons elected its first female President, orthopaedic surgeon Miss Clare Marx.* Slowly but surely, the number of women in medicine and surgery is reaching a par with men, and may soon overtake them.

The resistance continues, but the march goes on. Margaret Anne Bulkley, at the age of twenty, in a society in which a respectable young unmarried woman could not go out of doors without a chaperone, proved the lengths to which a person's determination can carry them, when she packed away her dresses and donned the persona of a young man. And she went on proving it, climbing over every obstacle, living a lie in order to live her ambition, until in the end the only force strong enough to unseat her was death.

---

* The RCS retains its historical disassociation with the MD degree; all fellows are Mr, Mrs or Miss.

Appendix A

James Barry and the Physical Examination

One of the many obstacles facing a woman trying to enter the British Army disguised as a man would surely be the physical examination that, one supposes, would have been part of the enrolment procedure. Some previous biographers of James Barry have speculated that some kind of subterfuge or patronage must have been involved. We know, for example, that the Earl of Buchan's intervention saved Barry on two occasions when his apparent age and delicacy came into question (at Edinburgh and again at Plymouth). Perhaps, therefore, the physical examination was waived due to similar influence – perhaps on the part of a professional patron such as Astley Cooper or Henry Cline?

This question originates with a biographical essay by Colonel Nathaniel J. C. Rutherford (1874–1960), published in the *Journal of the Royal Army Medical Corps* in 1939. Rutherford himself was an Army surgeon who had apparently served on selection boards during his career and had a detailed knowledge of procedures. He speculated that Barry must have obtained a certificate of fitness from a well-placed and friendly medical man, and that this, together with Barry's own audaciously insouciant manner, caused the Army Medical Board to waive the requirement for a naked physical examination. (Colonel Rutherford let his imagination run free, narrating the story of Barry's entrance interviews, complete with lengthy dialogue passages.[1] This was pure invention, shaped by the attitudes of Rutherford's era; he believed that James Barry had not been properly educated in medicine – since that would not be possible for a woman – and joined the Army in pursuit of a man with whom she was in love.)

In her 1958 biography, Isobel Rae disputed Rutherford's 'unwarranted assertion', on the grounds that procedures were less strictly observed in 1813 than they later became, and that Barry's physical examination might have been skipped due to laxity.[2] But this presupposes an unreasonable risk on Barry's part, since how could he rely on the authorities neglecting the examination? In a 1977 biography, June Rose suggested that Army physical examinations in Barry's day were probably 'perfunctory' and might not have discovered a person's sex.[3]

In fact, all of these biographers were mistaken. Whereas Rae and Rose were close to the truth, Rutherford's mistake was the greatest – he rashly assumed that the procedures of his day (the 1890s to the 1920s) would not have changed since 1813. In truth, they had altered substantially. In 1813 the admission procedure was very different indeed – and crucially, it *did not include a physical examination at all*, perfunctory or otherwise.

From the eighteenth century through to the mid-Victorian period, men entering the British Army at the commissioned officer level were regarded as gentlemen, and taken at their word. For regimental officers, indeed, commissions and even promotions were achieved by purchase more often than merit. Surgeons, by contrast, were appointed mainly on their qualifications (though social connections helped). No man entering the Army at this level was required to prove his physical fitness by stripping for a medical examination. It would have been viewed as an unseemly degradation.

This changed around 1870 (after Dr Barry's death and before Colonel Rutherford's birth), with the reforms overseen by Edward Cardwell, Secretary of State for War, which, among other things, reorganised the Army and abolished the purchase of commissions. Comparing the regulations before and after the Cardwell Reforms, we find a crucial difference. Fitness of medical officer candidates is covered by clause 2 of the regulations, which in 1873 – *after* the reforms – reads (emphasis added and racism noted):

2. The candidate must make a declaration that his parents are of unmixed European blood, and that he labours under no mental or constitutional disease, nor any imperfection or disability that can interfere with the most efficient discharge of the duties of a Medical Officer in any climate. His physical fitness will be determined by a Board of Medical Officers, who are required to certify that the candidate's vision is sufficiently

good to enable him to perform any surgical operation without the aid of glasses ... *The Board must also certify that he is free from organic or other disease, and from constitutional weakness or other disability* likely to unfit him for military service in any climate.[4]

A physical examination isn't explicitly described, but is implied by that last sentence. The equivalent clause in the 1865 regulations – *before* the reforms – reads simply:

2. The Candidate must make a declaration that he labours under no mental or constitutional disease, nor any imperfection or disability that can interfere with the most efficient discharge of the duties of a Medical officer in any climate. He must also attest his readiness to engage for general service immediately on being gazetted.[5]

In other words, the candidate's own sworn statement was sufficient. It is notable that Cardwell's reforms introduced not only rigour to the procedure but also a dose of explicit institutional racism.

As an afterthought, one wonders how different the story might have been if such an examination *had* been required in 1813 – would James have tried to game the system in the manner Rutherford conjectured? Or might Margaret have sent her alter ego on a different course, perhaps trying to establish him as a society practitioner in the mould of her mentors, as Dr Fryer apparently advised? She appears to have hesitated and considered this course but rejected it, perhaps due to fear of discovery, perhaps due to the call of adventure. Throughout history, men have sought both sanctuary and thrills in the armed forces, and the evidence suggests that in that respect at least, Margaret Bulkley was no different.

APPENDIX B

Who Discovered Dr Barry's Secret?

Previous biographies of James Barry have stated that the discoverer
of James Barry's biological sex was Sophia Bishop, the housemaid
at 14 Margaret Street; she is said to have laid out the body, and thus it
was she who disclosed the secret to Barry's doctor, Surgeon Major David
Reid McKinnon.[1]

This identification is based on the fact that Bishop is named on the
death certificate as having reported the death.[2] Yet the woman who told
Mr McKinnon of her astonishing discovery and subsequently reported
it publicly is *not named* by him in his account of the meeting – she is
merely 'the woman, who performed the last offices for Dr Barry'.[3] In
contemporary reports, the identity of the discoverer is hazy and subject to
speculation. *Saunders's News-Letter*, which broke the story, reported that
it had been 'two nurses' who had looked after Dr Barry in his last days.[4]
By the time Charles Dickens published his partially fictionalised account
in *All the Year Round* in 1867, the discoverer had become a 'charwoman'
tasked with laying out the body by Dr Barry's manservant; it is implied
that this charwoman was a periodic visitor to the house, not a live-in
servant.[5] Clearly the identity of the discoverer was subject to gossip and
uncertainty from the very beginning.

In fact, it is improbable that in 1865 a housemaid would be given the
job of laying out a body; either an undertaker would do it or, failing that,
one of the many women who worked as layers-out. In earlier centuries,
laying out the dead had been exclusively a job done by women, but as
the funeral business became more commercialised in the Victorian era,
these part-time professionals were largely supplanted by male undertakers.
Women continued in the trade well into the century, albeit no longer

considered respectable, and frowned upon by medical professionals; usually they performed laying out as an adjunct role, earning most of their living from private nursing and midwifery. This class of women was satirised by Charles Dickens in *Martin Chuzzlewit* (first published in 1843–4), in the character of Sarah Gamp, a garrulous, disreputable, hard-drinking old woman who 'went to a lying-in or a laying-out with equal zest and relish'. Mrs Gamp is said to be based on an actual woman who was hired by a friend of Dickens, and her kind was still sufficiently notorious by 1860 for Florence Nightingale to write in an unpublished draft of her *Notes on Nursing*: 'Mrs Gamps are not considered desirable now', going on to use that character as an illustration of bad, unregulated practice.[6]

The anonymous woman described in some detail by McKinnon could almost be Mrs Gamp to the life – confident, irascible and bold. Furthermore, this woman had argued with Mrs Anderson, the lodging house owner's wife, over 'some perquisites' (i.e. a tip or payment) for performing the laying out. Again this sounds more like a woman driving her trade than an employed servant.

But there is more. The layer-out, asked how she knew that Barry had borne a child, stated, 'I am a married woman, and the mother of nine children. I ought to know.' This in itself rules out Sophia Bishop, who was unmarried at the time and, as far as can be discerned from available records, had no children. She was a country girl, born in Weston Turville, Buckinghamshire, in 1834–5. At fifteen she and her (unmarried) mother were working as straw plaiters. By 1861 the twenty-six-year-old Sophia had moved to London and taken employment as live-in housemaid to Mr and Mrs James Anderson at 14 Margaret Street. She continued with them until at least 1865.[7] When Dr Barry died in the house, Sophia was thirty and still unmarried, and with no sign of children. Records show that by 1869 she had returned to Buckinghamshire and married a man called Paton, taking up the straw-plaiting trade again; still there is no evidence of children in her household.[8]

Since the only connection is her having signed the death certificate, we can quite confidently rule her out, and attribute the discovery to an unnamed outsider – Dickens's 'charwoman' is quite likely, especially since he knew the trade. It is strangely appropriate that it was a now nameless person who chanced upon the mystery of the late Dr James Barry.

Notes

Author's Note

1 www.measuringworth.com/ukcompare (retrieved 18 December 2015).

Prologue

1 Charles Dickens, *Martin Chuzzlewit*. In previous biographies, the identities of maidservant Sophia Bishop and the layer-out have been conflated; see Appendix B. The layer-out's name is not known.
2 She later gave her observations on Dr Barry's body to his doctor, David McKinnon, who'd had no knowledge of Barry's real sex (McKinnon to Graham, 24 August 1865, RJBa).

Chapter 1: A Family at War

1 Cordingly, *Billy Ruffian*, pp. 107–8.
2 Mary Anne Bulkley to James Barry RA, 11 April 1804, NLI.
3 Windele, *Historical and Descriptive Notices*, p. 39.
4 Mary Anne Bulkley to James Barry RA, 14 January 1805, NLI.
5 Marriage records, St Finbarr's (South) Church, Cork; a marriage is recorded between a Jeremiah Buckley (*sic*) and Mary Barry on 29 June 1782; at that time Mary Anne would have been aged about seventeen (she was born about 1765).
6 No record has been found of the births of either of the Bulkley children. Many of the records of St Finbarr's, St Peter's and St Paul's churches held in the Public Record Office were destroyed during the 1922 Civil War. Margaret's year of birth is inferred from her mother's description of her as being fifteen years old in mid-January 1805 (Mary Anne Bulkley to James Barry RA, 14 January 1805, NLI).
7 Mary Anne Bulkley to James Barry RA, 14 January 1805, NLI. Title in the house passed from her father to her brother James, but her mother, Juliana Barry, retained an interest that Mary Anne had to purchase from her. There seems to have been

an informal understanding that the house had been left to James on the condition
that he would sign it over to Mary Anne, but he did not do so. The whole situation
was complicated by debts and by the English laws of property at the time, whereby
the Barrys, as Roman Catholics, could only hold leases for up to thirty-one years.

8 Margaret refers to this fancy in a later letter to her brother, undated (probably late
1808), BFA.

9 James Gordon, *History*, p. 83.

10 The renewal of Longfield's appointment as Weigh-Master was passed during the
last sessions of the Irish parliament prior to its dissolution (Parliament of Ireland,
Statutes Passed, pp. 393–5). See also the entry for Mountifort Longfield, *History of
Parliament*.

11 Groups of nationalists under leaders such as James Corcoran, Robert Emmet and
Michael Dwyer continued to prick the sides of the British for several years. By
1804 the last rebel groups had been crushed and their leaders were dead.

12 Mary Anne Bulkley to James Barry, 11 April 1804, NLI.

13 Ibid.

14 Ibid.

15 This child is referred to in only three surviving documents. A letter from John
Bulkley to his father (undated, probably mid to late1803, BFA) closes with 'Give
my Love to my Dear Mother and Sisters'. A letter from Mary Anne Bulkley to
her brother James Barry (11 April 1804, NLI) refers to 'my two Daughters'. Five
years later, a letter from Jeremiah to Margaret mentions – as if it were a sensitive
subject – a dependent called 'Julian' (the name Juliana is sometimes rendered as
'Julian' in references to the late Juliana Barry – e.g. Mary Anne Bulkley to James
Barry, 14 January 1805, NLI). Given the context and the absence of evidence for
any other person with that name, it is likely that Julian(a) is the 'second daughter'
of the Bulkleys. Juliana Barry, Mary Anne's mother, had died in 1789, the year
Margaret was born.

16 Many Irish baptismal records were destroyed in 1922. Margaret's baby is likely to
have been born and baptised somewhere away from Cork. Pregnancies resulting
in live births are not unknown in girls as young as eleven or even ten, and more
common in girls aged twelve to thirteen. Margaret Bulkley must have been, at
most, thirteen years old at conception. Average age at the onset of puberty has
lowered significantly during the past two centuries – in the early 19th century it
was around seventeen years for girls, making Margaret's case very unusual. On
the other hand, present evidence shows that adolescent pregnancies cluster at
the younger end of the scale, since girls who mature early are immediately more
fertile than those who mature later (Scholl and Chen, 'Puberty and Adolescent
Pregnancy', p. 158). Furthermore, growing up in a household where there is stress
can bring on earlier puberty, and having few siblings can also advance the onset
of puberty (ibid.); both these applied to Margaret Bulkley.

17 Presently, about 90 per cent of sexual abuse of children is perpetrated by family
members or friends of the family, with the family itself accounting for about 30
per cent (Miller and Knudsen, *Family Abuse*, p. 157).

18 Patrick served under his mother's maiden name, Reardon (or Riordan). In 1789, the year their mother died, Patrick blamed Mary Anne and her husband for cruelly turning James against him (Patrick Barry to James Barry, 19 July 1789, BFA).

19 Redmond Barry to James Barry, 13 June 1777, BFA.

20 Redmond Barry to James Barry, 9 March 1781, BFA. Redmond served aboard HMS *Cumberland*, a seventy-four-gun ship of the line.

21 Patrick Barry to James Barry, 1 August 1789, BFA.

22 Redmond's portrait was drawn twice; as brother of James Barry, he came into contact with a number of artists, and the American-born painter Benjamin West used him as the model for the central 'sick man' in his *Christ Healing the Sick in the Temple* (painted 1800–11 and 1817). Some years later, when Redmond was living in poverty, a sketch of him was made (Subscription notice, 1825, BFA).

23 Patrick Barry to James Barry, 19 July 1789, BFA.

24 Redmond Barry to James Barry, 23 July 1802, BFA

25 Redmond Barry to James Barry, 2 May 1803, BFA.

26 Redmond Barry to James Barry, 23 July 1802, BFA. The encounter with the Bulkleys appears to have happened in early 1802; however, it is possible that the rift was *caused* in 1802 (by their attitude to him, plus Redmond's own unspecified 'behaviour') but that he went back in 1803, and it was on this occasion they ran him out of town and he returned to the Navy.

27 Mary Anne Bulkley to James Barry, 11 April 1804, NLI. Miss Ward (whose first name isn't recorded) was said (by Mrs Bulkley) to be the sister of General Thomas Ward (1748–94), who had been guillotined by the revolutionary government in France (given his date of birth, Miss Ward was more likely his daughter or niece than his sister).

28 John Bulkley to Jeremiah Bulkley, undated (probably mid to late 1803), BFA.

29 Ibid.

30 Mary Anne Bulkley to James Barry, 11 April 1804, NLI.

31 Ibid.

32 Ibid.

33 James Barry to Sleigh, 8 November 1769, in Fryer, *Works*, vol. I, pp. 164–6.

34 A self-portrait exists of James Barry RA as a relatively young man, painted between 1775 and 1780, when he was in his late thirties (now in the collection of the Victoria and Albert Museum, London). Compared with the miniature portrait of Margaret in the guise of James Barry MD, the resemblance is clear.

35 Mary Anne Bulkley to James Barry, 11 April 1804, NLI.

36 Margaret Anne Bulkley, postscript to letter, Mary Anne Bulkley to James Barry, 11 April 1804, NLI. This is the earliest known example of Margaret's hand.

37 Mary Anne Bulkley to James Barry, 11 April 1804, NLI.

Chapter 2: An Unprotected Girl

1   There is no evidence of what was done with the infant Juliana (aged between one and three years old) during this journey; she was probably left in the care of friends or relations.

2   On each of the occasions when Margaret is known to have visited James Barry, she went alone (Mary Anne Bulkley to James Barry, 14 January 1805, NLI); however, it is unthinkable that a respectable woman like Mrs Bulkley would let her unmarried daughter walk out without a chaperone. A servant (probably female) would have been paid to go with her.

3   The descriptions of Margaret's visits to her uncle are based in part on her mother's remarks (Mary Anne Bulkley to James Barry, 14 January 1805, NLI) and on the accounts given by other contemporary visitors, including the Irish lawyer William Henry Curran and the poet Robert Southey. The condition of the house is depicted in the contemporary pencil sketch by J. Bryant (B1977.14.17641, Paul Mellon Collection, Yale Center for British Art). Bryant's sketch was made after vandals attacked the house between October and December 1804 and left it in an even worse condition. Curran ('Barry the Painter', pp. 338–9) dates the scene of extreme dilapidation to 'early in the year 1804'; comparison with other sources indicates that he must have meant early 1805 (see later in this chapter).

4   Barry had been expelled in April 1799, by an almost unanimous vote, on the grounds of his inflammatory conduct. He remained until 2004 the only person ever to be expelled from the Royal Academy of Arts.

5   Curran, 'Barry the Painter', p. 338.

6   Ibid., p. 339.

7   Southey to Cunningham, 23 July 1829, in Southey, *Life*, vol. VI, p. 54.

8   Curran, 'Barry the Painter', p. 339.

9   Curran (ibid., pp. 340–2) observed that Barry was positively warm with old friends from Ireland, and enjoyed the company of an Irish Catholic woman who lived nearby in Portland Street and had an Irish priest as a lodger.

10 Ibid., p. 340.

11 The Royal Academy had forwarded Mary Anne's letter to a Mr Collop in Southampton Row, and it had eventually reached Little Castle Street (cover, Mary Anne Bulkley to James Barry, 11 April 1804, NLI).

12 Curran, 'Barry the Painter', p. 340.

13 Southey to Cunningham, 23 July 1829, in Southey, *Life*, vol. VI, p. 54.

14 Southey to Coleridge, 4 August 1802, in Southey, *Life*, vol. II, p. 191.

15 Redmond Barry to James Barry, 23 July 1802, BFA.

16 Margaret Anne Bulkley, obituary poem on James Barry, April 1807 tomo XVII, folio 139, AFM.

17 It isn't exactly certain what happened; Mrs Bulkley wrote that she and Margaret were 'Thrown out of house and home by a Husband & Son' (Mary Anne Bulkley to James Barry, 14 January 1805, NLI), but this is clearly figurative, meaning that

it was Jeremiah and John's reckless actions that had caused the two women to become homeless.

18 Peter Murray, *Cooper Penrose Collection*, pp. 18–20.

19 In 1806 Cooper Penrose's son William wrote that 'Jeremiah Bulkley (if alive) is in very indigent circumstances' (Penrose, Statement on behalf of Mary Anne Bulkley, 6 May 1806, BFA).

20 Mary Anne Bulkley to James Barry, 14 January 1805, NLI.

21 *Morning Chronicle*, 18 December 1804. The police referred to in the report, which pre-dates the foundation of the Metropolitan Police in 1829, were the law-enforcement officers employed by London boroughs, who worked with magistrates (a practice modelled on Fielding's Bow Street Runners).

22 Curran, 'Barry the Painter', pp. 338–9.

23 Based on the experience of Curran (ibid., p. 338).

24 Ibid., p. 339.

25 Southey to Cunningham, 23 July 1829, in Southey, *Life*, vol. VI, p. 54.

26 Barry to Buchan, 21 December 1804, NPG.

27 Southey to Cunningham, 23 July 1829, in Southey, *Life*, vol. VI, p. 55.

28 Barry to Buchan, 21 December 1804, NPG.

29 She receives a jar in the original legend; Pandora's 'box' is the result of a 16th-century translation error.

30 Barry began the painting in 1791, having produced several drawings in the preceding decades, and finished it in 1804. Several visitors, including William Henry Curran, saw it in the studio at this time. *The Birth of Pandora* is now in Manchester Art Gallery.

31 Buchan to Barry, 11 February 1805, in Fryer, *Works*, vol. I, pp. 292–3.

32 Mary Anne Bulkley to James Barry, 14 January 1805, NLI. A letter of attorney (another name for power of attorney) is a document authorising a person to act in legal matters on behalf of the grantor. In the early 19th century letters of attorney were sometimes used for the sale of property by absent owners.

33 Ibid.

34 Ibid.

35 Ibid.

36 Ibid.

37 A typical advertisement for a governess at this time stipulates: 'She must be capable of teaching the English and French Languages grammatically ... and understand sufficient of Music to be able to instruct in the absence of a Master' (*The Times*, 1 February 1806, p. 1). Families often required a governess's command of French to be 'perfect' and expected her to be experienced.

38 Penrose, Statement on behalf of Mary Anne Bulkley, 6 May 1806, BFA.

39 Curry, *Picture of Dublin*, pp. 125–6.

40 Jeremiah Bulkley to Margaret Anne Bulkley, 27 November 1809, BFA.

Chapter 3: Next of Kin

1   Edward Fryer, Thomas Clark, Francis Douce and Anthony Carlisle, draft press
    release on the death of James Barry, February 1806, NLI.

2   Southey to Cunningham, 23 July 1829, in Southey, *Life*, vol. VI, p. 54.

3   Ibid. Anthony Carlisle was a very eminent surgeon, anatomist and scientist. He
    had been a member of the Royal College of Surgeons when it was granted its
    royal charter in 1800, and in the same year was the co-discoverer (with William
    Nicholson) of electrolysis. A fellow of the Royal Society, he later became its
    Professor of Anatomy, and from 1820 he was surgeon to King George IV.

4   Farington, *Farington Diary*, vol. 3, pp. 153–4, 163. Joseph Farington RA was a
    landscape painter; he records hearing the story of James Barry's last days from the
    engraver John Landseer a few days afterwards. Further details of James Barry's last
    days are taken from a later index to Farington's diary (Newby, *Diary*, p. 2889) and
    a letter from Joseph Bonomi to the Earl of Buchan, 22 February 1806, JU/4/123,
    RAA.

5   Some sources say the shop was a pastry-cook's, others a fruiterer (Farington,
    Farington Diary, vol. 3, p. 163).

6   Farington, *Farington Diary*, vol. 3, p. 163.

7   *The Times*, 15 March 1806, p. 3.

8   Barry, *Account, passim*. The mural, which can still be seen in the Great Room, was
    begun in 1777 and completed in 1783.

9   Fryer, Clark, Douce and Carlisle, draft press release on the death of James Barry,
    February 1806, NLI; Farington, *Farington Diary*, vol. 3, p. 154.

10 Unknown author, note, 23 February 1806, BFA; Farington, *Farington Diary*,
    vol. 3, p. 163. Farington gives the sum as '£20 in cash & £20 in notes'; at this
    time, 'cash' usually meant coins. The anonymous note gives the figure as £41
    14s 9d.

11 Unknown author, attorney's notes on the administration of the James Barry estate,
    undated, BFA.

12 Farington, *Farington Diary*, vol. 4, p. 34 (Farington was given this information by
    Anthony Carlisle, who had a hand in the administration of the estate); Attorney's
    notes on the James Barry estate, undated, BFA.

13 Based on the depiction of the prison ship HMS *York* in Cooke, *Sixty-five Plates of
    Shipping*, pl. 27.

14 *The Times*, 15 March 1806, p. 3.

15 Attorney's notes on the James Barry estate, undated, BFA. It is probable that
    Redmond had been wounded at the Battle of Trafalgar, which had taken place
    on 21 October 1805. His last known posting was aboard HMS *Mars* (Redmond
    Barry to James Barry, 2 May 1803, BFA). *Mars* was severely damaged at Trafalgar,
    her stern raked by broadsides from two French ships; ninety-eight of her crew
    were killed or wounded, including the captain (Adkins, *Trafalgar*, pp. 152–3).
    Redmond Barry might well have been among them.

16 McLoughlin, 'Redmond Barry', in McLoughlin, *Correspondence*.

17 This letter is referred to in a letter from Mary Anne Bulkley to Daniel Reardon, 8 July 1806, BFA.

18 Deed of Trust between Redmond Barry and Alexander Poulden, 2 June 1806, BFA.

19 Horwood, *Plan*. Corbet Court is still there (although none of its old buildings survive), opposite Leadenhall Market, whose famously ornate edifice was constructed in 1881; in Margaret's time, the market was an untidy cluster of buildings and open spaces.

20 Mary Anne's mother, Juliana Barry, was born a Reardon (or Riordan). Daniel Reardon's friendship with Mary Anne apparently pre-dated his service to her as a lawyer. However, it seems that he did not know James Barry, for when Mrs Bulkley wrote to her brother in 1805 (Mary Anne Bulkley to James Barry, 14 January 1805, BFA), she mentioned Reardon as 'A Friend of mine ... (Mr Reardon, Aty)'. This seems odd if he was related, and doubly so given that Barry was inclined to be friendly with fellow Irish expatriates.

21 Penrose, Statement on behalf of Mary Anne Bulkley, 6 May 1806, BFA.

22 The exact date of their arrival in London is not known, but was probably some time in June 1806.

23 Unknown author, attorney's notes on the administration of the James Barry estate, undated, BFA.

24 Mary Anne Bulkley to Reardon, 8 July 1806, BFA.

25 If Daniel was related to the Barrys, it is striking that he was not apparently a Catholic (his surviving records of marriage and births of his children are recorded in the Anglican church of St Peter's, Cornhill). This was just as well, as the legal profession could be difficult for Catholics, and they had only been permitted to enter it since the Roman Catholic Relief Act of 1791.

26 Equity, a set of principles of justice, was held to be superior and antecedent to Law. Until the late 19th century, equity was a separate system by which disputed inheritances were settled, and the Court of Chancery was where it was practised. In general, attorneys handled law while solicitors (regarded as a cut above attorneys) specialised in equity; Daniel Reardon covered both. Equity was notoriously capricious and convoluted, parodied by Dickens in *Bleak House*.

27 Marriage record, Daniel Reardon and Elizabeth Payne, 18 February 1806, London Metropolitan Archives, St John Horselydown, Register of marriages, P71/JN, Item 019. Reardon's previous wife appears to have died young in 1805.

28 Philip Davis had been articled as a clerk to Daniel Reardon in 1802, and in 1807 he qualified; by 1813 he was a partner in the firm of Reardon and Davis (Articles of Clerkship for Philip Davis, 6 March 1802, and Michael Reardon, 22 April 1807, pieces 13 & 17, AOC).

29 List of valuables, undated, BFA. James Christie (1773–1831) was the son of the elder James Christie who had founded the auction house in 1766. James Christie the younger took over the business when his father died in 1803.

30 Jefcoate, 'Fryer'. Fryer is a mysterious figure; his family background is all but unknown, and no portrait or physical description of him has been found.

31 Mary Anne Bulkley to Reardon, 3 July and 18 November 1807, BFA.

32 A typical advertisement placed in *The Times*, 26 April 1808, announces an experienced lady 'in want of a Situation as a PRIVATE GOVERNESS' with expertise in 'Instructions in English, French, Drawing, Geography, and the Use of the Globes; History, Writing, and Arithmetic; and all kinds of Work'. ('Use of the globes' included the terrestrial and celestial spheres.) Some governesses offered skills such as needlework. An advertisement placed in *The Observer*, 14 April 1805, stipulated: 'Accomplishments are not so much the object as a person of education and information, by whose society her Pupils would be improved: of a good and cheerful temper, and above all, of strict religious principles.' In context, this last stipulation would be read as 'no Catholics'.

33 Somerville, *Personal Recollections*, pp. 45–6.

34 Ibid., p. 221.

35 Obituary, *The Times*, 12 January 1826, p. 4.

36 Fryer was described obliquely as a man of 'independent' values, and his involvement with Margaret underlines this. The Earl of Buchan published an essay in 1793 in which he argued that women were as intellectually capable as men 'in almost every respect' and deserved equal education (Buchan, *Essays*, I.28–30). Despite these advocates, women's education did not begin to advance until the 1840s (Simonton, 'Women and Education').

Chapter 4: A Small Fortune

1 Two of Miranda's biographers (Racine, *Francisco de Miranda*, p. 172 and Robertson, *Life of Miranda*, p. 4) give the date of his arrival at Portsmouth as 21 December 1807. However, Miranda left Tortola shortly after 15 November (Cochrane-Johnstone to Castlereagh, 15 November 1807, in Castlereagh, *Correspondence*, p. 405) and states that he endured 'a boisterous passage of forty-four days' (Miranda to Castlereagh, 3 January 1808 tomo XII, folio 123, AFM; reproduced in Castlereagh, *Correspondence*, p. 403), which would make the arrival date 29 December at the earliest. Furthermore, a local bellringing society celebrated his arrival with 'a Peal on the Bells' on New Year's Eve (Ringers of Portsmouth to Miranda, 31 December 1807 tomo XII, folio 103, AFM). Furthermore, the London *Morning Post* on 2 and 4 January 1808 recorded that General Miranda was awaiting leave to disembark on 31 December and received his 'passport' that evening (see also Miranda to Castlereagh, op. cit.).

2 Harvey, *Liberators*, p. 19.

3 Racine, *Francisco de Miranda*, p. 26.

4 Ibid., p. 142ff.

5 Ibid., pp. 150–4. Miranda's house survives, now 58 Grafton Way; the Venezuelan Consulate is next door at number 56, and there is a statue of Miranda at the corner of Grafton Way and Fitzroy Street. In 1803 this area was close to the northern limit of London's expanding sprawl, which was just beginning to infiltrate the countryside north of what was then called the New Road from Paddington (now Euston Road and Marylebone Road). As late as 1799 there was still a working

farm next to the junction of what is now Marylebone Road and Great Portland Street (Horwood, *Plan*).

6   There is no record of a marriage between Sarah Andrews and Francisco de Miranda. One biographer (Robertson, *Life of Miranda*, pp. 224–8) describes her as a kind of servant-concubine, whereas another (Racine, *Francisco de Miranda*, p. 154) suggests that they were legally married. Certainly their children bore his name, which was not usual with illegitimate children.

7   Biggs, *History*, p. 291. James Biggs was an American who served in the *Leander* expedition as a mercenary. One of his fellow Americans told Biggs that he 'believed the expedition would never succeed under Miranda; his indecision, caprice, petulance, meanness and duplicity render him unfit for any enterprise of magnitude' (Biggs, *History*, p. 179).

8   Ibid., p. 248.

9   Ellen Reardon was born on 10 October 1807 and baptised on 18 November (London Metropolitan Archives, St Peter's, Cornhill, Register of Baptisms 1775–1812 and burials 1775–1812, P69/PET1/A/002/MS08821; available online at www.ancestry.com; retrieved 30 March 2015).

10   Martin (pseudonym of Sarah Andrews) to Miranda, 1805–7 tomo VIII, AFM.

11   Miranda to Sarah Martin (pseudonym of Sarah Andrews), 4 January 1806 tomo 6, folio 194, AFM.

12   Andrews to Miranda, 18 June 1806, quoted in Pressly, *Life and Art of James Barry*, p. 198.

13   Sarah Martin (pseudonym of Sarah Andrews) to Miranda, 1 October 1806 tomo VIII, folio 156–7, AFM.

14   Ibid.

15   Robertson, *Life of Miranda*, p. 218.

16   Sarah Martin (pseudonym of Sarah Andrews) to Miranda, 9 February 1807 tomo IX, folio 211–12, AFM.

17   After the middle of 1807, Sarah's letters to Miranda cease, and so we have no confirmation of whether she employed Margaret. However, since General Miranda did subsequently agree to provide a reference, it is probable that Margaret had practised tuition on Leader.

18   Unknown author, attorney's notes on the administration of the James Barry estate, undated, BFA.

19   James Barry's furniture and effects had been auctioned by James Christie in October (Christie's catalogue, 22 October 1806, BFA). At this auction, Mrs Bulkley acquired her brother's sitter's chair (described in the catalogue as 'Lot 13. A mahogany elbow chair covered with red leather'), for which she paid £1 4s. This chair is believed to have been inherited by James Barry from Sir Joshua Reynolds (Pressly, 'Portrait', p. 138), in whose paintings it frequently appears; the chair now belongs to the Royal Academy.

20   Reardon, receipt for 15 guineas signed on behalf of Redmond Barry, 11 September 1806; Reardon, receipt for 1 guinea signed by Mary Barry, 21 November 1806, BFA. The wife's identity is a mystery; she may have been an Irishwoman whom

Redmond married in 1793 (McLoughlin, 'Redmond Barry', in McLoughlin, *The Correspondence of James Barry*, available online at www.texte.ie/barry/view?docId=Appendix_F_Redmond_Barry.xml; retrieved 4 March 2015); she earned a living intermittently as a low-grade seamstress (Report on the death of Redmond Barry, *The Times*, 17 June 1825).

21 Christie on behalf of Mary Anne Bulkley to Reardon, 1 December 1806, BFA.

22 Reardon, receipt for £200 of £380 received signed by Redmond Barry, BFA. (The £380 included money that Redmond had already received.)

23 Christie's auction catalogue, 10–11 April 1807, BFA.

24 James Christie's Great Room in Pall Mall was depicted in watercolours several times by Thomas Rowlandson between 1801 and 1810; many reproductions of these images survive, including copies by Pugin.

25 The previous October, Anthony Carlisle had taken the landscape painter Joseph Farington to Dr Fryer's house to view the *Pandora*. Farington was no admirer of Barry, and found the painting to be as he'd expected: 'Ingenuity in the Design, but nothing extraordinary & a great deal of Mythological circumstance attended to, but in respect of power of execution & colouring very deficient.' It was not fit to rival the Old Masters whom Barry had set himself to match, insisted Farington; under this stern disapproval, Carlisle found himself reluctantly agreeing (Farington, *Farington Diary*, vol. 4, p. 34).

26 Quoted in Farington, *Farington Diary*, vol. 4, p. 129.

27 Sarah Martin (pseudonym of Sarah Andrews) to Miranda, 21 May 1807 tomo IX, folio 180–1, AFM. The prices Sarah mentions (e.g. 104 guineas for *Pandora*) are incorrect according to Graves, *Art Sales*, p. 26, and the auction catalogue (BFA). The painter might have been even more deeply wounded had he known that the ungenerous purchaser of the *Venus Rising* was his supporter and his relatives' benefactor, Cooper Penrose, who also bought three other works (Dunne and Pressly, *James Barry*, p. 43). The knowledge that Penrose would be at the auction may have encouraged James Christie to expect good prices. To be fair to Penrose, he could hardly have bid against himself.

28 Barry's *Birth of Pandora* remained unsold until 1846, when Christie's disposed of it for the derisory sum of 11½ guineas; it found its way into the collection of Manchester Art Gallery in 1882.

29 The buyer of the engravings was the engraver Charles Warren (a renowned craftsman who had engraved Robert Smirke's illustrations for the popular 1802 edition of *Arabian Nights*). He had planned to publish prints of Barry's engravings, but realised that he couldn't afford the purchase (Warren to Reardon, 4 May 1807; Mary Anne Bulkley to Reardon, 21 May 1807, BFA).

30 The returns on the auction are taken from Pressly, 'Portrait of a Cork Family', p. 138. Mary Anne's half-share of the £1416 would have been £708, and she had spent £300 to buy Redmond's share.

31 Mary Anne Bulkley to Reardon, 21 May 1807, BFA.

32 It is assumed that Redmond and Mary Anne took equal shares of everything except the proceeds of the Christie's sale, giving Redmond £1257 17s. 4d. However,

there is no record of him receiving any sums beyond the £380 in receipts from Daniel Reardon. Since the bulk of the money was in investment funds, there would be no cash receipts.

33 Mary Anne Bulkley to Reardon, 19 November 1807, BFA. 'For my part,' Mrs Bulkley wrote, 'I have made every effort to get the cloths [sic] for him but I am certain it will not be possible to effect it, indeed the last & positively impertinent Answer I got from Mr Christie's Clerk was, what cloths he saw were such rags they were not worth the removal & he left them in the house.'

34 See Robertson, *Life of Miranda*, p. 217. Aside from his library, Miranda lived quite modestly for a man in his position, stipulating an annual sum of £200 to run his household; this had more impact on Sarah than on himself, as she was left with the responsibility of making the household function on too little money.

35 Margaret Anne Bulkley, addendum to letter to James Barry, 11 April 1804, NLI.

36 Hislop to Castlereagh, 20 October 1807, in Castlereagh, *Correspondence*, p. 404.

37 Cochrane-Johnstone to Castlereagh, 15 November 1807, in Castlereagh, *Correspondence*, p. 405. Cochrane-Johnstone had a post at the customs house at Tortola, as well as a seat in Parliament; a few years later he was exposed as an embezzler and fraud.

38 Miranda to Castlereagh, 10 January 1808, in Castlereagh, *Correspondence*, pp. 405–12.

39 Ibid.

40 Wellesley, memorandum, 8 February 1808, in Wellington, *Supplementary Despatches*, p. 64.

41 Ibid., pp. 65–6.

42 Wellesley, supplementary memorandum, 8 February 1808, ibid., pp. 67–8.

43 Biggs, *History*, p. 289.

44 Ibid. Miranda's height was five feet ten or eleven inches: enough to be considered tall. Biggs, as well as Miranda's hairdresser, a man named Harker, described him as 'stout', meaning sturdy rather than fat (Farington, *Farington Diary*, vol. 4, p. 30).

45 Biggs, *History*, p. 290.

46 Margaret Anne Bulkley, obituary poem on James Barry, April 1807 tomo XVII, folio 139, AFM.

47 Margaret Anne Bulkley, second obituary poem on James Barry, undated (probably 1807) tomo XVII, folio 140, AFM. Both poems remained in General Miranda's possession, and neither was used for Barry's epitaph. When a memorial bust was installed in St Paul's in 1818, it bore a simple epitaph written by Dr Fryer: 'Sacred to the memory of James Barry, who, to strong native powers of mind, added the intellectual riches (the only riches he ever needed or possessed) which spring from learning, philosophy and religion. Hence, both as a painter and a writer, a lofty conception, a moral tendency, and a Grecian taste, ennobled, sanctified, and adorned all his works' (Jefcoate, 'Fryer, Edward').

Chapter 5: A Revolutionary Plan

1   Charles Dickens, *The Life and Adventures of Nicholas Nickleby*, ch. 1.

2   Given the state of her relationship with Redmond, it cannot have been a friendly visit. The cause would probably be the sympathy felt towards Redmond by the friends of James Barry (see Chapter 18), which would have obliged Margaret to make a show of kinship.

3   Margaret's promise is alluded to by Redmond in a letter to Daniel Reardon, 29 October 1809, BFA.

4   Brook Street no longer exists. Its northern part is now Stanhope Street, and the southern half, where the Bulkleys lived at number 12, has disappeared under the office blocks of Triton Square.

5   Mary Anne Bulkley to Reardon, 25 December 1809; Reardon to Mary Anne Bulkley, 30 March 1810, BFA.

6   Various advertisements, *Morning Chronicle* and *Morning Post*, 1807–9.

7   *The Times*, 1 February 1808, p. 1.

8   *Morning Post*, 27 May 1808, p. 1.

9   *The Observer*, 18 July 1809, p. 1.

10 Margaret Anne Bulkley to Reardon, 21 May 1808, BFA.

11 Tipper in *The Satirist*, p. 592.1.

12 *The Morning Post*, 15 July 1808, p. 1. It was customary for both employers and applicants to use local shops as *post restantes* for their communications, and they invariably used their initials rather than their full names. This particular advertisement is the only one that can be found in the London papers of this period with the initials 'M.B.', and the fact that it closely matches Margaret's situation (lack of 'connections' and experience) is suggestive.

13 Wollstonecraft, *Thoughts on the Education of Daughters*, pp. 69–72.

14 Wollstonecraft, *Vindication*, pp. 238–40. One of the girls to whom Wollstonecraft was governess, Margaret King (1773–1835), grew up to be a radical; she disguised herself as a man in order to attend lectures in medicine and surgery at the University of Jena (see Chapter 8 and Gordon, *Vindication*, ch. 16; Gordon, 'Foreword' in Denlinger, *Before Victoria*, p. vii).

15 Mary Anne's letters to Daniel Reardon (29 June and 20 July 1808, BFA) indicate that they had given up their lodgings but intended, if Mrs Bulkley was well enough, to be back in London by early August.

16 *The Times*, 19 January 1808, p. 3.

17 Letter, *Kentish Gazette*, 6 February 1808, p. 2.

18 *Kentish Gazette*, 3 June 1808, p. 4; 17 June 1808, p. 2.

19 Mary Anne Bulkley to Reardon, 29 June and 20 July 1808, BFA. Records show a Benjamin Peel who ran a lodging house in Bilton Court (between the High Street and New Street) between 1801 and 1811, so this was presumably one of his properties (Edwards and Rowe, *General Valuation*, section 3: Margate Building Valuations 1801).

20 All of Mary Anne Bulkley's surviving letters (1804–12) appear to be in Margaret's

hand, including in most cases the signatures. The two letters written at Margate are the first to be signed in a different hand.

21 Receipts dated June 1808 from Joseph Booker of New Bond Street, Anthony Molteno of Pall Mall and an unidentified seller have survived (BFA), indicating modest stocks of four copies each.

22 Mary Anne Bulkley to Reardon, 9 February 1808, BFA.

23 Mary Anne Bulkley to Reardon, 20 July 1808, BFA. The practice of the time was for publishers to purchase the copyright (which then literally meant the right to make copies) in a work they wished to publish. Until the Copyright Act of 1842, copyright lasted only fourteen years from publication, after which it reverted to the author, provided he or she applied for an extension for a further fourteen years; once that period expired (or at the author's death, whichever was sooner), the copyright lapsed permanently.

24 Williams, *Whole Law*, p. 324.

25 *Bristol Journal*, 24 September 1808, p. 2; Register of HMS *Captivity*, CPH.

26 Register of HMS *Captivity*, CPH. Eventually, in April 1814, with a year still to run on his sentence, Redmond was set free.

27 Bone, *Dissertation*, p. 25, gives an account of the treatment of soldiers of the Royal York Rangers in the West Indies in 1818, when nearly one-third of the men died of disease.

28 Evidence of Major General Archibald Campbell in HMSO, *Report from His Majesty's Commissioners*, p. 96.

29 Report in *The Observer*, 4 September 1808, p. 4.

30 John Bulkley to Mary Anne Bulkley, 2 September 1808, BFA.

31 Margaret Ann Bulkley to John Bulkley, undated (probably September 1808), BFA.

32 *Hampshire Telegraph*, 3 October 1808, p. 3.

33 *Lincoln, Rutland and Stamford Mercury*, 28 October 1808, p. 1.

34 Margaret Reardon was born on 17 February 1809 and baptised on 27 March (London Metropolitan Archives, St Peter's, Cornhill, Register of Baptisms 1775–1812 and burials 1775–1812, P69/PET1/A/002/MS08821; available online at www.ancestry.com; retrieved 3 February 2015).

35 Opie, *Detraction Displayed*, pp. 251–3.

36 Barry, *Account*, pp. 73–4.

37 Barrell, *Birth of Pandora*, p. 165. A copy of Godwin's *On Political Justice* was included in Barry's estate sale.

38 Angelica Kauffman (1741–1807) and Mary Moser (1744–1819) were among the thirty-four founder members of the Royal Academy (the others, all male, included Joshua Reynolds and Thomas Gainsborough). The spirit of equality was not sustained, and it was 168 years before Dame Laura Knight became the third woman to be elected to the Academy in 1936.

39 Quoted by Joseph Farington, *Farington Diaries*, vol. 4, p. 35. When Carlisle went out of town to treat a patient, he charged an extra 1 guinea per mile travelled.

40 Obituary, *The Times*, 15 February 1841, p. 6. Both Carlisle and Cooper were

surgeons rather than physicians, and did not have the MD degree and therefore weren't entitled to be 'Dr'.

41   Farington, *Farington Diaries*, vol. 4, p. 182.

42   Christie, quoted in Robertson, *Life of Miranda*, p. 218.

43   Obituary, *The Times*, 12 January 1826, p. 4.

44   Gordon, *Vindication*, ch. 16; Denlinger, *Before Victoria*, pp. vii, 44–9.

45   Biggs, *History*, p. 289.

46   Ibid., pp. 290–1.

47   Booker to Mary Anne Bulkley, 21 January 1809, BFA.

48   Notes to Mary Anne Bulkley from Messrs Boydell and Anthony Molteno, January 1809, BFA.

49   Mary Anne Bulkley to Reardon, 12 March 1809, BFA.

50   Possibly £100, based on an entry in Reardon's statement of account, 3 April 1810, BFA.

51   Cadell and Davies to Mary Anne Bulkley, 14 July 1809, BFA.

52   It is inferred that Margaret had not taken permanent employment, either as a companion or a governess, since it left no mark in the historical record. Other than the letter concerning the lady in Camden Town in 1808 and the advertisement in July, no further direct trace of Margaret's career has been found. The only reference is in a letter from Jeremiah Bulkley to Margaret (27 November 1809, BFA) saying that he had heard from a mutual acquaintance that Margaret 'got your livelyhood by Teaching in a Family'.

53   Mary Anne Bulkley, will, 25 August 1809, BFA. The presence of Rosa Bonomi may imply that Mrs Bulkley had been moved to the Bonomi house to be nursed, like her brother before her.

54   Redmond Barry to Reardon, 29 October 1809, BFA.

55   Jeremiah Bulkley to Margaret Anne Bulkley, 27 November 1809, BFA.

56   This part of the letter is torn, and the words incomplete. The fate of Margaret's child is not known; nor do we know whether she ever sent any aid or love to her. Throughout her life, Margaret showed a consistent fondness for little children, so the parting from her own cannot have been lightly done. The only trace of Juliana's later life that has been discovered is in a Cork trade directory for 1826 and 1828 (see Pressly, 'Portrait of a Cork Family', p. 147), where a dressmaker called Miss Bulkley is listed as working at 17 George's Street (now Plunkett Street). Juliana Bulkley would be in her mid-twenties at that time, and the surname is uncommon enough in Cork that this is very probably her. After that brief appearance, she disappears again.

Chapter 6: Sanguine Expectations

1   On 30 November 1809, morning high tide at London Bridge was at 6.14 a.m. The smack would set sail about an hour later, when the light would be better and the tide ebbing (tide calculation by Tim Smith, UK Hydrographic Office, personal communication, 26 March 2013).

2 This was discovered only at the end of James Barry's life (see Chapter 34).

3 St Katharine's has been described as containing some of 'the most insanitary and unsalutary dwellings in London' (Broodbank, *History*, p. 154), although this view was claimed to be an exaggeration by those who opposed its later demolition (Weinreb et al., *London Encyclopaedia*, p. 779). The parish contained the vast Red Lion Brewhouse at the end of Lower East Smithfield, backing onto St Katharine's Street, casting the pungent reek of yeast over the whole district. There had been a brewery on the site since 1492 (Richmond and Turton, *Brewing Industry*, p. 182).

4 Weather data, Carey and Bancks, 'Meteorological Journal', p. 503.

5 The Leith smacks later became more comfortable, and by 1819 they were being advertised as 'equal in the point of convenience, and splendid decoration, to the first pleasure yachts', with staterooms 'replete with every possible convenience – even Piano Fortes have lately been introduced' (Reid, *Leith and London Smack Directory*, pp. 6–19). In 1809 the smacks were still little more than adapted fishing vessels.

6 Mary Anne Bulkley to Reardon, 14 December 1809, BFA.

7 December 1809 was unusually cold and snowy in Edinburgh, with temperatures rarely above freezing (*Edinburgh Annual Register*, pp. 488–9).

8 Barry to Reardon, 14 December 1809, BFA. In filing the letter, Reardon, perhaps acting out of habit, indiscreetly inscribed 'Miss Bulkley' on its leading edge. Discovered by Michael du Preez, this was the first piece of decisive evidence linking the identities of James Barry and Margaret Bulkley, a connection that had previously been conjectured but not proven (du Preez, 'Dr James Barry: The Early Years Revealed').

9 Normally, matriculation was a ceremonial occasion, held in the library in the presence of the principal (Rosner, *Medical Education*, pp. 44–5; Bower, *Student's Guide*, pp. 6–8). James Barry's first-year matriculation must have been less formal: the Winter Session began in November, and by the time he reached Edinburgh, he was a month late.

10 Price quoted by Rosner, *Medical Education*, p. 47. 'Natural philosophy' was the precursor to modern physics. The choice of courses was largely at the discretion of the student, though there were some (such as anatomy) that were required for the MD degree.

11 Sir Walter Scott's journal, quoted in Lockhart, *Memoirs*, vol. 4, pp. 204–5. At Buchan's funeral in 1829, Scott noted that the body was interred with the feet towards the west rather than the east, but chose not to correct it, because 'a man who had been wrong in the head all his life would scarce become right-headed after death'.

12 Barry to Reardon, 14 December 1809, BFA.

13 Ibid. The letter contains a strange word that the authors interpret differently. After describing the amount of studying, the letter reads, 'I am become also (& no doubt a very eligible) Member of the Philop_dian Society of Edinb'h and hope in due time to perfect all my plans.' One of us (du Preez) believes the mystery word is *Philopodian*, a neologism, perhaps invented by Margaret to mean a love of walking,

and therefore perhaps an ironic joke about the amount of legwork a medical student had to do between lectures and classes. The other author (Dronfield) believes the word is *Philopædian*, a very rare but extant word that means love of learning and knowledge. There was at least one Philopaedian Society in existence in the 19th century, a literary and debating club begun in 1841 at St Xavier College, Cincinnati (an institution founded in 1831 by Catholics). A search of Edinburgh University's records reveals no evidence of either a Philopodian or a Philopædian Society existing in 1809.

14 Barry to Miranda, 7 January 1810 tomo XVIII, folios 23–4, AFM.
15 Mary Anne Bulkley to Reardon, 25 December 1809, BFA.
16 Barry to Miranda, 7 January 1810 tomo XVIII, folios 23–4, AFM.
17 In 1819, as a doting patron of Sir Walter Scott, Buchan tried to arrange Scott's funeral, wrongly believing him to be dying, and had to be physically ejected from the ill writer's house by a servant, so determined was he to embrace the man one last time before he passed on (Lockhart, *Memoirs*, vol. 2, pp. 349–50).
18 Lockhart, *Memoirs*, vol. 4, p. 205.
19 Jeremiah Bulkley to Reardon, 24 February, 16 March, 9 April 1810, BFA.
20 Jeremiah Bulkley to Reardon, 9 April 1810, BFA.
21 Redmond Barry to Reardon, 18 March 1810, BFA.
22 Mary Anne Bulkley to Reardon, 11 May 1810, BFA.

Chapter 7: A Man of Understanding

1 Andrew Fyfe 'taught anatomy for some time in the Horse Wynd' (Struthers, *Historical Sketch*, pp. 75–6n), an alley behind the royal stables belonging to Holyrood House. It had once been prosperous, but was now declining. Most of its buildings were later pulled down during slum clearances. It is now the site of the Scottish Parliament.
2 Quoted in Darwin and Seward, *More Letters*, p. 7.
3 Darwin, *Life and Letters*, p. 47.
4 There were around 900 students in the Faculty of Medicine, of whom about two-thirds might have been studying anatomy, and only a few dozen of whom would ever graduate MD (Bower, *Student's Guide*, pp. 138–9; Struthers, *Historical Sketch*, p. 91). The anatomy theatre was housed in the building now known as Old College, in South Bridge. The building began construction in 1790, and by James Barry's day was still only half-complete (Fraser, *Building*, pp. 42–3).
5 Prior to 1829, these private courses were unregulated, and information about their administration is scarce. The three-month duration is inferred from later regulatory changes (Struthers, *Historical Sketch*, p. 92n). The price is quoted in a later guide (Bower, *Student's Guide*, p. 142). Barry later attested that he had taken '3 Courses of Dissections, in 1810, 1811, and 1812, with Mr. Fyfe' (War Office: RJBc).
6 Fyfe began as assistant to Monro *secundus* in 1777. He became a highly skilled dissector and anatomist, despite having no medical qualification, and wrote several volumes on the subject. The portrayal of Fyfe here is based in part on the

descriptions given by Bransby Cooper and his uncle Sir Astley (Cooper, *Life*, vol. 1, pp. 166, 172), as well as Struthers (*Historical Sketch*, pp. 74–5) and in part on Fyfe's own remarks in his *Compendium* (pp. 119–24). He was particularly known for his hesitant speech.

7   Aitchison, *Edinburgh and Leith*, p. 103.

8   The depiction of Fyfe's dissecting room is based in part on the description of the private room created by surgeon and anatomist Sir Astley Cooper in his own house (Cooper, *Life*, vol. 1, pp. 340–2), South's account of the dissecting room at St Thomas's Hospital in 1813 (South, *Memorials*, pp. 28–9) and on drawings such as Thomas Rowlandson's 'The Dissecting Room', which depicts the room of anatomist William Hunter (1718–83), and his 'Death in the Dissecting Room' (1815), as well as Hogarth's 'The Reward of Cruelty' (1751).

9   Under the Murder Act (1752), grave-robbing and dissection took place in a legal grey area. Stealing corpses was not a crime (since a corpse wasn't recognised as anyone's property), so the authorities tried to stop it by prosecuting for theft of the shroud. This went on until the Anatomy Act (1834), which allowed for the legal dissection of paupers and other unclaimed corpses.

10   London resurrectionist Joshua Naples mentions supplying cadavers to Edinburgh in his diary for December 1811 (quoted in Bailey, *Diary*, p. 142). Salting of cadavers is described in the case of an Edinburgh-bound shipment of thirty-three bodies seized by police in Liverpool docks in 1826; the preserving process was not wholly effective, and it was the 'horrible stench' coming from the casks in which the corpses were packed that alerted the ship's captain, who called in the police (Bailey, *Diary*, pp. 82–6; Hunt, 'Trade in Dead Bodies'). The prices paid for corpses are given by Naples in his diary (Bailey, *Diary*, pp. 139–76).

11   Description based on an 1801 edition preserved in the Rare Books collection of Cambridge University Library.

12   Various methods of dissecting the upper body were in use; the one described here is based on several (e.g. Fyfe, *Compendium*; Harrison, *Dublin Dissector*), but particularly that of Robert Knox (*Edinburgh Dissector*, pp. 198–206), who was a student contemporary with James Barry and went on to be a military surgeon and eminent anatomist. Some details (such as the unexpected toughness of the skin) are based on author Michael du Preez's own experience of human dissection.

13   Fyfe's remarks are taken almost verbatim from his *Compendium of the Anatomy of the Human Body* (pp. 119–24).

14   Arneth, 'Evidence of Puerperal Fever', p. 292.

15   Charles Darwin's uncle had been a medical student in Edinburgh, but died in 1778 from an illness believed to have been contracted during a dissection. He spent a day 'accurately dissecting the brain of a child which had died of hydrocephalus, and which he had attended during its life. That very evening he was seized with severe head-ach.' He got rapidly sicker, and died (Society in Edinburgh, 'Medical News', pp. 333–4).

16   Dr John Barclay (1758–1826) was a hugely successful lecturer with a 'genius for anatomy' (Struthers, *Historical Sketch*, p. 69). Despite his having no official post in

the university, attendance at his private lecture courses far outstripped the courses given by Monro. Surgeons' Square, where his house stood (ibid, p. 59), was within the bounds of the Royal Infirmary.

17 War Office: RJBc.

18 Rosner, *Medical Education*, p. 55.

19 War Office: RJBc; Rosner, *Medical Education*, pp. 60, 118; Bower, *Student's Guide*; Barry to Reardon, 14 December 1809, BFA.

20 Mary Anne Bulkley to Reardon, 29 January 1810, BFA. Mrs Bulkley was a keen student of the pianoforte, and had been taking lessons in London for several years.

21 Carphin in *The Lancet*, 19 October 1895.

22 Ibid. Janet Carphin knew Dr Jobson later in life, when he was practising as a physician in Kent; he told her about his student friendship after Barry died and the truth about his sex was made public. Jobson joined the Army as a hospital assistant in 1813, served with several regiments, and eventually returned to Edinburgh to finish his MD in 1819 (Johnston, *Roll*, p. 245).

23 Buchan to Anderson, 5 July 1810, LEB.

24 Scott, quoted in Lockhart, *Memoirs*, vol. 4, p. 204.

25 Buchan to Anderson, 15 October 1811, LEB.

26 Ibid.

27 Ibid.

28 Rose, *Perfect Gentleman*, p. 27; Rae, *Strange Story*, p. 11.

29 Mary Anne Bulkley, letters to Reardon, 11 February 1812, 28 April 1812, BFA.

30 At some point during the following decade, the university statutes were altered, and it became a requirement that all MD candidates be over twenty-one (Bower, *Edinburgh Student's Guide*). Whether this was a consequence of the Barry case is not known.

31 Rosner, *Medical Education*, pp. 72–85; Bower, *Student's Guide*.

32 Barry, *Disputatio*, pp. 4–5, JBE.

33 Duncan, 'Medical Department', p. 125. Infectious eye diseases became a serious problem in the Army after 1804, when a series of outbreaks of 'Egyptian ophthalmia' (trachoma) occurred among troops. In 1806 there were hundreds of cases in the 52nd Regiment alone, with ninety men losing one or both of their eyes (Lawrence, *Treatise*, p. 178).

34 Barry, *Disputatio*, title and dedication pages, JBE.

35 Buchan, *Essays*, vol. I, pp. 28–30.

36 Buchan to Anderson, 15 October 1811, LEB.

37 Slatta and de Grummond, *Simón Bolívar's Quest for Glory*, pp. 40–2.

Chapter 8: *'I Would Be a Soldier'*

1   Due to an ancient privilege, debtors had once been safe from their creditors in the Mint, and although the privilege was abolished in the early 18th century the area remained infested with poverty and crime (Hughson, *Walks*, p. 326).

2   The gates were closed at 9 p.m. and opened each morning at 10 (Golding, *Historical*

Account, pp. 201–2). Golding's book, although nominally a history, was mostly concerned with the running of the hospital at the time it was published (1819). St Thomas's (as it was called before it dropped the *s*) had stood in Southwark since 1215, but moved in 1862 to its present riverside location in Lambeth (McInnes, *St Thomas's Hospital*, pp. 102–13).

3 Gordon, *Vindication*, ch. 16; Denlinger, *Before Victoria*, pp. vii, 44–9.
4 St Thomas' Pupils, KCH.
5 Register, Cooper and Cline, KCH; South, *Memorials*, p. 31.
6 Advertisement, *The Times*, 4 September 1812, p. 1; South, *Memorials*, p. 27.
7 Golding, *Historical Account*, p. 223. In 1813 St Thomas's Hospital 'cured and discharged' 2713 in-patients and 6117 out-patients, and buried 117; as of April 1814, which was typical, there were 412 in-patients and 269 out-patients registered (*Morning Post*, 12 April 1814, p. 2). By custom, the Report of the City Hospitals (which gave these figures) was read out at a sumptuous Easter Monday banquet presided over by the Lord Mayor at his official residence, the Mansion House in the City.
8 Golding, *Historical Account*, p. 224.
9 Ibid., p. 232.
10 Those who were refused admission could apply to be treated as out-patients, in which case they could return on three successive Saturdays for examination and treatment.
11 Stanley, *For Fear*, pp. 137–9.
12 Golding, *Historical Account*, p. 222.
13 Ibid., p. 235; diet laid out on p. 237.
14 Ibid., p. 235. Golding, who was himself a surgeon, is quite specific about the absence of vegetables (he remarks that the governors had experimented with replacing part of the bread ration with potatoes, to give patients variety, but there were so many complaints that they quickly reverted). Given that some patients were in the hospital for months, one wonders how scurvy was avoided. At this time, it had been known for over sixty years that scurvy was prevented by fruit and vegetables. Possibly there was just enough vitamin C in the fresh meat (especially if beef liver was given) and milk, or even in the beer or wine, to prevent it.
15 Ibid., p. 240.
16 Quoted in *Medical History*, 'Introduction', p. 17.
17 McInnes (*St Thomas' Hospital*, pp. 91–2) gives an annual average income of £643 15s 1d for 1837–40, received by Richard Whitfield III, compared with between £239 and £488 for physicians and surgeons.
18 The garret was acquired after the church was built in 1703. Most of the old St Thomas's Hospital is now gone, but the 'Herb Garret' is still there above the church, now a museum, the only bit of the St Thomas's of Barry's time to survive. In the 1820s (after Barry's time), part of the roof space was given over to construction of a new operating theatre, which has also been preserved as part of the museum.
19 Golding, *Historical Account*, pp. 132–3.
20 Ibid., p. 136.

21 The old Guy's building is still there, and still a part of the hospital, now overlooked by the vast glass tower of the Shard skyscraper and the massive modern hospital.

22 Cooper, *Life of Sir Astley Cooper*, vol. 2, pp. 71–7.

23 Pettigrew, 'Sir Astley Paston Cooper', p. 3.

24 Cooper, *Life*, vol. 2, p. 77.

25 South, *Memorials*, pp. 34–5.

26 Cooper, *Life*, vol. 1, p. 314. Henry Cline (1750–1827) had been surgeon at St Thomas's since 1784. Cooper (1768–1841) became his apprentice on the recommendation of his uncle, William Cooper, surgeon at Guy's at the time (ibid., p. 87). Cooper received his baronetcy in 1820 as a reward for removing a lump from the head of King George IV; Henry Cline assisted with the operation. They had been called in by the royal physician, Sir Henry Halford – an eminent gentleman with whom Dr Barry would later come into conflict (see Chapter 21).

27 The discovery of the role of hygiene occurred in the 1840s in two independent obstetric studies: one by the American Dr Oliver Wendell Holmes Sr from 1843 onward, and another by Viennese Ignaz Semmelweis in 1847. Semmelweis suspected that the high rate of mortality from puerperal fever (also known as childbed fever) might be connected with students and doctors examining women after performing autopsies and dissections. He introduced a regime in which all had to scrub their hands with a solution of chloride of lime before entering the maternity ward. Mortality fell by about 80 per cent (Gallin, 'Historical Perspective', pp. 7–8). It took almost a decade for Semmelweis's and Holmes's results to be accepted by the medical profession, and for the wider implications to be recognised. In the 1850s surgeons were still wondering whether the mysterious 'morbific particles' that caused puerperal fever might also cause surgical fever (Simpson, *Obstetric Memoirs*, pp. 1–19).

28 Cooper, *Life*, vol. 2, pp. 78–9.

29 Golding, *Historical Account*, p. 128. The year after James Barry's period at the United Hospitals, work began on a new theatre, which was completed in 1814; it was large, well ventilated, and had attached to it a museum of specimens and a dissecting room that could accommodate up to 200 students all dissecting at once.

30 Cooper, *Lectures*.

31 South, *Memorials*, p. 32. John Flint South became a pupil at the United Hospitals in 1813, a few months after James Barry left.

32 Cooper, *Life*, vol. 1, p. 315.

33 Pettigrew, 'Sir Astley Paston Cooper', p. 3.

34 South, *Memorials*, p. 128.

35 Pettigrew, 'Sir Astley Paston Cooper', pp. 3–4.

36 Review of Bransby Cooper's *Life* in *The Times*, 14 April 1843, p. 5.

37 Mary Anne Bulkley to Reardon, 11 February and 28 April 1812, BFA.

38 Anderson to Mary Anne Bulkley, 3 November 1812, BFA. The letter is marked as having been delivered on Friday 6 November.

39 Fryer to Mary Anne Bulkley, 31 October 1812, BFA.

40 Pettigrew, 'Sir Astley Paston Cooper', p. 7. An often-told story of Cooper is that he performed a lithotomy on an elderly gentleman, removing a very large stone from the bladder; on being told afterwards that the fee was 200 guineas, the man pooh-poohed the sum and tossed Sir Astley his nightcap, which turned out to contain a cheque for a thousand.

41 Anderson to Mary Anne Bulkley, 17 November 1812, BFA. Mrs Bulkley's letter to Anderson has not survived; we only have his reply.

42 The *Pandora* was eventually knocked down for 11½ guineas in 1846.

43 Margaret Ann Bulkley to John Bulkley, undated (probably September 1808), BFA.

Chapter 9: Qualified to Serve

1   Army Medical Board Book of Candidates, June 1813, quoted in note appended to War Office: RJBb. The original Board Book has not been found; all we have is a note added to Barry's later records. In this document, Barry gave his date of birth as 'about 1799'. A later hand has added: 'If this is correct he must have entered the Service when he was *14* years of age', and then: 'But in the Board Book of Candidates Examinations in June 1813 he stated his Age to have been 18.'

2   The full procedure for surgical candidates is set out in Dunne, *Chirurgical Candidate*, pp. 47–52.

3   Based on a form sample in ibid., p. 48n.

4   The 1813 building, designed by George Dance the Younger, was largely demolished in 1833 and rebuilt, then was partially destroyed by bombing in the Second World War and rebuilt again. All that survives of the original is the pillared portico.

5   Cruikshank, Account of an examination, quoted in Puzzle-Pate, 'Medical Science Exemplified', p. 268. The fees are given in Dunne, *Chirurgical Candidate*, pp. 47–9.

6   Dunne, *Chirurgical Candidate*, pp. xiv–xv.

7   Ibid., p. xiv. Dunne appears to have had personal issues connected with qualification and respectability (which later became entangled in a libel case – see Dunne, *Mr. Dunne*), but the picture he draws is authentic.

8   Maclean, *Analytical View*, p. iii.

9   Ibid., pp. 37, 39.

10 Commissioners of Military Enquiry, *Fifth Report*.

11 See Ackroyd et al., *Advancing*, ch. 1.

12 Court of Examiners, 2 July 1813, RCS, f93. An earlier biography (Rae, *Strange*, p. 17) gives the date as 15 January 1813, an error deriving from a quirk in the RCS register. In the main alphabetical index of candidates, only one Barry is given – a Samuel Barry who was examined on that date. Rae, guessing that 'Samuel' was a clerical error, inferred that this was James. It wasn't. The problem was not a clerical error but a clerical aberration. The space set aside for the Bs in the index had filled up quickly, so subsequent Bs were entered in other places in the index book, apparently randomly, wherever space could be found. Thus, to find James Barry's entry took Michael du Preez the better part of a morning's searching through most of the index book. He eventually discovered it arbitrarily

written elsewhere, leading to the correct entry for James Barry in folio 93 of the register.

13 See Royal College of Surgeons, *General List*, p. 19; Leigh, *New Picture of London*, p. 171 for staff of the RCS. The procedure for examinations at the RCS retained some traditional features – including the ceremonial role of the costumed beadle – as late as 1963, when author Michael du Preez took his FRCS exam. The procedure in 1813 is described in part by Gibney (*Eighty Years*, pp. 91–2).

14 This room – and the Court of Examiners itself – is depicted in a cartoon by George Cruikshank, 'The Examination of a Young Surgeon', in satirical magazine *The Scourge* in October 1811.

15 The Court of Examiners on 2 July 1813 consisted of Mr Thompson Forster, Master; Sir Everard Home, governor; Sir William Blizard, governor; Sir James Earle; George Chandler; Thomas Keate; Sir Charles Blicke; David Dundas; Henry Cline; and William Norris. The youngest was Sir Everard Home, who was fifty-seven, with the average age being about sixty-five. Several of these men (including Cline, Home and Blizard) are recognisable in Cruikshank's cartoon.

16 Stanley, *For Fear*, p. 179.

17 South, *Memorials*, p. 46. John Flint South was examined at the RCS in 1819; many of the personalities were the same as in James Barry's year.

18 Ibid., p. 46.

19 Ibid., pp. 131–2.

20 Guthrie, 'Evidence', p. 42.

21 In 1813 the rates ranged between 70 and 95 per cent (Court of Examiners, f93, RCS). By the early 1830s the overall pass rate was still as high as 92 per cent, which incredibly was said to represent a doubling of rejections over preceding years (Guthrie, 'Evidence', p. 42). By Michael du Preez's day (1963), the figures had reversed, with only about one in ten candidates passing the final fellowship exam.

22 Cruikshank, Account of an examination at the Court of Examiners, quoted in Puzzle-Pate, 'Medical Science Exemplified', p. 268. There was pressure from the government to make the examination even easier. George James Guthrie, who served as a regimental surgeon in the Peninsular War and later became president and professor at the Royal College, recalled of his own examination in 1800 that it was 'very fair and reasonable' and that the candidate 'must have some knowledge of anatomy and surgery'. However, it had to have some slack in order to maintain a sufficient supply of qualified surgeons to the forces; indeed, 'the Government were under the necessity of refraining from having them examined at all' (Guthrie, 'Evidence', p. 1).

23 Court of Examiners, f93, RCS.

24 James Barry's certificate has not survived; this text is based on an 1806 example given by Dunne in *Mr. Dunne*, p. 8n.

25 Based on form letter in Dunne, *Chirurgical Candidate*, p. 50n. This letter, which counted as a certificate, was kept by the War Office, and the candidate had to obtain a copy on payment of yet another 5 shilling fee.

26 Dunne, *Chirurgical Candidate*, p. 51; Duncan, 'Medical Department', p. 125; Michael Crumplin, personal communication, 29 April 2015.

27 Ackroyd et al., *Advancing with the Army*, pp. 32–5; Kaufman, *Surgeons at War*, pp. 29–33.

28 War Office: RJBc.

29 See Appendix A. Military surgeon John Hennen (*Principles*, ch. 20) gives a detailed account of the thorough physical examination of recruits to the ranks.

30 There was no earthly reason why James should not have written to his friends and his 'aunt', and yet there is no evidence that he ever did so. It isn't impossible that Mrs Bulkley had been imprisoned for her debt, and that this helped force Margaret's decision to have James join the Army (as a means of raising money immediately and escaping London). On the other hand, the abruptness and completeness of the breach may point towards a falling-out between Margaret and her mother.

31 Adjutant General's Office, *General Regulations*, p. 219.

32 Grose, *Lexicon*. 'Dead Chelsea, by God!' is cited by Grose as 'an exclamation uttered by a grenadier at Fontenoy, on having his leg carried away by a cannon-ball'.

33 Ewart, in Gleig, *Veterans of Chelsea*, pp. 21–3. Named after the Duke of York, second son of George III, the hospital had formerly been the infirmary wing of the Chelsea Hospital (a new infirmary was later constructed under the direction of John Soane); the York, which was never fit for purpose, was demolished in 1819 and its facilities moved to Chatham (Faulkner, *Historical and Topographical Description*, p. 356; Select Committee on Medical Education, *Report*, p. 206; Ackroyd et al., *Advancing*, pp. 26–7). Graham Street (now Graham Terrace) was built on the site. Jews' Row is now part of Royal Hospital Road and Five Fields Row is now Ebury Street.

34 James Ewart's Story, in Gleig, *Veterans of Chelsea*, p. 23.

35 Pay rates at the York are given in Dupin, *A View*, p. 358, based on information gleaned in 1816.

36 Ackroyd et al., *Advancing*, p. 35.

37 Gibney, *Eighty Years*, pp. 93–4. Gibney cannot have recalled James Barry; he was writing his recollections some years after Barry's death and the revelation of his secret, and as he doesn't mention this, he had presumably failed to connect the name with the young man who had been one of the 'queer lot' at the York in 1813.

38 Ibid., p. 94

39 Ibid., p. 95.

40 Ibid., pp. 95–6.

41 War Office: RJBb; Buchan to Anderson, 20 November 1813, LEB.

42 The hospital was closed down after the First World War, and the building is now part of Devonport High School for Boys.

43 Skey had served in Barbados, and published a paper on the island's geology in the *Transactions of the Geological Society of London* in 1816.

44 Bradford, 'Reputed Female Army Surgeon'. The exact exchange has not survived; all we have is Skey's recollection, fifty years after the event, as told to fellow

military doctor Edward Bradford, who was a friend of Barry's in his later career. Bradford reports him as saying that he had referred the matter to 'the authorities', and received that terse reply; however, since James Barry did not have the powerful connections in the Army that he later acquired, and Buchan didn't have significant influence there, Bradford must have misunderstood, and 'the authorities' were in fact Lord Buchan himself.

45 Buchan to Anderson, 20 November 1813, LEB.

46 War Office: RJBb. Barry also stated, 'I entered the Army as a Medical Officer under the age of fourteen years' in a document written at the end of his career (War Office: RJBa).

47 *Royal Cornwall Gazette*, 16 April 1814, p. 2.

48 *Royal Cornwall Gazette*, 24 June 1815, p. 3; see also O'Keeffe, *Waterloo*, pt 2 ch. 3.

49 Bell to Horner, July 1815, in Bell, *Letters*, p. 247. Charles Bell is noted for the vivid watercolour sketches he made of the wounds he saw.

50 Edward Heeley, quoted in O'Keeffe, *Waterloo*, pt 1, ch. 3.

51 Cooper, *Lectures*, vol. 2, pp. 425–6, 428–9. The plaster was a sticky, oily (and toxic) compound of equal parts of *emplastrum thuris compositum* (plaster of frankincense, made from lead oxide mixed with lard, to which red iron oxide and frankincense were added) and *emplastrum saponis* (soap plaster, made from powdered soap and more of the lard/lead oxide mix) (ibid., vol. 1, pp. 185–6).

52 There was an alternative and much rarer method of amputation whereby, instead of a single circular incision, two cuts were used, one on each side of the limb, angled outwards, so as to create two long flaps that could be closed over the end of the stump; this method was used on the Earl of Uxbridge, whose knee was smashed by grapeshot at Waterloo. Proponents of this method were known as 'flappers', and there was a long-running dispute between 'flappers' and 'anti-flappers' over its efficacy (James Gregory, *Additional Memorial*, pp. 414–15).

53 Hennen, *Principles*, p. 253.

54 *Salisbury and Winchester Journal*, 10 July 1815, p. 3; also *Hampshire Chronicle*, 10 July 1815, p. 2. The thousands of French prisoners taken during the wars in the Peninsula and elsewhere had been released after Napoleon's defeat in1814; they formed the veteran core of his army in the Waterloo campaign.

55 *Salisbury and Winchester Journal*, 10 July 1815, p. 3.

56 Dr Barry 'sought every opportunity of making himself conspicuous, and wore the longest sword and spurs he could obtain' (Bradford, 'Reputed Female Army Surgeon'). Not only were Army surgeons expected to wear a sword, it was not unknown for them to have to wield it.

57 *The Times*, 25 July 1815, p. 2.

58 *The Times*, 1 August 1815, p. 3.

59 Maitland, *Surrender*, pp. 135–6.

60 *The Times*, 8 August 1815, p. 3.

61 'Boney Was a Warrior', quoted in Cordingly, *Billy Ruffian*, app. 2. Like many 'seventy-fours', HMS *Bellerophon* ended her life as a prison hulk; her name was

changed to *Captivity*, taking over from the lately broken-up ship of the same name in which Redmond Barry had been incarcerated from 1807 to 1814.

62 James Barry commission, 7 December 1815, RJBd; also War Office: RJBb.

63 This miniature is one of only three known images of James Barry taken from life, and the only one from his youth (there are two further claimed Barry portraits, but both are doubtful). The work is a true miniature on ivory, 45mm long by 32mm wide. There is a small vertical crack in the ivory at the upper edge.

Katherine Coombs, Curator of Paintings at the Victoria and Albert Museum (personal communication, 5 October 2005), considered that the work might be an amateur's, being quite slight and tentatively painted; if it was done by a professional there were four known miniaturists in the locality at that time, two of whom were women – Augusta and Jane Hamlyn, the former working from an address in Plymouth. Unfortunately, there is nothing on the back of the painting to offer any clue.

On the uniform, Mrs G. A. Brewer of the National Army Museum, Chelsea notes (personal communication): 'Surgeons and Assistant Surgeons wore plain red single-breasted coatees with no epaulettes or lacing, which is why there is so little ornament shown. From the size and shape of the collar, I would date the painting no later than 1816. From 1810 the coat had long imitation silk buttonholes across the chest, these were stopped in 1813 when plain coatees were again worn.' This places it at about the time of Barry's commission in 1815.

Chapter 10: *The Cape of Good Hope*

1 Typical East Indiamen were around 800 tons (although could be up to 1200 tons), while *Lord Cathcart*, built at Selby in 1807, was 362 tons (advertisement, *The Public Ledger and Daily Advertiser*, 16 April 1817, p. 4).

2 Williamson, *East India*, p. 28.

3 William Hickey, *Memoirs*, quoted in Parkinson, *Trade*, p. 270. Parkinson (ibid., p. 207) indicates that an assistant surgeon travelling to India in the East India Company's service paid £95 for passage; James Barry was only going halfway to India, so might have paid less, but as he wasn't a Company servant, his fare would be higher; therefore he probably paid between £70 and £100. It isn't clear whether the Army paid its officers' fares at this period.

4 Williamson, *East India*, pp. 32, 42.

5 Mary Ann Reid, 'Cursory Remarks', p. 346.

6 Marshall, *Epistles*, p. 208 (the author had been an officer in the East India Company's merchant marine, and included the anecdote for the amusement of his readers).

7 Renshaw, *Voyage*, p. 17. This particular incident took place on a warship, and there are no other references to nudity in the published literature of the time; however, Renshaw's was a popular book, and James Barry would quite likely have read it.

8 Burney, *Falconer's*, p. 139.

9 Teenstra (*Fruits*, pp. 302–8) gives a detailed description of the voyage to the Cape at this time.

10 Williamson, *East India*, p. 62.

11 Shipping Arrivals and Departures, Cape Town, 1816–1822, CO 6086, f8, WCA. This folio is damaged in such a way that the date of the *Lord Cathcart*'s arrival can only be inferred to lie between 23 and 26 October. The ship had departed from Gravesend on 9 August and joined the convoy at the Downs off the Kent coast on 10 August, making a voyage of eleven weeks, which was very good going.

12 The stacked boots are referred to by various 19th-century anecdotal sources, including the original author of Dickens, 'A Mystery Still'. The kapok stuffing was discovered early in Dr Barry's Cape career (see Chapter 11).

13 Picard, *Gentleman's Walk*, p. 150.

14 The letter from Lord Buchan has not survived. Its existence is known anecdotally, recalled half a century later by the anonymous informant of Dickens's 'A Mystery Still' (p. 492), who knew Barry and writes that when he first arrived at the Cape, he brought 'letters of introduction to the governor of that colony from a well-known eccentric Scottish nobleman'.
    Government House, now known as De Tuynhuys ('Garden House'), is nowadays the Cape Town office of the President of South Africa.

15 Millar, *Plantagenet*, p. 46.

16 Somerset to Beaufort, 20 January 1814, quoted in Millar, *Plantagenet*, p. 55.

17 Somerset to Beaufort, 16 September 1815, quoted in Millar, *Plantagenet*, pp. 75–6.

18 Ibid., p. 75. It would seem from Lord Charles's description that she had suffered from a peritonsillar abscess followed by fatal septicaemia. (In the same letter he wrote that 'the excessive swelling of the throat and glands alone caused uneasiness'.) This condition was well known at the time (commonly known as 'quinsy'), as were its potential complications. Available treatments – emetics, gargles etc. – were not particularly effective (Parr, *London Medical Dictionary*, pp. 116–19).

19 Dr Barry's reputation was well known in the Cape during his time there – to the point of fame (or infamy, depending on who one asked) – and is recalled in Dickens, 'A Mystery Still', p. 492.

20 A few years later Georgiana became sick again (after falling in love with a young officer and being forbidden by her father to marry him). Lord Charles again worried for her life, and took her back to England; by the time they reached St Helena she was already well again (Rose, *Perfect Gentleman*, pp. 45, 47).

21 When Napoleon left the Élysée Palace on 23 June 1815, he went in a small coach by a rear exit while Las Cases rode from the front in the imperial coach with two of Napoleon's aides-de-camp, braving the crowds; they rendezvoused on the outskirts of Paris and travelled on into exile (O'Keeffe, *Waterloo*, pt 4 ch. 2).

22 Desmond Gregory, *Napoleon's Jailer*, p. 125ff. One of Napoleon's party was an Irish doctor called Barry O'Meara, surgeon aboard HMS *Bellerophon*, who was appointed as Napoleon's personal physician during his exile; he involved himself in a campaign to undermine Lowe's authority. Lowe's biographer (ibid.) suggests that, given Napoleon's previous escape from Elba and the appalling consequences, Lowe's actions were understandable and even reasonable.

23 Lowe to Somerset, 28 December 1816, in RCC 11, pp. 232–5.

24 Las Cases, *Mémorial*, vol. 4.8, p. 94.

25 Ibid., pp. 95–6.

26 Ibid., p. 96.

27 Albemarle, *Fifty Years*, p. 204.

28 Las Cases, *Mémorial*, vol. 4.8, pp. 96–7.

29 Desmond Gregory, *Napoleon's Jailer*, p. 125.

30 Las Cases, *Mémorial*, vol. 4.8, p. 99.

31 Quoted in ibid., p. 109.

32 Ibid., p. 109.

33 Ibid., p. 112.

34 Ibid., p. 118.

35 Ibid., p. 121.

Chapter 11: 'Savage Neighbours'

1 Burchell, *Hints on Emigration*, pp. 6–7.

2 Somerset to Bathurst, 23 January 1817, in RCC 11, p. 256.

3 Somerset to Bathurst, 1 September 1816, in RCC 11, p. 150.

4 Alternatively known as the Gantouw Pass, the name given by the native Khoikhoi who first used it in pre-colonial times (*gantouw* means eland, a type of antelope). Later in the 19th century, this pass was abandoned and a new one, called Sir Lowry's Pass (after a later Governor), was created a little further south. This latter route is still in use today.

5 It is known that Barry spent a lot of time in the saddle during his colonial postings, although there is no evidence of when exactly he'd learned to ride. It is possible that Margaret was taught (side-saddle) as a girl in Ireland; this is improbable, as the Bulkleys were city-dwellers and not affluent enough to complete Margaret's ladylike accomplishments. However, James would almost certainly have ridden (and learned to do so in the male style) while a guest of the Earl of Buchan at Dryburgh Abbey in 1811.

6 Barry, 'Report Upon the Arctopus Echinatus', RJBe; see also Chapter 19.

7 *Cape Gazette*, October 1818, quoted in Millar, *Plantagenet*, p. 114. The fact that this proclamation was made during a period when Lord Charles was ill and under Dr Barry's care is significant.

8 Governor's proclamation, 14 March 1823, in RCC 15, pp. 320–1. Eland and bontebok still live wild in South Africa to this day thanks to Somerset's intervention.

9 Brenton, *Memoir*, pp. 543–4.

10 Ibid., pp. 548–9.

11 Ibid., p. 550; Millar, *Plantagenet*, p. 94.

12 Thompson, *Travels*, p. 4.

13 Latrobe, *Journal*, pp. 150–1.

14 Ibid., p. 157.

15 Storrar, *George Rex*.

16 William Harrison, 'George III and Hannah Lightfoot', p. 117.

17   Metelerkamp, *George Rex*, pp. 87–9. Metelerkamp refutes the popular alternative story, which is that the 'kapok' part of the nickname was given on account of Dr Barry's pale complexion.

18   Rogers to Brereton, 4 September 1818, in RCC 12, p. 43. The farm subsequently grew into a town, called Somerset East (to distinguish it from Somerset West, near Cape Town).

19   Somerset to Bathurst, 24 April 1817, in RCC 11, pp. 303–4.

20   Report by Lt Col. Graham, 2 January 1812, in RCC 8, p. 236.

21   Cradock to Lord Liverpool, 7 March 1812, in RCC 8, p. 355.

22   Beck, *History*, pp. 56–8.

23   Somerset to Bathurst, 24 April 1817, in RCC 11, p. 303.

24   Somerset to Bathurst, 23 January 1817, in RCC 11, pp. 252–3.

25   Ibid.

26   Ibid., p. 254.

27   Governor's proclamation, April 1817, in RCC 11, pp. 294–5.

28   There were 4500 troops stationed at the Cape at this time, including artillery, three regiments of infantry, one of dragoons, and the local Cape Regiment. In addition to those listed, there was also the 60th Regiment of Foot, the Royal Americans (Return of Troops, in RCC 11, p. 261).

29   A detailed account of this meeting and the subsequent conference is given by Colonel Bird, reproduced in RCC 11, pp. 310–15.

30   Cradock to Lord Liverpool, 7 March 1812, in RCC 8, p. 355.

31   Bird, conference minutes, April 1817, in RCC 11, p. 311.

32   Bird, conference minutes, April 1817, in RCC 11, p. 314.

33   Williams, quoted in Cory, *Rise*, p. 306.

34   Somerset to Bathurst, 24 April 1817, in RCC 11, p. 303.

35   Somerset to Bathurst, 22 May 1819, in RCC 12, pp. 193–202.

Chapter 12: A Prodigy in a Physician

1   Las Cases, *Mémorial*, vol. 4.8, p. 122.

2   Somerset to Bathurst, 18 August 1817, in RCC 11, p. 369.

3   Las Cases, *Mémorial*, vol. 4.8, p. 133.

4   Ibid., p. 135.

5   Ibid., pp. 139–40.

6   Somerset to Bathurst, 18 August 1817, in RCC 11, p. 369.

7   Barry to Somerset, 21 June 1817, CO 81 f107, WCA.

8   Somerset to Bathurst, 18 August 1817, in RCC 11, p. 370.

9   Las Cases, *Mémorial*, vol. 4.8, p. 147.

10   Brenton, *Memoir*, p. 455.

11   Ibid.

12   Dillon, *Narrative*, p. 408.

13   Ibid.

14   Plasket and Miller, *Proclamations*, p. 403.

15 Hay to Merry, 15 February 1826, in RCC 26, p. 29.

16 Cradock, memorandum, 21 April 1812, in RCC 8, p. 384; also various letters and proclamations, ibid. *passim*; see also Burrows, *History*, pp. 98–9.

17 Burrows, *History*, pp. 97–102.

18 Governor's proclamation, 17 March 1812, in RCC 8, p. 360.

19 List of Offices, 25 October 1824, in RCC 19, p. 56.

20 Ackroyd et al., *Advancing*, pp. 48–9.

21 Newspaper account (date not recorded, probably late 19th century) based on report of Mrs Bales, granddaughter of Mrs Cloete, MFC.

22 John Reid, *Treatise*, p. 133.

23 Ibid., p. 134.

24 Ibid., p. 136ff; Thomas, *Modern Practice*, p. 145.

25 Thomas, *Modern Practice*, p. 146.

26 Newspaper account (date not recorded, probably late 19th century) based on report of Mrs Bales, granddaughter of Mrs Cloete, MFC.

27 Ibid. The original account implies that Dr Barry left immediately after letting in fresh air and scolding the family, without even examining the patient; this would have been thoroughly unprofessional, and is highly unlikely.

28 Newspaper account (1880s, title not recorded) by Lois Chance, granddaughter of the patient, quoted in Rose, *Perfect Gentleman*, pp. 39–40.

29 Bird to Bathurst, 29 September 1818, in RCC 12, p. 45.

30 Working from Dr Barry's diagnosis (q.v.) and the known general progression of Lord Charles Somerset's illness, the symptoms have here been reconstructed.

31 Bird to Bathurst, 29 September 1818, in RCC 12, p. 46. Bird had been promoted from deputy to full colonial secretary that August.

32 Thomas, *Modern Practice*, p. 40.

33 '[Dysentery] frequently occurs about the same time with autumnal intermittent and remittent fevers,' wrote Robert Thomas in his 1819 *Modern Practice of Physic* (p. 40), 'and with these it is often complicated. It is likewise frequently combined with typhus.' Dr Barry's double diagnosis is given in Bird to Bathurst, 29 September 1818, in RCC 12, p. 46.

In fact, cases conventionally diagnosed as 'typhus with dysentery' in the early 19th century were almost certainly typhoid fever, which was not recognised prior to the 1850s. Whereas typhus is an infection of the entire system by *Rickettsia* bacteria transmitted by lice, fleas and other parasites, typhoid fever (which is named for the resemblance of some of its symptoms to typhus) is a bacterial infection primarily infecting the bowel, caused by ingestion, which later may spread systemically.

34 Bird to Bathurst, 29 September 1818, in RCC 12, p. 46.

35 Thomas, *Modern Practice*, pp. 289–90. The treatments described here are taken from Thomas.

36 Ibid., p. 44.

37 Bird to Bathurst, 1 October 1818, in RCC 12, p. 46.

38 Somerset to Bathurst, 17 October 1818, in RCC 12, pp. 49–50.

39 Somerset, quoted in Millar, *Plantagenet*, p. 113.
40 Somerset to Sir Hudson Lowe, date and source not given, quoted in Millar, *Plantagenet*, p. 92. As Lady Lowe's illness appears to have occurred in early 1819 (Desmond Gregory, *Napoleon's Jailer*, pp. 135–6), this would be the approximate date.

Chapter 13: The Most Wayward of Mortals

1   Fenton, *Journal*, p. 324.
2   Newspaper account (1880s, title not recorded) by Lois Chance, granddaughter of one of Barry's lady-friends, quoted in Rose, *Perfect Gentleman*, pp. 39–40.
3   Mimosa, 'Het Kapokdoktertje'.
4   Ibid.
5   Ibid.
6   *South African Advertiser and Mail*, 30 October 1865, p. 2.
7   Albemarle, *Fifty Years*, p. 204.
8   Ibid.
9   Ibid.
10 This consistent failure to shed her femininity is one of the strands of evidence against the idea that Margaret/James had a transgender personality. She may have been bigender, but we have no evidence for this; she lived one part of her life exclusively as female, and the other (with limited success) as male. By modern definitions, it is not altogether certain that she counts even as a transvestite, since the decision to live as a man was apparently motivated more by ambition than identity.
11 Albemarle, *Fifty Years*, p. 204.
12 Memoir of William Cattell, WLC.
13 Ibid. Cattell (1829–1919) states that the officer was posted to Tristan da Cunha. This is doubtful, since although the island had been garrisoned from the Cape in 1816, it was abandoned in 1817, leaving behind just a tiny population of settlers. The posting would more likely be St Helena or perhaps Mauritius.
14 There is a portrait of Captain Josias Cloete as a young man (probably by Georg Koberwein: Museum Africa, item 1966-905) which bears a strong, almost brother–sister resemblance to the miniature of James Barry.
15 Cloete's birth is usually given as 1794; however, his Army record gives his age as twenty-one in 1813 (list of captains, 21st Light Dragoons, 1812–15 in 'War Office: Campaign Medal and Award Rolls 1793–1949 (General Series)': National Archives microfilm publication WO 100: available online at www.ancestry.com; retrieved 1 October 2015).
16 Somerset to Bathurst, 24 October 1816 and 7 June 1817, in RCC 11, pp. 202–4, 350–1; Cloete to Somerset, 24 April 1817, ibid., pp. 300–3.
17 Somerset to Bathurst, 21 June 1817, in RCC 11, p. 355; Buckingham to Banks, 1 August 1819, in Buckingham, *Travels*, p. 645. Cloete sailed from Calcutta in early August 1819 intending to sail to England, but instead stopped at the Cape. The Calcutta–Cape Town voyage would take roughly one and a half months.

18 Cloete memoir, quoted in R. C. Bellenger to Major-General A. MacLennan, 17 November 1969, WLC. Mr Bellenger was an antiquarian book dealer who came into possession of Captain Cloete's papers, including this memoir, and quoted this passage from it in a letter to General MacLennan, who was researching James Barry. It is not known what happened to these papers subsequently; all attempts by author Michael du Preez to trace them have drawn a blank.

19 This incident – including expressions and dialogue – was recounted by Cloete in a conversation with General Sir William Mackinnon (1830–97), Director General of the British Army Medical Service, copied in Rogers, letter to the editor, *The Lancet*.

20 The business might be guessed. During 1819, Lord Charles Somerset was approached by Mrs Redelinghuys, newly married wife of a wealthy landowner, who had inherited lands of her own on the death of her previous husband. She wanted the Governor to grant her the purchase right to a tract of government land, and also wanted to purchase a valuable horse – Sorcerer's Colt – from him. Lord Charles negotiated a deal whereby he sold the land to Mrs Redelinghuys's husband, and gave them Sorcerer's Colt at a favourable price of 10,000 rixdollars (about £750) – an improper mixture of private and public business and a distinct conflict of interests that led to an accusation of corruption and an official investigation (see 'Report of the Commissioners of Enquiry to Earl Bathurst', 12 October 1824, in RCC 18, pp. 442–93).

21 Cloete, quoted in Rogers, letter to the editor, *The Lancet*.

22 Englishmen were supposed to turn the other cheek and withdraw with dignity after receiving a blow, and only duel as a last resort. The Irish code of honour was much more violent: 'There is no part of the world,' wrote one contemporary expert, 'in which duelling has been productive of such serious evil as in the Emerald Isle. It was formerly practised there, to a most extraordinary extent, and even yet there is scarcely a single hour elapses without a hostile meeting in some part of the island' (Hamilton, *Only Approved Guide*, p. 220). Even in England and Europe, the causes of duels could be amazingly trivial; Hamilton (ibid., p. 94ff) cites examples including: a dispute over the loan of a handkerchief; a difference of opinion over training horses; and a misunderstanding over anchovies and capers. Usually the trigger was one person imputing the truthfulness, honour or competence of another.

23 The identity of Dr Barry's second is a mystery. An account obtained verbally from the Cloete family in 1932 by Colonel N. J. C. Rutherford ('Dr James Barry', p. 174) gives the name as Foss and describes him as a surgeon. But there were no surgeons (military or civilian) of that name at the Cape at that time, and the only officer with a similar name and comparable rank was Charles Richard Fox (a name that renders as Vos in Dutch), who is known to have become a captain in the Cape Corps in 1820; but despite his commission, Fox did not arrive until July 1821, long after the duel (*London Gazette*, 19 August 1820, p. 1589; entry for General Sir Charles Richard Fox (1796–1873) in *History of Parliament: the House of Commons 1820–1832*, ed. D. R. Fisher; available online at www.historyofparliamentonline.

org/volume/1820-1832/member/fox-charles-1796-1873; retrieved 3 October 2015). Rutherford presumably misheard and/or mistranscribed the name. 'Foss' could be W. H. Lys, an Army staff surgeon who was James Barry's colleague at the Vaccine Institution and might well have acted for him.

24 Hamilton, *Only Approved Guide*, p. 14.

25 Ibid., pp. 18–19.

26 Ibid., p. 246.

27 Ibid., pp. 215–16.

28 Ibid., p. 217.

29 The interval between the flash in the pan and the firing of the ball could be as little as one-tenth of a second or as long as two seconds, depending on the make of the weapon and the quality of the powder; duels were often decided by who could maintain his aim and his nerve while the pistol discharged (Roger Ingle, Durban Blackpowder and Historical Gun Club, personal communication, 14 September 2012).

30 Cloete memoir, quoted in Bellenger to MacLennan, 17 November 1969, RAMC/238/1, WLC; Rutherford, 'Dr James Barry', p. 174. Rutherford fictionalised his account of James Barry very heavily in areas where he had no source material (which in his day, before Dr Barry had been thoroughly researched, was most of the story). Here, however, he is reliable, as he had the main points of the duel from the Cloete family during a visit to Alphen in 1932 (even though he got the name of the second wrong – see note 23 above).

31 Donkin to Moresby, 3 April 1820 and Bathurst, 22 May 1820, in RCC 13, pp. 103, 140. The settlement became Port Elizabeth.

32 War Office, *A List of the Officers*, 1821, pp. 511–12. Many other surplus light dragoon regiments were frozen at the same time.

Chapter 14: A Change of Circumstances

1 Saunders, 'Between Slavery and Freedom', pp. 36–7.

2 Somerset to Bathurst, 19 May 1817, in RCC 11, pp. 342–3.

3 For instance, 'Return of Troops', 25 May 1819, in RCC 12, p. 210, lists seventy-one 'Prize Negroes', listed separately from the regiments.

4 Editor's commentary, in Brenton, *Memoir*, p. 602.

5 Ibid., p. 604. By the 1840s it was reported that Hermes had settled again in the Colony and become a respectable citizen.

6 Somerset to Bathurst, 25 April 1819, and to Goulburn, 12 April 1820, in RCC 12, p. 176 and vol. 13, p. 107.

7 By the time their ship touched St Helena, Miss Somerset was much improved (Millar, *Plantagenet*, p. 127).

8 Millar, *Plantagenet*, pp. 123–7.

9 Donkin to Bathurst, 31 January 1820, in RCC 13, pp. 12–13.

10 Acting Governor's proclamation, 1 February 1820, in RCC 13, pp. 14–15.

11 Bathurst to Donkin, 17 May 1820, in RCC 13, pp. 132–3.

12 War Office, RJBb.

13 Kinnis, 'Observations', pp. 28–9. This quarantine was probably the reason for the long delay in the news reaching Cape Town – more than a month elapsed between the outbreak and HMS *Hardy* setting sail.

14 See Gillkrest and Fergusson, *Letters* for a contemporary discussion of cholera epidemiology.

15 Kinnis, 'Observations', p. 29.

16 War Office, *A List of the Officers*, 1821, p. 383.

17 Kinnis, 'Observations', p. 2.

18 Ibid., p. 3.

19 Ibid.

20 Hays, *Epidemics*, ch. 22. Cholera is believed to have originated in the Indian subcontinent, and was little known beyond that region until the 1817–24 pandemic. The cholera bacteria might have evolved following the effects of the Mount Tambora eruption and 'volcanic winter' of 1816.

21 Brenton, undated memorandum (late 1820), in RCC 13, pp. 322–9.

22 War Office: RJBb.

23 Somerset to Bathurst, 13 December 1821, in RCC 14, pp. 209–11.

Chapter 15: Heaven and Earth

1 The baby, Poulett Somerset, was born on 19 June 1822, so presumably had been conceived aboard during September.

2 Donkin to Bathurst, 20 September 1821, in RCC 14, p. 118.

3 Government advertisement, 21 September 1821, in RCC 14, pp. 118–19; War Office, *A List of the Officers*, 1805, p. 289; 1821, p. 379.

4 Bird to Barry, 18 March 1822, in RCC 14, pp. 315–16.

5 Plasket and Miller, *Proclamations*, p. 549.

6 Barry to Bathurst, 6 December 1825, in RCC 24, p. 67.

7 Governor's proclamation, 26 September 1823, in RCC 16, pp. 307–11.

8 Hay to Merry, 15 February 1826, in RCC 26, p. 29.

9 Burrows, *History of Medicine*, p. 81.

10 Barry to Bird, 24 March 1822, CO 159/12, WCA.

11 Barry to Bird, 19 April 1822 and 20 May 1822, CO 159 items 14 and 21; Barry to Brink, 25 August 1824, CO 204/55, WCA.

12 Records of the trial of William Gebhard, in RCC 18, pp. 281–325.

13 Lind, deed of accusation, 18 September 1822, in RCC 18, pp. 282–3.

14 Shand, chirurgical certificate on the slave Joris, in RCC 18, p. 286.

15 Tardieu, autopsy report, 24 September 1822, MC 15, WCA.

16 Somerset to Barry, 22 October 1822, MC 27, WCA.

17 Barry to Somerset, 22 November 1822, MC 27, WCA.

18 Barry to Bird, 7 May 1822, CO 159/18, WCA.

19 Barry to Bird, 18 March 1823, CO 180/6, WCA.

20 Governor's proclamation, 18 August 1807, in RCC 6, pp. 192–3.

21 Governor's proclamation, 26 September 1823, in RCC 16, p. 309.

22 Notice for recapture, *Cape Town Gazette and African Advertiser*, 8 June 1822, copy in CCP 8/1/17, WCA. Estimates of Danzer's (also known as James Danster or Salomon) age vary, but according to James Barry himself he was twelve at this time (Barry to Bourke, 27 August 1828, CO 3936, WCA).

23 Teenstra, *Fruits*, p. 323.

24 Governor's proclamation, 14 February 1817, printed in *Cape Town Gazette and African Advertiser*, 22 February 1817, CCP8/1/11, WCA.

25 Leprosy is caused by infection by the bacteria *Mycobacterium leprae* and spreads from person to person through respiratory droplets (usually released through coughing). Contrary to popular belief, the rate of infection through contact with infected persons is extremely low and incubation is very long (sometimes decades). The main visible symptom is multiple disfiguring granulomas, and the loss of extremities is due to secondary infections, often resulting from untreated injuries to the enervated skin.

26 Barry to Bird, 4 November 1822, MC 27, p.18, WCA.

27 Barry to Bird, 12 November 1822, CO 159/36, WCA.

28 Ibid.

29 Ibid.

30 Ibid.

31 Somerset to Bathurst, 1 July 1823, in RCC 16, p. 106.

32 Leitner to Deane, 12 August 1823, attached to Barry to Bird, CO 180/26, WCA.

33 Barry to Bird, 21 August 1823, CO 180/26, WCA.

34 Barry to Bird, 25 September 1823, CO 180/43, WCA.

35 Barry to Brink, 8 March 1824, CO 204/14, WCA.

36 Brink to Burgher Senate, 30 April 1824, in RCC 17, p. 281.

37 Barry to Brink, 2 November 1824, CO 204/72, WCA.

38 Report of the Commission Investigating the State of the Somerset Hospital, 24 February 1825, CO 226/13, WCA.

39 Ibid.

Chapter 16: 'If Rumour Speaks Truth'

1 Rae (*Strange Story*, p. 22). Joseph 'Pea-Green' Hayne was a noted dandy who became famous in 1824 when he was sued for breach of promise by his fiancée, Maria Foote (Knight, 'Foote, Maria (1797–1867)', *Oxford Dictionary of National Biography* online edition, www.oxforddnb.com/view/article/9807; retrieved 28 Oct 2015). The source of Hayne's nickname was a mystery in his own lifetime; one opinion was that it referred to inexperience, while others called this 'a vulgar newspaper mistake'; rather 'he first came out in a pea green coat, which he threatened to turn to yellow in the autumn' ('Examination of a Young Pretender', *The London Magazine*, May 1825, pp. 47–8).

2 *The London Magazine*, April 1825, p. 520.

3 Millar, *Plantagenet*, p. 69.

4 Barry to Somerset, 16 April 1824, in RCC 17, pp. 245–6.

5 Ibid., p. 245.

6 Ibid., p. 246.

7 Ibid.

8 Ibid. Denyssen's letter has not been traced, and its content is inferred from Dr Barry's comments.

9 Brink to Barry and Denyssen, 30 April 1824, in RCC 17, p. 280.

10 Barry to Brink, 20 July 1824, CO 204/41, WCA.

11 Ibid.

12 Ibid.

13 War Office: RJBb. This may have been at Lord Charles's instigation, as it is extremely unlikely that Dr Barry would have time to do Army work.

14 Somerset to Bigge, 23 April 1824, quoted in Millar, *Plantagenet*, pp. 177–8.

15 Deane, evidence to inquiry, 4 June 1824, in RCC 18, pp. 72–3.

16 Findlay, evidence to inquiry, 4 June 1824, in RCC 18, pp. 74–5.

17 Inquiry minutes, CJ 3352, WCA. In the transcript of the inquiry published in RCC, the text of the placard is redacted. It appears, in Dutch, in the copy of the original minutes in the WCA. The Dutch court clerk, struggling with some of the English words, rendered the vital verb, with many corrections, as 'bugjgeuring'. The translation used here is by Michael du Preez.

18 Inquiry minutes, CO 3352, WCA. The part marked 'illegible' is illegible in the record, not apparently in Captain Findlay's recollection of the placard.

19 Hammond, evidence to inquiry, 11 June 1824, in RCC 18, p. 103; Van der Sandt, evidence to inquiry, 4 June 1824, ibid., p. 86.

20 Samuel Hudson diary, 2 June 1824, A602 v3, WCA.

21 Ibid., 3 June 1824.

22 Denyssen to Somerset, 7 July 1824, in RCC 18, p. 65.

23 Anon to Barry, 4 June 1824, in RCC 18, p. 72. The letter begins, 'Sir, I did what I promised you yesterday [3 June, the day after the Placard's appearance], and now beg leave to suggest …' and goes on to set out precise instructions for their questioning the suspects in court, but without giving reasons for suspicion. There are no other traces of James Barry's dealings with this person, and when he passed the letter on to the Fiscal, he didn't identify the source.

24 Greig to Somerset and enclosed prospectus, 20 December 1820, in RCC 16, pp. 469–71.

25 Denyssen to Somerset, 5 May 1824, in RCC 17, p. 293; also public notices of 5 and 8 May 1824 and warrant for suppression, ibid., pp. 295, 299–301.

26 Edwards to Somerset, 8 March, and to Bathurst, 15 March 1824, in RCC 17, pp. 135–6, 145–7.

27 Record of trial of William Edwards, May 1824, in RCC 17, pp. 373–423.

28 Lee, evidence to inquiry, 9 June 1824, in RCC 18, p. 89.

29 Burnett, *Reply*, pp. 277–8.

Chapter 17: Dr Barry's Nemesis

1 RCC 26, p. 178.
2 Liesching, statement to the Governor, 14 August 1824, in RCC 18, p. 229.
3 Ibid., p. 228.
4 Governor's proclamation, 26 September 1823, in RCC 16, p. 308.
5 It may have originated in some spat over qualifications. Liesching's father had no recognised diplomas, but was permitted to practise because of his long standing and good professional reputation. James would certainly have disapproved of him as an artefact of the older, unregulated system, and might well have commented on this, perhaps in the hearing of young Karl. If Karl were rash enough to defend his father by making a comparable accusation against James (whom some would see as an upstart, promoted far beyond his natural seniority by favouritism), that would be sufficient to cause an explosion. Whatever James said to Liesching, it was enough to terrify the young man.
6 Brink to Barry, 3 August 1824, in RCC 18, p. 207.
7 Barry to Brink, 23 August 1824, CO 204 items 55 and 56, WCA.
8 Liesching, statement to the Governor, 14 August 1824, in RCC 18, p. 230.
9 Barry to Brink, 24 September 1824, in RCC 18, p. 321.
10 Ibid.
11 Bailey et al., memorandum to Brink, 24 September 1824, CO 204/64, WCA.
12 Denyssen to Plasket, 29 November 1824, in RCC 19, pp. 182–3.
13 Plasket to Barry, 14 December 1824, in RCC 19, p. 312.
14 Barry to Plasket, 31 December 1824, in RCC 19, p. 381. In her biography of James Barry (Scanty Particulars, p. 124), Holmes states that Barry stormed to Newlands and had it out with Lord Charles, quoting (without identifying it) a source that says: 'a long, stout arm seized the little man who was near the window and the same arm suddenly thrust the yelling Surgeon through the window, dangling him over a bed of hydrangeas until he prayed for mercy.' In fact this passage is taken from a work of fictionalised history, Cape Currey (ch. 6, p. 80) by René Juta published in 1920. In that book (which is essentially a novel in which Barry is a comical character), the scene is rendered as Lord Charles's dressing-down of Barry following the Cloete duel, and has nothing to do with Liesching. In short, the incident almost certainly never happened. Going back still further it has roots in Charles Dickens's fanciful article ('A Mystery Still', p. 492), which has Barry receiving this treatment as a punishment for an insolent remark. It may have some basis, but has become too detached from history to be reliable.
15 Report of examining board, 25 January 1825, CO 226/7, WCA.
16 Barry to Plasket, 31 December 1824, CO 204/94, WCA.
17 Ibid.
18 Barry to Brink, 2 November 1824, CO 204/73, WCA.
19 Barry to Plasket, 31 December 1824, CO 204/94, WCA.
20 Carnall diary, 23 October 1824, in RCC 21, p. 202.

21 Carnall diary, 22 October 1824, in RCC 21, p. 202.
22 Barry to Brink, 26 March 1825, CO 226/15, WCA.
23 Ibid.
24 Barry to Bathurst, 6 December 1825, in RCC 24, p. 67.
25 Bird and Colebrooke, *State of the Cape*, p. 19.
26 Liesching, certificate on Arthur (*sic*) Smith, 18 August 1825, RJBf.
27 Denyssen to Plasket, 18 August 1825, RJBf.
28 Barry to Plasket, 25 August 1825, RJBf.
29 Ibid.
30 Plasket to Denyssen, 1 September 1825, RJBf.
31 Liesching, report on the Tronk, 12 September 1825, RJBf.
32 Barry to Plasket, 12 September 1825, RJBf.
33 Plasket to Denyssen, 13 September 1825, RJBf.
34 Wernicke-Korsakoff Syndrome (WKS) or Alcoholic Encephalopathy occurs in chronic alcoholics and is the result of poor nutrition, specifically dietary deficiency of thiamine, a vitamin usually found in cereals, wholewheat flour, yeast and a number of other naturally occurring foodstuffs, including oranges and asparagus. This complex disorder combines various mental disturbances, including confusion, apathy and disorientation, certain changes involving the eyes and unsteadiness of gait and posture, psychotic states and unpleasant hallucinations.
35 Barry to Somerset, 16 September 1825, CO 226/58, WCA, and to Bigge and Colebrooke, 14 November 1825, in RCC 35, p. 212.
36 Barry to Bigge and Colebrooke, 14 November 1825, in RCC 35, p. 212.
37 Ibid.
38 Bird and Colebrooke, *State of the Cape*, p. 17.
39 Barry to Bigge and Colebrooke, 14 November 1825, in RCC 35, p. 213.
40 Barry to Somerset, 16 September 1825, CO 226/58, WCA.
41 Barry to Bigge and Colebrooke, 14 November 1825, in RCC 35, p. 213.
42 Bird and Colebrooke, *State of the Cape*, p. 17.
43 Denyssen to Plasket, 19 September 1825, RJBf.
44 Denyssen to Plasket, 17 September 1825, RJBf.
45 Barry to Bigge and Colebrooke, 14 November 1825, in RCC 35, p. 214.
46 Ibid. The whole of this meeting – including its context, verbal remarks and sequel – is described in Barry's letter.
47 In his account of this exchange (op. cit.) Barry, who shared the casual antisemitism that was endemic at this time, said 'cut off both his ears, his Jew's ears off'. This is not only offensive but odd, since Daniel Denyssen, born and baptised into the Dutch Reformed Church, was not Jewish (Harmen Snel, archivist, Amsterdam city archives, personal communication, October 2012).
48 Barry to Bigge and Colebrooke, 14 November 1825, in RCC 35, p. 215.
49 Ibid.
50 Bigge and Colebrooke to Bathurst, 14 March 1826, in RCC 26, p. 164.
51 Denyssen to Plasket, 29 September 1825, RJBf.
52 Plasket to Barry, 30 September 1825, RJBf.

53 Barry to Plasket, 3 October 1825, RJBf; original in CO 226/67, WCA.
54 Plasket to Barry, 4 October 1825, RJBf.

Chapter 18: 'Blighting My Fair Prospects'

1   *The Times*, 17 June 1825, p. 4. An original copy of the subscription notice (initiated by Charles Warren the engraver) survives in the BFA archive. It includes a pen portrait of Redmond, aged and blind, in which the Barry features are even more pronounced than in the earlier depiction by West.
2   Ibid.
3   Ibid.
4   Barry to Plasket, 10 October 1825, RJBf; original in CO 226/69, WCA.
5   Barry to Somerset, 13 October 1825, RJBf; original in CO 226/70, WCA; and Somerset to Barry, 14 October 1825, RJBf.
6   Barry to Somerset, 13 October 1825, RJBf; original in CO 226/70, WCA.
7   Somerset to Barry, 14 October 1825, RJBf.
8   Ibid.
9   Brink to Barry, 17 October 1825, RJBf.
10 Plasket to Barry, 29 October 1825, RJBf.
11 Barry to Plasket, 29 October 1825, RJBf.
12 Governor's proclamation, 1 November 1825, in RCC 23, pp. 357–8.
13 War Office: RJBc.
14 Somerset to Bathurst, 1 November 1825, in RCC 23, p. 357.
15 Commissioners' report on Dr Barry, 14 March 1826, in RCC 26, p. 184.
16 Plasket to Bigge and Colebrooke, 27 November 1825, in RCC 23, pp. 486–7.
17 Bigge and Colebrooke to Plasket, 7 December 1825, in RCC 24, p. 109.
18 He had moved by 14 November 1825, when he wrote to the Commissioners from his new address.
19 Barry to Bathurst, 6 December 1825, RJBf; copy in RCC 24, pp. 67–70.
20 In 1864 the Somerset Hospital moved from its original location on Chiapinni Street (off Strandstraat) to new purpose-built premises on what is now Beach Road. That building is still the core of the modern hospital. The New Somerset was the main teaching hospital of the University of Cape Town until 1937, when it was superseded by the new Groote Schuur Hospital (where author Michael du Preez was a consultant urologist from 1968 to 1994).
21 Burnett, *Reply*.
22 Plasket to Wilmot-Horton, 28 September 1825, in RCC 23, p. 176.
23 Plasket to Wilmot-Horton, 1 November 1825, in RCC 23, pp. 359–61.
24 Perceval to Lady Bathurst, 19 January 1826, quoted in Millar, *Plantagenet*, p. 225. Perceval was the son of the assassinated Prime Minister Spencer Perceval.
25 Perceval to James Stephen, 3 March 1826, quoted in Millar, *Plantagenet*, pp. 230–3.
26 The procession and embarkation are described in the *South African Chronicle*, 7 March 1826, copy in National Library of South Africa, and *Cape Town Gazette and African Advertiser*, 10 March 1826, copy in CCP 8/1/21, WCA.

27 Anon., quoted in Millar, *Plantagenet*, p. 191.

28 *South African Chronicle*, 7 March 1826, copy in National Library of South Africa.

Chapter 19: A New Life

1 Johannes Albertus Munnik was born in 1818 (George, *Descendants*, p. 202), and is now apparently forgotten by the family; it is presumed that he did not survive infancy.

2 Barry took three courses in midwifery while a student at Edinburgh (War Office: RJBc).

3 Dr Barry wrote no report of the operation himself, and the details of the case (such as they are) come from the oral tradition of the Munnik family.

4 Locher, 'History', p. 17.

5 Further details of the conduct of a contemporary caesarean are given in Deward et al., Statements.

6 Locher, 'History', pp. 17–18.

7 Ibid., p. 19.

8 Baptismal notices, *South African Commercial Advertiser*, 22 August 1826.

9 There was a twist. Barry Hertzog (as J. B. M. Hertzog was known) grew up to be a lawyer, a soldier and an Afrikaner nationalist; at the turn of the century he served successfully as a general in the Boer War against the British, and after 1910 was Minister of Justice in the new Union of South Africa, and from 1924 was its prime minister; he strove for independence from Britain, consolidation of white power, and was instrumental in bringing about Apartheid in South Africa. What Dr James Barry, who detested oppression, would have thought of his name – at however many removes – descending to this end might only be imagined.

10 Pressly, 'Portrait of a Cork Family', p. 147.

11 Bradford, 'Reputed Female Army Surgeon'. Bradford was a military surgeon who first became acquainted with James Barry in Jamaica in 1832.

12 Ibid.

13 Barry to Bathurst, 1 November 1826, CO 48/97, TNA.

14 Barry to Hay, 20 November 1826, RJBf.

15 Barry, memorandum, 31 July 1826, in RCC 27, pp. 199–200.

16 Arthur, 'Report', RHT.

17 Ballingall, *Outlines of Military Surgery*, pp. 450–8.

18 O'Shea, 'Two Minutes with Venus', p. 392.

19 Barry, Report Upon the Arctopus, RJBe.

20 Barry, Report Upon the Arctopus, RJBe.

21 Arthur, 'Report', RHT.

22 War Office: RJBb.

23 Particulars Regarding the Trial of Salomon alias James Danster, 2 August 1827, CJ 821/24, WCA.

24 Memorial of James, a Bosjesman, a Prisoner in the Town Prison, 17 August 1827, CO 3934/169, WCA (Danzer was also known as James Danster).

25 Plasket to landdrost, 25 August 1827, CO 4887/295, WCA.

26 Barry to Pedder, 11 February 1828, CO 357/19, WCA.

27 Barry to Bourke, 27 August 1828, CO 3936, WCA.

28 *Kaapse Courant, of De Verzamelaar*, 10 September 1828.

29 Register of shipping, arrivals and departures at Cape Town: departure of *Eliza Jane*, 26 September 1828, CC 2/12, WCA; and Report of Passengers on the English Ship *Eliza Jane*, Z2D3/203-9/10/1828, no. 288, NAM.

Chapter 20: A Precipitate Departure

1   Fenton, *Journal*, pp. 279, 280.

2   War Office: RJBb; and Report of Passengers on the English Ship *Eliza Jane*, Z2D3/203-9/10/1828, no. 288, NAM. On the list of disembarking passengers, Danzer is listed as 'Peter Danstar', aged twenty-three; John Smith was thirty-six.

3   War Office, *Army List for July 1829*, p. 65.

4   Colville, quoted in Rose, *Perfect Gentleman*, p. 89.

5   War Office, *Army List for July 1829*, pp. 69–70; Fenton, *Journal*, pp. 281–2.

6   Butler Kell, 'Annual Return', RHT.

7   Collier, 'Annual Return', RHT.

8   Fenton, *Journal*, p. 323.

9   Ibid., p. 310. Fenton calls him Robinson, but in fact he was P. Robertson (War Office, *Army List for July 1829*, p. 30).

10 War Office, *Army List for July 1829*, p. 53.

11 Fenton, *Journal*, p. 323.

12 Ibid.

13 Mrs Fenton (*Journal*, p. 324) says there was 'some notice of removal to Dr Barry, the particulars of which I forget'.

14 Quoted in Rae, *Strange Story*, p. 62.

15 Fenton, *Journal*, p. 323.

16 Clarke, *Autobiographical Recollections*, p. 347.

17 Montgomery and Barry, 'Case of Carotid Aneurism', p. 421. The paper was credited primarily to Montgomery as operating surgeon, but written entirely by Barry.

18 Montgomery and Barry, 'Case of Carotid Aneurism', p. 422.

19 U. Sohum, National Archives of Mauritius, personal communication, 7 October 2011. Some maintain that Barry's motive for going to England was to counter in person the damage done to him by the official reports sent to Horse Guards (Rae, *Strange Story*, p. 62); this assumes that he sought to defend himself against allegations of military unfitness by going absent without leave, an irony that stretches credulity even with Barry's temperament. In an account by Barry himself (contained in RJBa) written decades later, he stated that he 'was recalled in consequence of the serious illness of Lord Charles Somerset'.

Chapter 21: An Indefatigable Friend

1 Register of Shipping, Arrivals and Departures at Cape Town, CC 2/12, WCA.
2 *Windsor and Eton Press*, 4 July 1829, p. 3; *Morning Chronicle*, 13 August 1829, p. 3.
3 *Morning Chronicle*, 21 November 1829, p. 1.
4 *The Examiner*, 24 January 1830, p. 50.
5 Dickens, 'A Mystery Still', p. 493.
6 Somerset to McGrigor, 14 January 1830; McGrigor to Barry, 20 January 1830, WLC.
7 Dr Derrick Burns writes that 'cardiac failure is the most likely underlying health problem, but he is also likely to have suffered chronic pulmonary problems which were so common then – most likely associated chronic bronchitis … This raises the question of the cause of the heart failure, i.e. left ventricular failure due to ischaemic or hypertensive heart disease being most likely or cor pulmonale secondary to chronic chest disease. Although severe oedema is more likely in right sided CCF associated with cor pulmonale (and there is reference to very swollen legs) his chest disease does not sound to be a dominant problem and so the most likely diagnosis is probably ischaemic heart disease (with or without hypertensive disease) … Then there is the arthritis (swollen joints – more than arthralgia). Although osteoarthritis is likely, so is chronic gout, which is quite possible considering his heart disease'. (Derrick Burns, consultant physician (retired), Groote Schuur Hospital, Cape Town, personal communication, 28 October 2010).
8 Montgomery and Barry, 'Case of Carotid Aneurism'.
9 *The Pilot*, 26 February 1830, p. 2; *Saunders's News-Letter and Daily Advertiser*, 3 April 1830, p. 1.
10 *Morning Post*, 10 April 1830, p. 3 and 6 July 1830, p. 3; *Brighton Gazette*, 26 August 1830, p. 2.
11 *Berkshire Chronicle*, 22 May 1830, p. 1. The then common expression 'might and main' (meaning great exertion) is rarely used nowadays.
12 Somerset to Beaufort, 11 October 1830, DOB.
13 *Morning Post*, 12 November 1830, p. 3; Somerset to Beaufort, 26 November 1830, DOB. Snettisham Hall was then the property of a Mr Henry L. Styleman, who sold it a few years later. The Earl (later Duke) of Darlington's family seat was Raby Castle in County Durham.
14 Somerset to Beaufort, 26 November 1830, DOB.
15 *Morning Post*, 18 November 1830, p. 3.
16 Ibid.; *The Times*, 25 November 1830, p. 2; *The Pilot*, 24 November 1830, p. 2.
17 Somerset to Beaufort, 31 December 1830, DOB.
18 Clarke, *Autobiographical Recollections*, p. 343.
19 Ibid., pp. 349–50. Wardrop's sobriquet for Halford is recorded by Clarke.
20 Ibid., p. 417.
21 Quoted in Morris, 'Sir Henry Halford', p. 431.
22 Somerset to Beaufort, 31 December 1830, DOB.
23 Somerset to Beaufort, 6 January 1831, DOB.

24   Somerset to Beaufort, 8 January 1831, DOB.

25   Somerset to Beaufort, 6 January 1831, DOB.

26   Ibid.

27   Somerset to Beaufort, 8 January 1831, DOB.

28   Ibid.

29   Ibid.

30   Somerset to Beaufort, 23 January 1831, DOB.

31   Somerset to Beaufort, 4 February 1831, DOB.

32   *Morning Advertiser*, 19 February 1831, p. 3.

33   Will of Lord Charles Somerset, quoted in Millar, *Plantagenet*, p. 256.

34   St Andrew's Chapel, designed in 1827 by Sir Charles Barry (no relation), in Waterloo Street, is not the same as St Andrew's Church, Hove. The funeral is described in the *Morning Post*, 5 March 1831, p. 3; *Morning Advertiser*, 5 March 1831, p. 3; *Sussex Advertiser*, 7 March, p. 3; Rose, *Perfect Gentleman*, p. 94.

35   *Morning Post*, 1 March 1831, p. 3.

36   *Brighton Gazette*, 3 March 1831, p. 3.

37   Barry to Fitzroy, 5 February 1831 (*sic* – probably 25 February), in Eriksen, 'A Letter by Dr James Barry'. This letter was found among the papers of Henry Plantagenet Somerset (1852–1936), grandson of Lord Charles, who became a politician in Australia. It is shorter than it originally was – a second page of text, apparently inside the letter cover, has been lost to a cover collector.

38   Barry to Fitzroy, 5 February 1831 (*sic* – probably 25 February), in Eriksen, 'A Letter by Dr James Barry'.

Chapter 22: Fever Island

1   Macaulay, *Anti-Slavery Monthly Reporter*, *passim*.

2   War Office: RJBb.

3   *Watchman and Jamaica Free Press*, 15 June 1831.

4   Up Park was the main base throughout the period of British rule, and is still the headquarters of the Jamaica Defence Force.

5   *Dublin Evening Packet*, 15 February 1831, p. 4; *Drogheda Journal*, 28 May 1831, p. 2.

6   War Office, *Army List for July 1829*, pp. 69–70.

7   Marshall and Tulloch, *Statistical Report*, p. 45.

8   Draper, 'Annual Report', RHT.

9   Ibid.; also George Gregory, *Elements*, pp. 51–65.

10   Quoted in Dunn, *Tale*, p. 342.

11   *Watchman and Jamaica Free Press*, 2 January 1832.

12   *Watchman and Jamaica Free Press*, 4 January 1832.

13   Dunn, *Tale*, p. 348.

14   *Watchman and Jamaica Free Press*, 7 January 1832.

15   Wilson, quoted in Rogers, letter to the editor, *The Lancet*.

16   Bradford, 'The Reputed Female Army Surgeon'.

17 What caused James Barry to name his dogs after her is a mystery. It may have
    been a reference to the heroine of Greek legend, or to the mind, the soul, or the
    'pneuma psychikon' (animal spirit or soul) in Galenic medicine.

18 Strangely, this man's name was never properly recorded (or perhaps not so
    strangely, since he was a black man and a servant, and therefore regarded as of
    little consequence). However, Charles Dickens, in his account of the life of 'Doctor
    James' ('A Mystery Still', p. 493), called him 'Black John', and since his piece was
    derived from an informant who had known them both, this may well have been so.

Chapter 23: The Past Revisited

1   There is no surviving correspondence – nor any reference to contact of any kind
    – between Mrs Bulkley and her daughter (or her alter ego) after 1813.

2   The England census, 1851, lists Esther Bulkley (then sixteen) as born in Deptford.

3   Convict ship *Medina* sailed from Deptford in July 1823 and called at Cork in late
    August, where she took on board 180 male prisoners. The journal of the ship's
    surgeon, John Rodwell RN, records Jeremiah Bulkley on 29 November having
    sustained a 'severe contusion to the Wrist, in consequence of a fall'; this occurred
    when the ship was about 1000 miles southeast of Madagascar, in the region where
    high seas were often encountered (Director General of the Medical Department
    of the Navy: Medical Journals: ADM 101, 804 bundles and volumes: National
    Archives, Kew; available online at www.ancestry.com; retrieved 19 November
    2015). No record of Jeremiah's crime or his arrival in Australia has been discovered,
    despite the extensive convict records.

4   Lewis, *Topographical Dictionary*, p. 427.

5   Evidence of Justin McCarty on the 'Nature and Extent of the Disturbances in
    Ireland', in House of Lords, *Sessional Papers*, pp. 389–96.

6   Reproduced in *Belfast Commercial Chronicle*, 25 May 1835, p. 3; *Waterford Mail*, 27
    May 1835, p. 1; etc.

7   Letter in *The Times*, 2 June 1835, p. 5.

8   War Office: RJBb. James's service in Jamaica came to an end in February 1835, and
    it would have taken him about a month or two to reach Britain. Interestingly, this
    is one of only two transitions in his post-Cape career for which he did not enter
    precise dates (just 'Feb/35'), the other being another return home that occurred in
    unusual circumstances a few years later (see Chapter 25). There may have been a
    hiatus between postings caused by upheavals in the government and the handover
    of St Helena from the East India Company.

9   Reports by Stockenström and ship's surgeon, CO 447/34–58, WCA. Lela claimed to
    have been vaccinated against smallpox, but vaccines are not absolutely prophylactic
    in individuals.

10 Report of a meeting of the Colonial Medical Committee, CO 447/34 et seq.,
    WCA.

11 Barry to D'Urban, 21 August 1836, CO 4372/5, WCA.

12 Ibid.

13 Ibid.

14 D'Urban to Barry, 26 October 1836, CO 4372/5 bis, WCA.

15 Death Register, MOOC 6/3, vol. 4, pp. 78–9, WCA.

16 J. George, *Descendants of Count Jacob van Reenen*. Catherina Cornelia Sandenberg (widow of Hercules Sandenberg) was the daughter of Sebastian van Reenen (or Renen), as was Wilhelmina Munnik. Mrs Cloete was likewise a Van Reenen by birth.

17 Barry to Munnik, 18 December 1837, MFC.

18 According to Munnik family tradition.

Chapter 24: An Officer and a Gentleman

1 Las Cases, *Mémorial*, vol. 1.2, p. 216.

2 He was eventually disinterred in 1840 and taken back to France for burial.

3 Darwin, *Journal*, p. 486.

4 War Office, *A List of the Officers*, 1835, p. 370.

5 Darwin, *Journal*, p. 488.

6 Paragraph 64, Act for the Abolition of Slavery throughout the British Colonies, 28 August 1833. Ceylon and all East India Company territories were also exempted. Abolition finally reached those territories in 1843.

7 Governor's proclamation, 27 February 1836, CO 247/42, TNA.

8 For example, Glenelg to Middlemore, 27 November 1846, CO 247/44, TNA; and Editorial, 'Colonial Misgovernment', *Blackwood's Magazine*, November 1838, p. 624ff.

9 Stephen to Spearman, 31 December 1836, CO 247/42, TNA.

10 Statistics from Porter, *Tables*, pp. 106, 108.

11 Barry, quoted in Rose, *Perfect Gentleman*, p. 106; War Office: *A List of the Officers*, 1833, p. 281.

12 Barry to Alexander, 13 September 1836, Colonial Secretary's Entry Book 1, SHA.

13 Alexander to Seale, 13 September 1836, Colonial Secretary's Entry Book 1, SHA.

14 Glenelg to Middlemore, 27 November 1846, CO 247/44, TNA.

15 Barry to Middlemore, 15 November 1836, Colonial Secretary's Entry Book 1, SHA.

16 Middlemore to Glenelg, 22 June 1837, SHA; Legislative Council minutes in George, *Dr James Miranda Barry*, pp. 6, 21.

17 Seale to Barry, 26 September and 7 October 1836, Colonial Secretary's Entry Book 1, SHA.

18 Barry to McGrigor, 15 November 1836, SHA.

19 McGrigor to Barry, 27 October 1836, SHA.

20 Glenelg to Middlemore, 29 September 1836, CO 247/42, TNA.

21 Middlemore to Glenelg, 28 October 1836, CO 247/42, TNA.

22 Seale to Hopkins, 10 October 1836, SHA.

23 Barry, Report on the Proceedings of the Board, 7 November 1836, General Orders Book, p. 24, SHA.

24 Barry, quoted in Rose, *Perfect Gentleman*, p. 109, gives an account of the incident that ensued having begun while 'bathing in the morning'. Rose dates this as 13 November; however, this does not fit with the dates of other evidence for the incident that followed. Since it took place on a Sunday, it must have been the 20th, which fits perfectly with the sequence of other evidence.

25 Dumat, 'The Famous Dr James Barry'; and Dickens, 'A Mystery Still', p. 493. Dickens claimed to have derived his life of 'Doctor James' from a person who had known him in St Helena.

26 Darwin, *Journal*, p. 487.

27 Ibid., p. 486.

28 Barry, quoted in Rose, *Perfect Gentleman*, p. 109.

29 Knowles had been stuck in this rank since 1816 (War Office, *List of the Officers*, 1835, p. 363; 1841, p. 206).

30 Knowles to Barry, 11 November 1836, CO 247/52, TNA.

31 Barry to Glenelg, 14 November 1836.

32 Barry, quoted in Rose, *Perfect Gentleman*, p. 110.

33 General Orders, 21 November 1836, p. 31, SHA.

34 Knowles, quoted in Rose, *Perfect Gentleman*, p. 111.

35 Barry, quoted in ibid., p. 111.

36 General Orders, 7 December 1836, CO 247/52, TNA.

37 Barry, undated note, CO 247/52, TNA.

38 Ibid.

39 General Orders, 7 December 1836, CO 247/52, TNA.

40 Middlemore to Somerset, 7 December 1836, Governor's Despatches, p. 34, SHA.

41 Middlemore to Somerset, 14 December 1836, Governor's Despatches, p. 36, SHA.

Chapter 25: Homeward Bound

1 Dumat, 'The Famous Dr James Barry'.

2 Barry to Glenelg, 16 August 1838, CO 247/49, TNA.

3 The epidemic seems to have affected the black population (of whom there were about 1600) more heavily than the whites (numbering about 400). The subsequent shortage of labour was a serious problem, and, in 1810 the East India Company began importing Chinese labourers from the its factory at Canton, simply to keep the island's economy going; eventually there were around 400 Chinese on St Helena, doing all kinds of agricultural work, from driving carts to ploughing fields, for a shilling a day (Beatson, *Tracts*, pp. 186–7, 328).

4 Barry to Seale, 30 December 1836, Colonial Secretary's Entry Book 2, SHA.

5 Minutes of the Legislative Council, January 1837–1842, SHA.

6 Barry to Seale, 28 July 1837, Colonial Secretary's Letters Book 1, SHA.

7 Barry to Seale, 28 July 1837, Colonial Secretary's Letters Book 1, SHA.

8 Minutes of the Legislative Council, January 1837–1842, SHA.

9 Phillips, *Profligate Son*, pp. 29–45, 103.

10 *Derby Mercury*, 29 October 1828, p. 1; *Cambridge Chronicle*, 21 May 1830, p. 2.

11 *Brighton Gazette*, 3 February 1848, p. 2; *Carlisle Patriot*, 28 May 1859, p. 1. In
    justice to Helps, there were many people who ended up in crippling lifelong debt
    through no fault of their own (ill-advised investments, the collapse of banking
    houses etc.). But the pattern of his debts indicate an inveterate and profligate
    borrower and spender.
12 Middlemore to Somerset, 21 June 1837, Governor's Despatches Book 1, SHA.
13 Barry to Seale, 2 May 1837, Colonial Secretary's Letters Book 1, SHA.
14 Barry to Seale, 8 May 1837, Colonial Secretary's Letters Book 1, SHA.
15 Reed to Middlemore, 9 May 1837, Colonial Secretary's Letters Book 1, SHA.
16 Reed to Middlemore, 16 May 1837, Colonial Secretary's Letters Book 1, SHA.
17 Seale to Barry, 20 May 1837, Colonial Secretary's Letters Book 1, SHA.
18 Seale to Churchwardens, 20 May 1837, Colonial Secretary's Letters Book 1, SHA.
19 This is due to research by Barbara George, local St Helena historian, who located
    the sole surviving records in the St Helena Archives (see George, *Dr James Miranda
    Barry*).
20 Court of Inquiry, in General Orders, 16 October 1837, SHA.
21 Middlemore to Somerset, 1 November 1837, Governor's Despatches, SHA.
22 Middlemore, General Orders, 21 March 1838, SHA.
23 Ibid.
24 Ibid.
25 Middlemore to Glenelg, 2 April 1838, CO 247/46, TNA; Rae, *Strange Story*, p.
    81.
26 Middlemore to Glenelg, 15 April 1838, Governor's Despatches, SHA.
27 Dickens, 'A Mystery Still', p. 493.
28 Middlemore to Glenelg, 2 April 1838, CO 247/46, TNA.

Chapter 26: Friends in High Places

1   'Her Majesty's Levee', *Morning Chronicle*, 19 July 1838, p. 5.
2   The relevant records – including the mass of material sent to Horse Guards by
    General Middlemore – are not in the files. The only extant records are those
    unearthed in St Helena.
3   For example, *Southern Reporter and Cork Commercial Courier*, 15 March 1838, p. 1.
4   Anti-Slavery Office, *Reasons*.
5   The bill became a reality the following year: *The Times*, 3 May 1839, p. 3.
6   For example, *The Times*, 6 May 1839, p. 3; 11 May 1839, p. 3.
7   Hart, *New Army List, August 1839*, p. 209.
8   Day, *Five Years*, vol. 1, p. 9.
9   Ibid., p. 10.
10 Ibid., pp. 64–6.
11 Ibid., vol. 2, pp. 267–8.
12 Marshall and Tulloch, *Statistical Report*, p. 35.
13 Ibid.
14 Ibid.

15 Thome and Kimball, *Six Months' Tour*, p. 4.

16 Ibid.

17 Ibid., p. 11.

18 Buckley, *British Army*, pp. 203–47.

19 James, *Regimental Companion*, quoted in Crumplin, *Men of Steel*, pp. 170–1.

20 Ballingall, *Outlines*, pp. 478–83.

21 Barry to Laboutiere, 26 July 1839, CO 247/52, TNA.

22 War Office: RJBb; Hart, *New Annual Army List, 1840*, p. 309; *New Army List, January 1841*, p. 209.

23 War Office: RJBb. The records of the Windward and Leeward Islands command for this period are unfortunately missing from the National Archives, so we do not have the full details of Dr Barry's period there.

24 Day, *Five Years*, vol. 1, p. 171.

25 During this whole period, James Barry is the only member of the Army Medical Department who has 'Trinidad' listed as his station; all other Trinidad personnel, including regiments, are listed under 'Barbados' (Hart, *New Annual Army List, 1840* et seq.; and Distribution of the British Army, NMG).

26 Hart, *New Annual Army List, 1843*, p. 323.

27 Marshall and Tulloch, *Statistical Report*, pp. 17–18.

28 Quoted in Ballingall, *Outlines*, p. 144.

29 Fergusson in *United Services Magazine*, 1838, p. 92; also Fergusson, *Notes*, pp. 71–6

30 Marshall and Tulloch, *Statistical Report*, pp. 9, 48–9.

31 McGrigor, circular no. 12378, 9 March 1841, WO 334/174, TNA. McGrigor's inquiry was an effort to build upon the work of Andrew Blake, a regimental surgeon who had produced a landmark study of delirium tremens in 1830 (*A Practical Essay on Delirium Tremens*, London: Burgess and Hill). Blake's clinical observations were very precise, and are entirely relevant to this day, noting clear stages in the evolution of delirium tremens that closely accord with present criteria.

32 Barry to Bone, 9 May 1842, WO 334/174, TNA.

33 Barry, report, 1 April to 31 December 1841, WO 334/174, TNA.

34 Ibid.

35 In the early 19th century, 'simulants' and 'depressants' were classified differently; alcohol was a stimulant, while opium was a combined stimulant and narcotic (e.g. Guy, *Dr Hooper's Vademecum*, p. 158). The stimulant/depressant classification was based on the effect on pulse rate/strength (bleeding, for example, was a depressant), whereas now the distinction is based on the effect on neurotransmission.

36 Ibid.

37 *The Times*, 11 March 1842, p. 4; 5 April 1842, p. 4; 6 April 1842, p. 6.

38 Bradford, 'The Reputed Female Army Surgeon'.

39 McCowan, 'Late Dr Barry'.

40 'Captain', letter to the editor, *The Lancet*.

41 This diagnosis is based on the fact that Barry had a relatively quick convalescence, which would not be the case with yellow fever. If his illness was malaria, it would have to be the *Plasmodium falciparum* type, as he is not known to have experienced

any recurrence of the illness in later life, and of the various types of malaria, this is the only one that does not recur.

42 The following events are based on accounts given after James Barry's death by the then General Robert Lowry, Sir Thomas Longmore, a senior Army surgeon who in 1845 was an assistant with the 19th Regiment, and a Colonel de Montmorency. Some of the accounts were published by Lieutenant Colonel E. Rogers in 1895 (see Rogers, letter to the editor, *The Lancet*); one appears in an archive (Longmore, undated note, WLC), and another in a newspaper (McCowan, 'Late Dr Barry').

43 Hart, *New Annual Army List, 1843*, p. 210; *New Annual Army List, 1845*, p. 311.

44 Lowry, verbal account quoted by Rogers, letter to the editor, *The Lancet*.

45 About a decade later, having served in the Crimea, O'Connor vanished from the Army List, having either died or resigned (War Office, *Army List, 1846*, p. 83; General Orders, *The Times*, 18 June 1854, p. 7; Hart, *New Annual Army List, 1854*, p. 311); he cannot have retired, as he does not appear on the half-pay list. Montmorency, speaking about the Barry episode decades later (verbal account quoted in Rogers, letter to the editor, *The Lancet*), said, 'As a matter of fact, I have never till now mentioned the subject.' Lowry also appears to have kept quiet.

46 Dr Barry refers to his 'serious attack of yellow fever contracted at Trinidad' in a memorandum on his service (War Office: RJBa).

47 Longmore, undated note, WLC.

48 War Office: RJBb.

Chapter 27: The Navel of the Mediterranean

1 *The Times*, 5 February 1846, p. 5.

2 *Morning Post*, 19 February 1846, p. 5.

3 Entry for William, Viscount Lowther MP (1787–1872) in *The History of Parliament: the House of Commons 1820–1832*, ed. D. R. Fisher; available online at www.historyofparliamentonline.org/volume/1820-1832/member/lowther-william-1787-1872#footnoteref25_s894n1k (retrieved 28 November 2015).

4 Benjamin Disraeli, *Tancred* (1847).

5 *The Times*, 24 February 1846, p. 6.

6 *London Evening Standard*, 25 February 1846, p. 4.

7 Register of Arrivals at the Great Harbour of Valetta f 981, 16 November 1846, NMA.

8 Distribution of the British Army, 31 January 1846, 3 April 1847, NMG. Fencible (short for 'defencible') regiments were local militias raised for the defence of British territories during the French Revolutionary and Napoleonic Wars.

9 Savona-Ventura, 'Dr James Barry', pp. 42–4.

10 Ibid., p. 42. In that paper, the church is wrongly identified as the Catholic Collegiate church. In fact, it was the Protestant church of St Paul, where the English Chaplain Reverend John Cleugh officiated.

11 *Malta Mail and United Service Journal*, 31 December 1846.
12 Dr John Gardiner, consultant neurologist, Cape Town, personal communication, 2014. Multiple sclerosis was first described in 1868 by Jean-Martin Charcot, the father of modern neurology.
13 Distribution of the British Army, 3 April 1847, NMG.
14 Barry to Stuart, quoted in Savona-Ventura, 'Dr James Barry', p. 43.
15 Ibid.
16 Distribution of the British Army, 3 April 1847, 29 July 1848, NMG; Hart, *New Annual Army List, 1848*, p. 221; *1849*, p. 195.
17 Register of Clearance and Departure (passenger list), Valetta Harbour 1st April 1851 f 285, NMA; Distribution of the British Army, 29 July 1848, NMG.
18 Barry, Annual Report, WO 334/16, RHT.
19 Dr John Gardiner, consultant neurologist, Cape Town, personal communication, 2014.
20 Barry, Annual Report, WO 334/16, RHT.
21 Ibid.
22 Savona-Ventura, 'Dr James Barry', p. 43.
23 Quoted in Mitchel, *Last Conquest*, p. 96.

Chapter 28: A Question of Numbers

1 Barry, 'Statement of a Professional Investigation of the Cases Reported as Cholera Asiatica in Casal Curmi', 14 October 1848, CO 158, TNA.
2 Sanitary Committee to Lushington, 12 September 1848, CO 158, TNA.
3 O'Ferrall to Grey, 19 October 1848, CO 158, TNA.
4 Admiralty, *Navy List 1848*, p. 132.
5 O'Ferrall to Grey, 19 October 1848, CO 158, TNA. Other members of the board were Edward Caldwell of the receiving ship *Ceylon*, Dr Edward Robertson of the 44th Regiment, and Daniel Armstrong, also of the 44th.
6 Barry, 'Statement', 14 October 1848, CO 158, TNA.
7 Ibid.; Barry to Pipon, 2 October 1848, CO 158, TNA.
8 Board of Health reports, 27 and 28 September 1848, quoted in O'Ferrall to Grey, 19 October 1848, CO 158, TNA.
9 Today most of these conditions are classified as gastroenteritis or dysentery, qualified by the name of the exact causal agent once it has been identified by a bacteriologist. In Dr Barry's day the discovery of bacteria was still in the future and the miasma – or foul, 'vitiated' air – theory held fast.
10 Review of inaugural discourse by Dr T. Chetcuti, *British and Foreign Medico-Chirurgical Review*, vol. 2 (July 1848), pp. 239–40.
11 *The Colonist*, 17 June 1828; War Office, *A List of the Officers, 1827*, p. 280.
12 Barry to Pipon, 2 October 1848, CO 158, TNA.
13 Ibid.
14 Richardson, autopsy report, 12 October 1848, CO 158, TNA.
15 Quoted in Savona-Ventura, 'Dr James Barry', p. 44.

16 List of medical officers present at the autopsy of 7 October 1848; O'Ferrall to Ellice, 11 October 1848, CO 158, TNA.

17 O'Ferrall to Ellice, 11 October 1848, CO 158, TNA.

18 Barry to Pakenham, 13 October 1848, CO158/143, TNA.

19 Ibid.; George Gregory, *Elements*, pp. 522–35.

20 *Malta Times*, 3 October 1848, p. 3.

21 *London Medical Gazette*, 12 July 1850, p. 83.

22 *London Medical Gazette*, 19 July 1850, p. 171.

23 *London Medical Gazette*, 2 August 1850, p. 215.

24 Snow, *On the Mode*, p. 11.

25 *London Medical Gazette*, 7 September 1849, p. 470.

26 Minutes of the Governor's Council, 11 September 1848, Gov 138/121, NMA. The total cost was £2349 11s 7¾d.

27 *London Medical Gazette*, 9 August 1850, p. 253.

28 Barry to Pipon, 3 September 1850, Gov 138, NMA.

29 Ibid.

30 Ellice, annotations on Barry to Pipon, 3 September 1850, Gov 138, NMA.

31 Ellice to QMG, 12 October 1850, Gov 138, NMA.

32 *London Medical Gazette*, 23 August 1850, pp. 348–9.

33 *London Medical Gazette*, 27 September 1850, p. 557.

34 More O'Ferrall to Ellice, 10 October 1850, Gov 138, NMA.

35 Barry to Pakenham, 2 December 1850, Gov 138, NMA.

36 Barry to Pakenham, 2 December 1850, Gov 138, NMA.

37 Memorandum of the Services of Dr James Barry, January 1860, RJBa.

38 Register of Clearance and Departure (passenger list), Valetta Harbour 1st April 1851 f 285, NMA.

39 Quoted in Savona-Ventura, 'Dr James Barry', p. 45.

Chapter 29: The Most Kind and Humane Gentleman

1 War Office: RJBb; Hart, *New Annual Army List, 1851*, p. 309; *1852*, p. 309.

2 Hart, *New Annual Army List, 1845*, p. 309; *1851*, p. 309. Initially Andrew Smith was ranked 'Superintendent' and confirmed as Director General the following year.

3 Hart, *New Annual Army List, 1852*, p. 313.

4 Ibid.

5 Distribution of the British Army, 1 March 1851, NMG.

6 *Medico-Chirurgical Review*, Review, pp. 411–17.

7 This is entirely plausible; the drawing is crude, but in style and character is not at all unlike Lear's rough sketches.

8 F. E. Salter, cited in Rae, *Strange Story*, p. 96.

9 J. C. P., unidentified newspaper, late 19th century, RAMC/238/3, WLC.

10 Anonymous, cited by Hutchison, unidentified newspaper, late 19th century, RAMC 238/3, WLC.

11 Ibid.
12 Ibid.
13 War Office: RJBb.
14 *Carlisle Journal*, 1 October 1852, p. 3.
15 A. M. S., letter to the editor, *The Lancet*.
16 Sarah Horniman, unpublished memoir, MFC.
17 *The Times*, 15 September 1852, p. 5.
18 *The Times*, 16 September 1852, p. 5.
19 *Whitehaven News*, 24 August 1865, p. 5; England census, 1851.
20 *Carlisle Journal*, 1 October 1852, p. 3.
21 Ibid.
22 *London Gazette*, 12 October 1852, p. 2663.
23 *The Times*, 7 December 1852, p. 3.
24 *The Times*, 19 November 1852, p. 5.
25 Classified adverts, *The Times*, 9 November 1852, p. 1.
26 *The Times*, 19 November 1852, p. 5.
27 John Murray, *Handbook*, p. 1.
28 Ibid., p. 171.
29 Ibid., p. 177.
30 Ibid., p. 191.
31 Weigall, 'Dr James Barry'.
32 Ibid.

Chapter 30: Prodigality and All Wickedness

1   Figes, *Crimea*, ch. 4.
2   Ibid., p. 123.
3   *The Times*, 15 February 1854, p. 5.
4   *The Times*, 13 February 1854, p. 12.
5   Distribution of the British Army, 3 April 1852, 2 April 1853, NMG.
6   *The Gentlemen's Magazine*, September 1853, p. 304.
7   Charteris, 'Corfu', p. 84.
8   *Limerick and Clare Examiner*, 9 March 1853, p. 3.
9   The incident that follows is based partly on a contemporary report (*Cork Examiner*, 23 November 1853, p. 3) and partly on a recollection by R. F. Hutchison, a soldier, in an unidentified Jamaican news cutting (RAMC 238/3, WLC). The two versions differ somewhat; where they do, the contemporary report is deemed more reliable (on one or two points demonstrably so).
10 For example, *Cork Examiner*, 23 November 1853, p. 3.
11 *Belfast Commercial Chronicle*, 21 October 1854, p. 4.
12 Distribution of the British Army, 3 March 1855, NMG.
13 Kaufman, *Surgeons at War*, p. 142.
14 Hall, diary, 27 January 1855, RAMC 524/15/5-6 and PC1/7-8, WLC.
15 Memorandum of the Services of Dr James Barry, January 1860, RJBa.

16 Ibid.; Hart, *New Annual Army List, 1854*, p. 243.
17 Memorandum of the Services of Dr James Barry, January 1860, RJBa.
18 Ibid.
19 Shepherd, *Crimean Doctors*, vol. 2, p. 343.
20 Rae, *Strange Story*, p. 97; Charteris, 'Corfu', p. 85.
21 Charteris, 'Corfu', p. 85.
22 Ibid.
23 *The Times*, 5 December 1854, p. 4.
24 Shepherd, *Crimean Doctors*, vol. 2, p. 457; Rae, *Strange Story*, p. 98.
25 Macintosh to Raglan, 7 May 1855, quoted in Rae, *Strange Story*, pp. 98–9.
26 Ibid.
27 Raglan to Macintosh, 21 May 1855, quoted in Rae, *Strange Story*, pp. 99–100.
28 Quoted in Shepherd, *Crimean Doctors*, p. 510.

Chapter 31: The Land of Mornise

1 *The Times*, 27 August 1855, p. 8.
2 Soyer, *Culinary Campaign*, pp. 214–16. Crimean fever is now recognised as brucellosis, an infection picked up from unpasteurised dairy products.
3 Barry to Henderson, 5 October 1854, JBE.
4 Linton to Hall, 6 November 1855, RAMC 801/6, WLC; Rogers, letter to the editor, *The Lancet*.
5 Nightingale to Verney, undated (after Barry's death), MS 9001/145, WLC. The recipient was Nightingale's sister, Frances Parthenope Verney.
6 *Association Medical Journal*, 4 May 1855, p. 425.
7 Cumming to Hall, 16 October 1855, RAMC 238/3 FCO 19, WLC.
8 Barry to Henderson, 5 October 1855, JBE.
9 McCormick, *Visit*, p. 34.
10 Alexander, *Passages*, p. 150.
11 Ibid., p. 3.
12 Ibid., p. 5.
13 Memorandum of the Services of Dr James Barry, January 1860, RJBa.
14 Money and Money, *Sevastopol*, pp. 231–2.
15 Ibid., p. 232.
16 Roberts, Item 838, in Commissioners of Inquiry (Crimea), *Report*, p. 184.
17 Memorandum of the Services of Dr James Barry, January 1860, RJBa.
18 General Orders, *The Times*, 18 June 1855, p. 7. Details of this kind – as well as troop movements – were routinely reported in the newspapers.
19 General Orders, *The Times*, 8 November 1855, p. 7; 10 January 1856, p. 5.
20 Anonymous, cited by Hutchison, unidentified newspaper, late 19th century, RAMC 238/3, WLC. The story (repeated in several biographies) was that the medical board happened in Corfu immediately after the citadel incident, and that Denny never went to the Crimea.
21 Distribution of the British Army, 5 July 1856, 9 May 1857, NMG.

22 *The Times*, 1 December 1856, p. 10.

23 *The Times*, 3 October 1857, p. 7.

24 Memorandum, WO 138/1, TNA; *Medical Times and Gazette*, 25 April 1857, p. 425.

25 Unannotated item from 'Report on Foreign Stations of the Army', 1863, WLC.

Chapter 32: 'This Vorld of Voe, this Wale of Tears'

1   This implies that Margaret's disguise might not have been wholly motivated by expediency, and that she enjoyed at least some aspects of being a man. On the other hand, she did sometimes overact James's male traits (the dispute with Cloete, for instance), and this might be another example.

2   *Whitehaven News*, 1 October 1857, p. 3; also *Lincolnshire Chronicle*, 2 October 1857, p. 5.

3   *Whitehaven News*, 1 October 1857, p. 3.

4   Ibid.

5   Barry to Bell, 3 August 1857, RAMC 1026, WLC.

6   England and Wales census, 1851.

7   Burials in the parish of St Matthew, Bethnal Green, Board of Guardian Records, 1834–1906, and Church of England Parish Registers, 1813–1906, London Metropolitan Archives.

8   No record of Mrs Bulkley's death has been discovered.

9   Hall, *Observations*, p. 26.

10 Barry to Hall, 25 September 1857, RAMC 397/FCO15–18, WLC.

11 Sutherland, *Reply*, p. 5.

12 Hall, *Rejoinder*, p. 18.

13 *Carlisle Journal*, 2 October, p. 8.

14 *Westmorland Gazette*, 9 September 1857, p. 4. Dickens and Collins turned the holiday and the accident into a short story – 'The Lazy Tour of Two Idle Apprentices' (first published in *Household Words* in October 1857).

15 Barry to Hall, 25 September 1857, RAMC 397/FCO15–18, WLC; *Kendal Mercury*, 10 October 1857, p. 8.

16 Commission, 26 September 1857, RJBa; War Office: RJBb.

17 In September 2015, exactly 158 years after James Barry's commission, Major General Susan Ridge became the first (officially) female general in the British Army, as head of the Army Legal Service.

18 Memorandum of the Services of Dr James Barry, January 1860, RJBa.

19 War Office: RJBb.

20 Barry to Hall, 25 September 1857, RAMC 397/FCO15–18, WLC.

21 Barry to Bell, 3 August 1857, RAMC 1026, WLC.

22 Hurwitz and Richardson, 'Inspector General James Barry', p. 302.

23 Harrison, 'Hall, Sir John (1795–1866)', *Oxford Dictionary of National Biography* online edition, www.oxforddnb.com/view/article/11974; retrieved 11 Dec 2015).

24 Barry to Bell, 3 August 1857, RAMC 1026, WLC.

25 War Office: RJBb.

26 Distribution of the British Army, 3 July 1858, NMG.

27 Hart, *New Annual Army List, 1858*, pp. 388, 408.

28 Barry, Report, WO 334/22, RHT.

29 Ibid. He was correct; coal emits toxic substances including methane, ethane, sulphur dioxide and various oxides of nitrogen, lead and arsenic.

30 Hart, *New Annual Army List,1858*, pp. 388–92.

31 Barry, Report, WO 334/22, RHT.

32 Memoir of Sydney Bellingham, pp. 169–70, LAC; Bannerman, 'Double Life'.

33 Andrée Vincent, Club Saint-James Montreal, personal communication, 24 April 2014.

34 Robert C. Daley, 'Bellingham, Sydney Robert', *Dictionary of Canadian Biography* online edition, www.biographi.ca/en/bio/bellingham_sydney_robert_12E.html (retrieved 12 December 2015).

35 Memoir of Sydney Bellingham, pp. 169–70, LAC.

36 Ibid.

37 War Office: RJBb.

38 Bannerman, 'Double Life'; Mackenzie, 'Dr James Barry'.

39 Mackenzie, 'Dr James Barry'.

40 Barry to Rollo, 25 January 1859, PRO 30/46/19, TNA.

41 Bethune to Eyre and Bishop of Montreal to Eyre, 24 January 1859, PRO 30/46/19, TNA. The scene of this incident is unclear; Bethune specifies 'St John's Chapel', but no such place exists now in Montreal, and no other contemporary references to it have been found. There is a St John's Church, but it wasn't founded until 1861.

42 Bethune to Eyre, 24 and 26 January 1859, PRO 30/46/19, TNA.

43 Barry to Rollo, 25 January 1859, PRO 30/46/19, TNA.

44 Hart, *New Annual Army List, 1846*, p. 193.

45 Ibid., p. 211; obituary, *British Medical Journal*, 2/2548 (30 October 1909), p. 1322.

46 Rollo to Eyre, 18 February 1859, PRO 30/46/19, TNA.

47 Quoted in ibid.

48 Ibid.; Hart, *Annual Army List, 1848*, p. 221. The then Captain Cole's time in Malta with the 69th (1847 onward) might have slightly overlapped with Captain Rollo's time there with the 42nd (1846–7), both within James Barry's period on the island.

49 Rollo to Eyre, 18 February 1859, PRO 30/46/19, TNA.

50 Rollo to Eyre, 28 February 1859, PRO 30/46/19, TNA.

51 Hart, *New Annual Army List, 1860*, pp. 77, 92.

52 Eyre to Yorke, 21 February 1859, PRO 30/46/19, TNA.

53 Draft memorial of Dr James Barry, 1860; and Memorandum of the Services of Dr James Barry, January 1860, RJBa.

54 Campbell, quoted in Bannerman, 'Double Life'. Dr Campbell later became a professor of medicine at McGill University, and would describe his experience to his students as an object lesson in how 'you should never let yourself be too impressed by any colleague to treat him just like any other patient'.

55 St James's Club records, quoted in Rose, *Perfect Gentleman*, p. 147.

Chapter 33: This Life and No Other

1 Memorandum of the Services of Dr James Barry, January 1860, RJBa.

2 Ibid.

3 Draft memorial of Dr James Barry, 1860, RJBa.

4 Ibid.

5 Memorandum of the Services of Dr James Barry, January 1860, RJBa.

6 Obituary, *The Lancet*, 7 March 1868, pp. 331–2.

7 Hart, *Annual Army List, 1860*, pp. 439–40; *1861*, pp. 422–3, *1862*, p. 422.

8 War Office: RJBb. It was the end for Sir William Eyre too. His health had been broken in the Crimea, and just after James Barry's departure from Canada Eyre fell seriously ill and was forced to resign; he died that September.

9 Unidentified newspaper cutting, c. 1865, included in museum accession note, RJBd. This single loss has hampered James Barry's biographers ever since. A tiny number of items were recovered from the wreck site, and only one of those is still in existence (see Chapter 34).

10 B. Mosse, letter in *Sunday Express* cutting, RAMC 801/6/5, WLC; Johnston, *Roll*, p. 359. Perhaps Barry took to Mosse because he perceived an outstanding talent or personality; if so, his judgement was sound, as the young man made Surgeon Major within six years and Deputy Surgeon General nine years after that.

11 B. Mosse, letter, *Sunday Express* cutting, RAMC 801/6/5, WLC. Miss Mosse was Deputy Surgeon General Mosse's granddaughter. On the back of the photograph is printed 'Duperly Bros, No. 3, Church Street, Water Lane, Kingston, Jamaica'.

12 J. C. M'Crindle, letter, *Glasgow Herald* cutting, 1949, RAMC 238/1, WLC.

13 Ibid. In later years, the writer of this letter, who was M'Crindle's son, recalled the name in the inscription being 'Marion'; clearly an error of memory. Once the truth about James Barry came out, the family speculated that this might have been his real name.

14 Rogers, letter to the editor, *The Lancet*; Rogers, letter, unidentified Jamaican newspaper, RAMC 238/3, WLC. Lieutenant (later Lieutenant Colonel) Ebenezer Rogers later became one of the principal early historians of James Barry's career.

15 *Annual Register*, 1857, p. 280.

16 *London Daily News*, 2 July 1861, p. 3; Hart, *New Annual Army List, 1861*, p. 473; *1862*, p. 473.

17 Hart, *New Annual Army List, 1855*, p. 172; Clerke obituary, *Lancaster Gazette*, 30 December 1891, p. 3. This regiment was later renamed the 21st Royal Scots Fusiliers.

18 Johnston, *Roll*, p. 325; Hart, *New Annual Army List, 1861*, p. 269; Distribution of the British Army, 31 March 1860, NMG.

19 Gannon, 'The Inspector'; Clerke, cited in Rogers, letter to the editor, *The Lancet*.

20 *London Daily News*, 2 July 1861, p. 3.

21 *Whitehaven News*, 24 August 1865, p. 5.

22 A snapshot of the household is given in the England census, 1861.

23 England census, 1861. The letters in Daniel Reardon's possession revealing the
    identity of James Barry and Margaret Anne Bulkley probably didn't pass through
    his daughters' hands; they would more likely have remained in the keeping of the
    firm.
24 Joan Self, Exeter Meteorological Library and Archive, personal communication,
    2011.
25 Ibid.
26 *The Lancet*, 29 July 1865, p. 135.
27 Johnson, *Notes on Cholera*, p. 87.
28 Ibid., pp. 86–7.
29 Ibid., pp. 91–4.

Chapter 34: A Perfect Female

1   Tomo XVII, folio 139, AFM.
2   McKinnon to Gibson, 25 July 1865, RJBa.
3   Kensal Green Cemetery records, via Barry Smith, trustee, Friends of Kensal Green
    Cemetery.
4   Death certificate, James Barry; McKinnon to Graham, 24 August 1865, RJBa.
5   J. C. M'Crindle, letter, *Glasgow Herald* cutting, 1949, RAMC 238/1, WLC; Rose,
    Perfect Gentleman, p. 151. The visit by the footman (or two) was attested by more
    than one source, but M'Crindle is the only witness to the existence of the black
    box. He was told of its removal by the footman when John visited him on his
    return to Jamaica. One obvious explanation for John's apparent absence at the
    time of James Barry's death could be that he had gone to notify the owner of the
    box.
6   Verran to Rutherford, April 1955, RAMC 801/6, WLC.
7   Dr R. T. McCowan, letter, *Whitehaven News*, 7 September 1865, p. 4. McCowan
    claimed to have known Barry 'intimately' in Trinidad and to be a friend of Dr
    O'Connor; if so, he must have been a civilian, as there is no trace of him in the
    Army Lists.
8   Kensal Green Cemetery records, via Barry Smith, trustee, Friends of Kensal Green
    Cemetery.
9   Adjutant General's Office, *Queen's Regulations*, pp. 35–6. Had James Barry received
    a military funeral, as a non-combatant officer he would not have had a salute fired
    over his grave.
10 David McKinnon gave a detailed description of this encounter, including the
    remarks exchanged; see McKinnon to Graham, 24 August 1865, RJBa. For the
    identity of the layer-out, see Appendix B.
11 McKinnon to Graham, 24 August 1865, RJBa.
12 *Saunders's News-Letter and Daily Advertiser*, 14 August 1865, pp. 1–2. The Irish
    venue appears to have been a coincidence; there was no contemporary knowledge
    of a connection between Dr James Barry and Ireland, other than his surname.
13 *Cork Examiner*, 26 August 1865, p. 3.

14 *Whitehaven News*, 24 August 1865, p. 5.

15 Albemarle, *Fifty Years*, p. 205.

16 *Medical Times and Gazette*, 26 August 1865, p. 228.

17 Graham to McKinnon, 23 August 1865; McKinnon to Graham, 24 August 1865, RJBa.

18 James Barry commission, 7 December 1815 and museum acquisition note, RJBd.

19 Verran to Rutherford, April 1955, RAMC 801/6, WLC.

Epilogue

1 War Office, *Army List, 1939*, p. 1349. There had been many more reforms, the Royal Army Medical Corps had been brought into existence and doctors now had standard Army ranks.

2 Rutherford, 'Dr James Barry', p. 106.

3 Ibid., p. 109.

4 Advertisement, *The Times*, 18 July 1919, p. 5.

5 *The Times*, 23 July 1919, p. 10.

6 *The Observer*, 27 July 1919, p. 9.

7 *Manchester Guardian*, 23 July 1919, p. 8.

8 Rae, *Strange Story*.

Appendix A: James Barry and the Physical Examination

1 Rutherford, 'Dr James Barry', pp. 112–18.

2 Rae, *Strange Story*, pp. 17–18.

3 Rose, *Perfect Gentleman*, p. 29.

4 Army Medical Department, 'Qualifications of Candidates' (1873), p. 289.

5 Army Medical Department, 'Qualifications and Examination of Candidates' (1865), p. 307.

Appendix B: Who Discovered Dr Barry's Secret?

1 For example, Rose, *Perfect Gentleman*, pp. 12, 14; Holmes, *Scanty Particulars*, p. 258. Isobel Rae (*Strange Story*, pp. 113–14) is circumspect, confining herself to a summary of the contradictory gossip.

2 Death certificate of James Barry, 26 July 1865, RJBa.

3 McKinnon, letter to Graham, Registrar General, 24 August 1865, RJBa.

4 *Saunders's News-Letter and Daily Advertiser*, 14 August 1865, pp. 1–2; see also Rae, *Strange Story*, pp. 113–14.

5 Dickens, 'A Mystery Still', p. 494.

6 Skretkowicz, *Florence Nightingale's Notes on Nursing*, p. 19.

7 England censuses, 1851, 1861.

8 England censuses, 1871, 1881; marriage record of Sophia Bishop, Aylesbury, July 1869, General Register Office.

Bibliography

Archives and unpublished materials
(alphabetically by abbreviation)

AFM   Archivo del Francisco de Miranda (El Archivo Colombeia): Section Negociaciones: Archivo General de la Nación de Venezuela, Caracas; available online at www.franciscodemiranda.org/colombeia/ (retrieved 24 December 2014)

AOC   Articles of Clerkship; Court of King's Bench: Plea Side: Affidavits of Due Execution of Articles of Clerkship, Series I; Class: KB 105

BFA   Barry Family Albums (correspondence and papers of Dr James Barry and the Bulkley family): The Lewis Walpole Library, Yale University, Farmington, Connecticut

CPH   Home Office: Convict Prison Hulks: Registers and Letter Books, 1802–1849. Microfilm, HO9, piece 8: National Archives, Kew, England

DOB   Beaufort Family Archives, in possession of the 11th Duke of Beaufort, Badminton Estate, England

JBE   Barry, James (Margaret Bulkley), *Disputatio Medica Inauguralis: De Merocele vel Hernia Crurali* (Inaugural Medical Dissertation on Merocele or Femoral Hernia), 1812, translated by Nigel Coulton on behalf of Dr Edward Myers, 2002: Att.83.7.15/4; Barry to Henderson, 5 October 1855, Gen 1730: Edinburgh University Library, Edinburgh

KCH   St Thomas's Pupils and Dressers Cash Book, 1811–1837: TH/FP7/1 f 5; St Thomas's Pupils, Dressers, 1723–1819: TH/FP1/IN; Register of Anatomy Pupils of Cooper and Cline, 1808–1814; Register of Course of Surgery by Cooper and Cline, Autumn 1812: TH/FP1/1: 1808–1814 f 33: Archives of King's College Hospital, London

LAC   Library and Archives Canada, Wellington Street, Ottawa

LEB   Letters of David Steuart Erskine, 11th Earl of Buchan: Adv.MS.22.4.13: National Library of Scotland

MFC   Munnik family collection of papers and artefacts relating to James Barry: private collection in possession of Dr J. B. Munnik, South Africa

NAM   National Archives of Mauritius, Port Louis, Mauritius

NLI   National Library of Ireland MS 2069: National Library of Ireland, Dublin

NMA   National Archives of Malta, Triq l-Isptar, Rabat, Malta

NMG   Data from *The Naval and Military Gazette* and *East India and Colonial Chronicle*: Combined Arms Research Library Digital Library: Nafziger Collection: available online at cgsc.contentdm.oclc.org/cdm/landingpage/collection/p15040coll6 (retrieved 28 November 2015)

NPG   National Portrait Gallery Archive autograph letters (uncatalogued): National Portrait Gallery, London

RAA   Royal Academy of Arts Collections: James Barry: Royal Academy of Arts, London

RCC   see Books and Articles (below)

RCS   Royal College of Surgeons: Court of Examiners, 15 January and 2 July 1813, ff 71–2 and f 93, Examination Book Volumes 1 and 2, RCS-EXA/2/2/1/1, 1800–1820: Library of the Royal College of Surgeons of England, London

RHT   Reports on health of troops: Annual Return and Report (Mauritius), 1825–6 by James Butler Kell and Report (Cape Colony), 1825–6 by John Arthur, in WO 334/3; Annual Return and Report (Mauritius), 1829–30 by Charles Collier and Annual Return and Report (Jamaica), 1829–30 by Thomas Draper, in WO 334/5; Annual Report (Malta), 1847–8 by James Barry, in WO 334/16; Annual Report (Canada), 1857–8 by James Barry, in WO 334/22: National Archives, Kew, England

RJBa   Records of Dr James Barry, Inspector General of the Army Medical Department, WO 138/1: National Archives, Kew, England

RJBb   Records of Dr James Barry: War Office, 'Statement of the Home and Foreign Services: James Barry', WO 25/3899 f 614: National Archives, Kew, England

RJBc   Records of Dr James Barry: War Office, 'Return of the services and professional education of James Barry, MD', 7 April 1824, WO 25/3910 f 3: National Archives, Kew, England

RJBd   Records of Dr James Barry: Commission as Assistant Surgeon to the Forces, MA 1987-188: Museum Africa, Johannesburg, South Africa

RJBe   'Report Upon the Arctopus Echinatus or Plat Doorn of the Cape of Good Hope' by James Barry MD, Assistant Surgeon to the Forces, in RHT

RJBf   Colonial Office, Case of Dr Barry; Abolition of Office of Medical Inspector, CO 48/97: National Archives, Kew, England

SHA   St Helena Archives, Jamestown, St Helena; most of the cited documents are included in George, *Dr James Miranda Barry* (q.v.)

TNA   The National Archives, Kew, England

WCA   Records of the Government of the Cape Colony; Western Cape Archives and Records Service, Cape Town

WLC   Wellcome Library collection, RAMC/373/39: Papers on the life and
           career of James Barry; RAMC/238/1: Papers relating to Dr James Barry;
           RAMC/283/33: Note by Sir Thomas Longmore relating to Dr James
           Barry: Wellcome Library, London

                              Books and articles
                                Abbreviations

RCC   Theal, *Records of the Cape Colony*

Ackroyd, Marcus et al., *Advancing with the Army: Medicine, the Professions, and Social
     Mobility in the British Isles, 1790–1850* (Oxford: Oxford University Press, 2006).
Adjutant General's Office, Horse Guards, *General Regulations and Orders for the Army*
     (London: W. Clowes, 1811).
Adjutant General's Office, Horse Guards, *The Queen's Regulations and Orders for the
     Army, December 1859* (London: W. H. Allen, 1860).
Adkins, Roy, *Trafalgar: The Biography of a Battle* (London: Little, Brown, 2004).
Admiralty, *The Navy List, 20 June 1848* (London: John Murray, 1848).
Aitchison, Thomas, *The Edinburgh and Leith directory to July 1801* (Edinburgh: 1800).
Albemarle, George Thomas, Earl of, *Fifty Years of My Life*, 3rd edn (London: Macmillan,
     1877).
Alexander, James Edward, *Passages in the Life of a Soldier*, vol. 2 (London: Hurst and
     Blackett, 1857).
A. M. S., Letter to the editor, *The Lancet*, 19 October 1895, p. 1021.
Anti-Slavery Office, *Reasons for Temporarily Suspending the Constitution of Jamaica* (London:
     Hatchard, 1839).
Army Medical Department, 'Qualifications and Examination of Candidates for
     Commissions in the Army Medical Service', *The Medical Times and Gazette* vol.
     II for 1865, pp. 306–7.
Army Medical Department, 'Qualifications of Candidates for Commissions in the
     Army Medical Service', *The Medical Times and Gazette* vol. II for 1873, pp. 289–90.
Arneth, F. H., 'Evidence of Puerperal Fever Depending Upon the Contagious
     Inoculation of Morbid Matter', *The Retrospect of Practical Medicine & Surgery* 23
     (July 1851), pp. 292–5.
Bailey, James Blake, *The Diary of a Resurrectionist, 1811–1812* (London: Swan
     Sonnenschein, 1896).
Ballingall, George, *Outlines of Military Surgery*, 3rd edn (Edinburgh: Adam and Charles
     Black, 1844).
Bannerman, James, 'The Double Life of Dr. James Barry', *MacLean's, Canada's National
     Magazine*, 1 December 1950, p. 24ff.

Barrell, John, *The Birth of Pandora and the Division of Knowledge* (London: Palgrave Macmillan, 1991).

Barry, James, RA, *An Account of a Series of Pictures in the Great Room of the Society of Arts* (London: William Adland, 1783).

Barry, James, RA, *A Series Of Etchings By James Barry, Esq. From His Original And Justly Celebrated Paintings, In The Great Room Of The Society Of Arts* (London: Colnaghi, 1808).

Beatson, Alexander, *Tracts Relative to the Island of St Helena; Written During a Residence of Five Years* (London: Nicol, 1816).

Beck, Roger B., *The History of South Africa*, 2nd edn (Santa Barbara: ABC-CLIO, 2013).

Bell, Sir Charles, *Letters of Sir Charles Bell* (London: John Murray, 1870).

Biggs, James, *The History of Don Francisco de Miranda's Attempt to Effect a Revolution in South America* (Boston: Oliver and Munroe, 1809).

Bird, William Wilberforce and Henry Thomas Colebrook, *State of the Cape of Good Hope, in 1822* (London: John Murray, 1823).

Bone, Dr George F. (Assistant Surgeon to the Forces), *Inaugural Dissertation on Yellow Fever*, quoted in a review, *London Medical Gazette* vol. III (1846), p. 677.

Bower, Alexander, *The Edinburgh Student's Guide: or an Account of the Classes of the University* (Edinburgh: Waugh & Innes, 1822).

Bradford, Edward, 'The Reputed Female Army Surgeon', *The Medical Times and Gazette* vol. II for 1865, p. 293.

Brenton, Jahleel, *Memoir of the Life and Services of Vice-Admiral Sir Jahleel Brenton*, ed. Henry Raikes (London: Hatchard, 1846).

Broodbank, Sir Joseph G., *History of the Port of London* (London: O'Connor, 1921).

Buchan, David Steuart Erskine, 11th Earl of, *The Anonymous and Fugitive Essays of the Earl of Buchan* (Edinburgh: Ruthven, 1812).

Buckingham, James Silk, *Travels Among the Arab Tribes Inhabiting the Countries East of Syria and Palestine* (London: Longman, 1825).

Buckley, Roger N., *The British Army in the West Indies* (Gainesville: University Press of Florida, 1998).

Burchell, William J., *Hints on Emigration to the Cape of Good Hope* (London: J. Hatchard, 1819).

Burchell, William J., *Travels in the Interior of Southern Africa* (London: Longman, 1822).

Burnett, Bishop, *A Reply to the 'Report of the Commissioners of Inquiry at the Cape of Good Hope'* (London: Cheese, Gordon and Co., 1826).

Burney, William (ed.), *Falconer's Marine Dictionary*, expanded edn of *A New Universal Dictionary of the Marine* by William Falconer (London: Cadell and Davies, John Murray, 1819).

Burrows, Edmund H., *A History of Medicine in South Africa* (Cape Town: A. A. Balkema, 1958).

'Captain', Letter to the editor, *The Lancet*, 26 October 1895, p. 1087.

Carey, John and Robert Bancks, 'Meteorological Journal kept at London, 1809', *Edinburgh Annual Register* 1809, pp. 493–505.

Carphin, Janet, Letter to the Editor, *The Lancet*, 19 October 1895, p. 1021.

Castlereagh, Viscount, *Correspondence, Despatches, and Other Papers of Viscount Castlereagh, Second Marquess of Londonderry: Second Series: Military and Miscellaneous*, vol. VII, ed. Charles William Vane (London: William Shoberl, 1851).

Charteris, Mr, 'Corfu', *The English Presbyterian Messenger*, 1854, pp. 84–5.

Clarke, J. F., *Autobiographical Recollections of the Medical Profession* (London: Churchill, 1874).

Commissioners of Inquiry (Crimea), *Report of the Commissioners Appointed to Inquire into the Regulations Affecting the Sanitary Condition of the Army, the Organization of Military Hospitals, and the Treatment of the Sick and Wounded*, append. 79 (London: HMSO, 1858).

Commissioners of Military Enquiry, *Fifth Report of the Commissioners of Military Enquiry: Army Medical Department* (London: HMSO, 1808).

Cooke, E. W., *Sixty-five Plates of Shipping and Craft* (London: Cooke, 1829).

Cooper, Sir Astley, *The Lectures of Sir Astley Cooper, Bart FRS on the Principles and Practice of Surgery*, 3 vols, ed. Frederick Tyrrell (London: Thomas and George Underwood, 1824–5; W. Simpkin and R. Marshall, 1827).

Cooper, Bransby Blake, *The Life of Sir Astley Cooper*, 2 vols (London: Parker, 1843).

Cordingly, David, *Billy Ruffian: The Bellerophon and the Downfall of Napoleon* (London: Bloomsbury, 2003).

Cory, G. E., *The Rise of South Africa*, vol. 1 (London: Longmans, 1910).

Crumplin, Michael K. H., *Men of Steel* (Shrewsbury: Quiller, 2007).

Curran, William Henry, 'Barry the Painter' in *The New Monthly Magazine and Literary Journal volume VII: Original Papers*, pp. 338–42 (London: Henry Colburn, 1823).

Curry, William (publisher), *The Picture of Dublin, or, Stranger's Guide to the Irish Metropolis* (Dublin: William Curry Jun. & Co., 1835).

Darwin, Charles, *Journal of Researches into the Natural History and Geology of the Countries Visited During the Voyage of HMS Beagle Round the World*, 2nd edn (London: John Murray, 1845).

Darwin, Charles, *The Life and Letters of Charles Darwin*, ed. Francis Darwin (London: John Murray, 1887).

Darwin, Francis and A. C. Seward (eds), *More Letters of Charles Darwin: A Record of his Work in a Series of Hitherto Unpublished Letters*, vol. 1 (London: John Murray, 1903).

Day, Charles William, *Five Years' Residence in the West Indies*, 2 vols (London: Colburn, 1852).

Denlinger, Elizabeth, *Before Victoria: Extraordinary Women of the British Romantic Era* (New York: Columbia University Press, 2005).

Deward, Elizabeth et al., Statements in evidence on a Caesarean birth, *The Lancet*, 19 January 1833, pp. 537–9.

Dickens, Charles (ed.), 'A Mystery Still', *All the Year Round* XVII, 18 May 1867, pp. 492–5.

Dillon, Sir William Henry, *A Narrative of My Professional Adventures (1790–1839)*, vol. 2, ed. Michael A. Lewis (Greenwich: Navy Records Society, 1956).

Dumat, H. Aylmer, 'The Famous Dr James Barry', *South African Medical Record*, 8 July 1911, p. 192.

Duncan, Andrew (ed.), 'Medical Department of the Army', *Edinburgh Medical and Surgical Journal* vol. 13 (1817), pp. 124–5.

Dunn, Richard S., *A Tale of Two Plantations: Slave Life and Labor in Jamaica and Virginia* (Cambridge, MA: Harvard University Press, 2014).

Dunne, Charles, *The Chirurgical Candidate or, Reflections on Education: Indispensable to Complete Naval, Military, and Other Surgeons* (London: Samuel Highley, 1808).

Dunne, Charles, *Mr. Dunne, Mr. Justice Best and Serjeant Spankie, or, the Opinion of the Chief Justice of the Common Pleas on the subject's right of petitioning Parliament* (London: C. Dunne, 1825).

Dunne, Tom and William L. Pressly, *James Barry, 1741–1806: History Painter* (Farnham: Ashgate, 2010).

Dupin, Charles, *A View of the History and Actual State of the Military Force of Great Britain*, vol. 1, transl. by 'An Officer' (London: John Murray, 1822).

du Preez, H. M., 'Dr James Barry: The Early Years Revealed', *South African Medical Journal* 98/1 (2008), pp. 52–8.

du Preez, H. M., 'Dr James Barry (1789–1865): The Edinburgh Years', *Journal of the Royal College of Physicians of Edinburgh* 42 (2012), pp. 258–65.

Edwards, Jane and Arthur Watson Rowe (eds), *A General Valuation of the lands and Tenements in the Parish of St John the Baptist, in the Isle of Thanet*, manuscript copy of 1801 original in Margate Library, available online at www.margatelocalhistory. co.uk/DocRead/Margate%20Valuation%201801%20notes.html (retrieved 20 April 2015).

Eriksen, E. O., 'A Letter by Dr. James Barry Concerning the Death of Lord Charles Somerset', *Africana Notes and News* 28 (1988–9), pp. 253–6.

Farington, Joseph, *The Farington Diary*, vol. 3: September 14, 1804 to September 19, 1806 and vol. 4: September 20, 1806 to January 7, 1808, ed. James Greig (London: Hutchinson, 1924).

Faulkner, Thomas, *An Historical and Topographical Description of Chelsea*, vol. 2 (Chelsea: T. Faulkner, 1829).

Fenton, Elizabeth, *The Journal of Mrs Fenton* (London: Edward Arnold, 1901).

Fergusson, William, *Notes and Recollections of a Professional Life* (London: Longman, 1846).

Figes, Orlando, *Crimea: The Last Crusade* (London: Penguin, 2011).

Fraser, A. G., *The Building of Old College* (Edinburgh: Edinburgh University Press, 1989).

Fryer, Edward (ed.), *The Works of James Barry, Esq., Historical Painter*, 2 vols (London: Cadell & Davies, 1809).

Fyfe, Andrew, *A Compendium of the Anatomy of the Human Body, Intended Principally for the Use of Students*, 2nd edn, vol. II (Edinburgh: Pillans, Guthrie, 1801).

Gallin, John I., 'A Historical Perspective on Clinical Research' in *Principles and Practice of Clinical Research*, eds John I. Gallin and Frederick P. Ognibene (London: Academic Press, 2012).

Gannon, Michael, 'The Inspector Was a Woman', *London Evening News*, 29 October 1954.

George, Barbara B., *Dr James Miranda Barry on St Helena* (St Helena: Busy Bee Books, 2006).

George, J., *The Descendants of Count Jacob van Reenen* (Lulu, 2012).

Gibney, William, *Eighty Years Ago: or The Recollections of an Old Army Doctor* (London: Bellairs & Co., 1896).

Gillkrest, James and Sir William Fergusson, *Letters on the Cholera Morbus* (London: Nichols, 1831).

Gleig, George Robert (ed.), *The Veterans of Chelsea Hospital*, vol. 3 (London: Richard Bentley, 1842).

Golding, Benjamin, *An Historical Account of St Thomas's Hospital, Southwark* (London: Longman, 1819).

Gordon, James, *History of the Rebellion in Ireland, in the Year 1798* (Dublin: Porter, 1801).

Gordon, Lyndall, *Vindication: A Life of Mary Wollstonecraft* (London: Virago, 2005).

Graves, Algernon, *Art Sales from Early in the Eighteenth Century to Early in the Twentieth Century vol. 1* (Bath: Kingsmead Reprints, 1973).

Gregory, Desmond, *Napoleon's Jailer: Lt Gen. Sir Hudson Lowe: A Life* (London: Associated University Presses, 1996).

Gregory, George, *Elements of the Theory and Practice of Medicine*, 4th edn (London: Baldwin and Cradock, 1835).

Gregory, James, *Additional Memorial to the Managers of the Royal Infirmary* (Edinburgh: Murray & Co., 1803).

Grose, Francis, *Lexicon Balatronicum: A Dictionary of Buckish Slang*, updated and enlarged edn (London: C. Cassell, 1811).

Guthrie, G. J., 'Evidence before the Select Committee on Medical Education', 30 April 1834 in *Report from the Select Committee on Medical Education: Part I, Royal College of Physicians, London* (London: HMSO, 1836).

Guy, Augustus, *Dr Hooper's Physician's Vademecum: or A Manual of the Principles and Practice of Physic* (London: Renshaw, 1846).

Hall, John, *Observations on the Report of the Sanitary Commissioners in the Crimea* (London: W. Clowes, 1857).

Hall, John, *Sir John Hall's Rejoinder to Dr Sutherland's Reply* (London: W. Clowes, 1858).

Hamilton, Joseph, *The Only Approved Guide through All the Stages of a Quarrel: Containing the Royal Code of Honor; Reflections upon Duelling; and the Outline of a Court for the Adjustment of Disputes* (London: Hatchard, 1829).

Harrison, Robert, *The Dublin Dissector, or System of Practical Anatomy*, 5th edn, vol. I (London: Simpkin, Marshall, 1847).

Harrison, William, 'George III and Hannah Lightfoot', *Notes and Queries* 2nd series, vol. XI (February 1861), p. 117.

Hart, H. G., *The New Army List: August 1839* (London: Smith, Elder and Co., 1839).

Hart, H. G., *The New Annual Army List: 1840* et seq. (London: John Murray, 1840 et seq.).

Hart, H. G., *The New Army List: January 1841* et seq. (London: John Murray, 1841 et seq.).

Harvey, Robert, *Liberators: Latin America's Struggle for Independence* (Woodstock NY: Overlook, 2000).

Hays, J. N., *Epidemics and Pandemics: Their Impacts on Human History* (Santa Barbara: ABC-CLIO, 2005).

Hennen, John, *Principles of Military Surgery*, 2nd edn (Edinburgh: Archibald Constable and Co., 1820).

HMSO, *Report from His Majesty's Commissioners for Inquiring into the System of Military Punishments*, vol. I (London: HMSO, 1836).

Holmes, Rachel, *Scanty Particulars: The Life of Dr James Barry* (London: Viking, 2002).

Horwood, Richard, *Plan of the Cities of London and Westminster, the Borough of Southwark and Parts Adjoining, Shewing Every House* (London: Horwood, 1795–9).

House of Lords, *The Sessional Papers: 1801–1833*, vol. 190: 1825 (London: HMSO, 1825).

Howell, Thomas Bayly and Thomas Jones Howell (eds), *A Complete Collection of State Trials and Proceedings for High Treason and Other Crimes and Misdemeanors vol. XXXI* (London: Hansard, 1823).

Hughson, David, *Walks through London: Including Westminster and the Borough of Southwark* (London: Sherwood, Neely and Jones, 1817).

Hunt, Leigh, 'Trade in Dead Bodies', *The Examiner* 1826, p. 666.

Hurwitz, Brian and R. Richardson, 'Inspector General James Barry MD: Putting the Woman in her Place', *British Medical Journal* 298/6669 (4 February 1989), pp. 299–305.

Jefcoate, Graham, 'Fryer, Edward (1761–1826)', *Oxford Dictionary of National Biography* (Oxford: Oxford University Press, 2004); available online at www.oxforddnb.com/view/article/10215 (retrieved 26 March 2015).

Johnson, George, *Notes on Cholera, Its Nature and Its Treatment* (London: Longmans, 1866).

Johnston, Colonel William, *Roll of Commissioned Officers in the Medical Service of the British Army* (Aberdeen: Aberdeen University Press, 1917).

Kaufman, Matthew H., *Surgeons at War: Medical Arrangements for the Treatment of the Sick and Wounded in the British Army during the Late 18th and 19th Centuries* (London: Greenwood Press, 2001).

Keane, J. R., 'Pituitary Apoplexy Presenting with Epistaxis', *Journal of Clinical Neuro-Ophthalmology* 4 (March 1984), pp. 7–8.

Kinnis, John, 'Observations on Cholera Morbus and other Diseases, which Prevailed Epidemically among the Soldiers of the 56th Regiment, Stationed at Port Louis, Mauritius, in the End of the Year 1819', *Edinburgh Medical and Surgical Journal* 17 (1821), pp. 1–29.

Knox, Robert, *The Edinburgh Dissector: or System of Practical Anatomy: for the Use of Students in the Dissecting Room*, publ. anon. by a 'Fellow of the Edinburgh College of Surgeons'; attribution by Lonsdale, 197 (Edinburgh: Rickard, 1837).

Laidler, P. W. and M. Gelfand, *South Africa: Its Medical History 1652–1898* (Cape Town: Struik, 1971).

Las Cases, Emmanuel, Comte de, *Mémorial de Sainte Hélène* (London: Henry Colburn, 1823).

Latrobe, C. I., *Journal of a Visit to South Africa, in 1815, and 1816* (London: L. B. Seeley, 1818).

Lawrence, W., *A Treatise on the Diseases of the Eye* (London: John Churchill, 1833).

Lecky, W. E. H., *A History of Ireland in the Eighteenth Century*, vol. 3 (Cambridge: Cambridge University Press, 2010; orig. publ. 1892).

Leigh, Samuel (publisher), *Leigh's New Picture of London* (London: Samuel Leigh, 1818).

Lewis, Samuel, *A Topographical Dictionary of Ireland*, vol. 1 (London: S. Lewis, 1837).

Locher, J. J., 'History of a Case of Caesarean Operation', *Medico-Chirurgical Transactions* 9/1 (1818), pp. 11–25.

Lockhart, John G., *Memoirs of the Life of Sir Walter Scott*, 4-vol. edn (Paris: Baudry, 1838).

Macaulay, Zachary (ed.), *Anti-Slavery Monthly Reporter*, vol. 2: June 1827–May 1829 (London: Society for the Mitigation and Abolition of Slavery, 1829).

McCormick, Richard Cunningham, *A Visit to the Camp Before Sevastopol* (New York: Appleton, 1855).

McCowan, R. T., 'The Late Dr Barry', *The Whitehaven News*, 24 August 1865.

McInnes, E. M., *St Thomas's Hospital* (London: Allen and Unwin, 1963).

MacKenzie, Ridley, 'Dr James Barry', *Canadian Medical Association Journal* 21 (1929), pp. 85–6.

Maclean, Charles, *An Analytical View of the Medical Department of the British Army* (London: J. J. Stockdale, 1810).

McLoughlin, Tim (ed.), *The Correspondence of James Barry*, online archive, www.texte.ie/barry (retrieved 4 March 2015).

Maitland, Frederick Lewis, *The Surrender of Napoleon* (London: William Blackwood, 1904).

Marshall, George, *Epistles in Verse, Between Cynthio and Leonora* (Newcastle: George Marshall, 1812).

Marshall, H. and A. M. Tulloch, *Statistical Report on the Sickness, Mortality and Invaliding Among the Troops in the West Indies* (London: HMSO, 1838).

Medical History (ed.), 'Introduction', *Medical History* 31 (1987) supplement S7 ('A Medical Student at St Thomas's Hospital, 1801–1802: The Weekes Family Letters'), pp. 1–30.

Medico-Chirurgical Review (ed.), Review of *Statistical Reports on the Sickness, Mortality and Invaliding among the Troops* by Tulloch and Balfour (1853), *British and Foreign Medico-Chirurgical Review* 13 (April 1854), pp. 405–25.

Metelerkamp, Sanni, *George Rex of Knysna* (Cape Town: Howard Timmins, c. 1956).

Millar, Anthony Kendal, *Plantagenet in South Africa: Lord Charles Somerset* (London: Oxford University Press, 1965).

Miller, JoAnn and Dean D. Knudsen, *Family Abuse and Violence: A Social Problems Perspective* (Lanham: AltaMira Press, 2007).

Mimosa, 'Het Kapokdoktertje' ('The Little Kapok Doctor'), *Ons Tijdschrift* 3 (1898–9), p. 287. English translation by Michael du Preez, 2015.

Mitchel, John, *The Last Conquest of Ireland (Perhaps)* (Glasgow: Washbourne, 1861).

Money, A. and G. H. Money, *Sevastopol: Our Tent in the Crimea* (London: Bentley, 1856).

Montgomery, Mr and James Barry, 'Case of Carotid Aneurism Successfully Treated', *The Lancet*, 29 June 1833, pp. 421–2.

Morris, John S., 'Sir Henry Halford, President of the Royal College of Physicians', *Postgraduate Medical Journal* 83 (2007), pp. 431–3.

Murray, John (pub.), *Handbook for Travellers in Southern Germany* (London: John Murray, 1850).

Murray, Peter, *The Cooper Penrose Collection* (Cork: Crawford Art Gallery, 2008); previously printed in *Irish Arts Review* Summer 2008, pp. 120–3.

Newby, Evelyn (ed.), *The Diary of Joseph Farington: Index* (New Haven: Yale University Press, 1998).

O'Keeffe, Paul, *Waterloo: The Aftermath*, ebook edn (London: The Bodley Head, 2014).

Opie, Amelia, *Detraction Displayed* (London: Longmans, 1828).

O'Shea, J. C. ' "Two Minutes with Venus, Two Years with Mercury": Mercury as an Antisyphilitic Agent', *Journal of the Royal Society of Medicine* 83 (1990), p. 392.

Parliament of Ireland, *Statutes Passed in the Parliaments Held in Ireland, vol. XII: 1799–1800* (Dublin: Grierson, 1801).

Parliament of Ireland, *The Statutes at Large, Passed in the Parliaments Held in Ireland, 1310–1800 vol. XX* (Dublin: Grierson, 1801).

Parkinson, C. Northcote, *Trade in the Eastern Seas: 1793–1813* (Cambridge: Cambridge University Press, 1937).

Parr, Bartholomew, *The London Medical Dictionary* (London: J. Johnson et al., 1809).

Pettigrew, Thomas Joseph, 'Sir Astley Paston Cooper, Bart.', in *Medical Portrait Gallery: Biographical Memoirs of the Most Celebrated Physicians, Surgeons, etc. etc.*, vol. 1 (London: Fisher, 1838).

Phillips, Nicola, *The Profligate Son: Or, a True Story of Family Conflict, Fashionable Vice, and Financial Ruin in Regency England* (Oxford: Oxford University Press, 2013).

Picard, H. W. J., *Gentleman's Walk* (Cape Town: C. Struik, 1968).

Plasket, Sir Richard and T. Miller, *Proclamations, Advertisements and other Official Notices Published by the Government of the Cape of Good Hope* (Cape Town: Government Press, 1827).

Porter, G. R., *Tables of the Revenue, Population, Commerce, &c. of the United Kingdom and Its Dependencies*, pt 7 (1837) (London: HMSO, 1839).

Pressly, William L., *The Life and Art of James Barry* (New Haven and London: Yale University Press, 1981).

Pressly, William L., 'Portrait of a Cork Family: The Two James Barrys', *Journal of the Cork Historical and Archaeological Society* 90/249 (1985), pp. 127–49.

Puzzle-Pate, Peter, 'Medical Science Exemplified', *The Scourge* 2 (October 1811), pp. 263–8.

Racine, Karen, *Francisco de Miranda: A Transatlantic Life in the Age of Revolution* (Wilmington, DE: 2003).

Rae, Isobel, *The Strange Story of Dr James Barry* (London: Longmans, Green, 1958).

Reid (publisher), *Reid's Leith and London Smack Directory* (W. Reid, 1819).

Reid, John, *A Treatise on the Origin, Progress, Prevention, and Treatment, of Consumption* (London: Richard Phillips, 1806).

Reid, Mary Ann, 'Cursory Remarks on Board the *Friendship*', *Asiatic Journal and Monthly Register for British India and Its Dependencies* VIII (July–December 1819), pp. 237–9, 344–7.

Renshaw, Richard, *Voyage to the Cape of Good Hope, Indian Ocean, and Up the Red Sea*, 2nd edn (Manchester: M. Wilson, 1813).

Richmond, Lesley and Alison Turton (eds), *The Brewing Industry: A Guide to Historical Records* (Manchester: Manchester University Press, 1990).

Robertson, William Spence, *The Life of Miranda*, vol. 2 (Chapel Hill: University of North Carolina Press, 1929); available online at http://penelope.uchicago.edu/Thayer/E/Gazetteer/People/Francisco_de_Miranda/ROBMIR/home.html (retrieved 15 March 2015).

Rogers, Ebenezer, Letter to the editor on the duel between Captain Cloete and Dr Barry, *The Lancet*, 2 May 1896, p. 1264.

Rose, June, *The Perfect Gentleman* (London: Hutchinson, 1977).

Rosner, Lisa, *Medical Education in the Age of Improvement* (Edinburgh: Edinburgh University Press, 1991).

Royal College of Surgeons, *A General List of the Members of the Royal College of Surgeons in London* (London: T. Bayley, 1812).

Rutherford, N. J. C., 'Dr James Barry: Inspector-General of the Army Medical Department', *Journal of the Royal Army Medical Corps* 73/2–4 (1939), pp. 106–20, 173–8, 240–8.

Saunders, Christopher, 'Between Slavery and Freedom: The Importation of Prize Negroes to the Cape in the Aftermath of Emancipation', *Kronos* 9 (1984), pp. 36–43.

Savona-Ventura, C., 'Dr James Barry: An Enigmatic Army Medical Doctor', *Maltese Medical Journal* 8/1 (1996), pp. 41–7.

Scholl, Theresa O. and Xinhua Chen, 'Puberty and Adolescent Pregnancy' in *Women & Health*, 2nd edn, eds Marlene B. Goldman, Rebecca Troisi and Kathryn M. Rexrode, pp. 151–62 (London: Academic Press, 2012).

Select Committee on Medical Education, *Report from the Select Committee on Medical Education: Part II: Royal College of Surgeons* (London: House of Commons, 1834).

Shepherd, John, *The Crimean Doctors* (Liverpool: Liverpool University Press, 1991).

Simonton, Deborah, 'Women and Education' in *Women's History: Britain, 1700–1850*, eds Hannah Barker and Elaine Chalus, pp. 33–56 (Abingdon: Routledge, 2005).

Simpson, James Y., *The Obstetric Memoirs and Contributions of James Y. Simpson*, eds W. O. Priestley and H. R. Storer (Edinburgh: Adam and Charles Black, 1856).

Skretkowicz, Victor (ed.), *Florence Nightingale's Notes on Nursing: Commemorative Edition with Historical Commentary* (New York: Springer, 2010).

Slatta, Richard W. and Jane Lucas de Grummond, *Simón Bolívar's Quest for Glory* (College Station, TX: Texas A&M University Press, 2003).

Snow, John, *On the Mode of Communication of Cholera* (London: John Churchill, 1849).

Society in Edinburgh, 'Medical News', *Medical and Philosophical Commentaries*, vol. 5/1 (1778), pp. 321–7.

Somerville, Mary, *Personal Recollections, from Early Life to Old Age, of Mary Somerville*, ed. Martha Somerville (London: John Murray, 1873).

South, John Flint, *Memorials of John Flint South*, ed. Charles Lett Feltoe (London: John Murray, 1884).

Southey, Robert, *The Life and Correspondence of Robert Southey*, ed. Charles Cuthbert Southey (London: Longmans, 1849).

Soyer, Alexis, *Soyer's Culinary Campaign: Being Historical Reminiscences of the Late War* (London: Routledge, 1857).

Stanley, Peter, *For Fear of Pain: British Surgery, 1790–1850* (Amsterdam: Rodopi, 2003).

Storrar, Patricia, *George Rex: Death of a Legend* (Johannesburg: Macmillan, 1974).

Struthers, John, *Historical Sketch of the Edinburgh Anatomical School* (Edinburgh: Maclachlan & Stewart, 1867).

Sutherland, John, *Reply to Sir John Hall's 'Observations'* (London: Harrison, 1857).

Teenstra, M. D., *The Fruits of My Labours*, transl. by Van Riebeeck Society from *De vruchten mijner werkzaamheden* (Cape Town: Van Riebeeck Society, 1943, orig. pub. 1830).

Theal, George McCall (ed.), *Records of the Cape Colony, 1793–1831: Copied for the Cape Government, from the Manuscript Documents in the Public Record Office, London*, 36 vols (Cape Town: Government of the Cape Colony, 1897–1905).

Thomas, Robert, *The Modern Practice of Physic* (London: Longman, 1816).

Thome, James A. and J. Horace Kimball, *Emancipation in the West Indies: A Six Months' Tour in Antigua, Barbadoes, and Jamaica* (New York: Anti-Slavery Society, 1838).

Thompson, George, *Travels and Adventures in Southern Africa* (London: Henry Colburn, 1827).

Thorne, R. (ed.), The History of Parliament: The House of Commons 1790–1820, ed. R. Thorne; online edition: www.historyofparliamentonline.org/volume/1790-1820/member/longfield-mountifort-1746-1819 (retrieved 26 November 2014).

Tipper, Samuel, *The Satirist, or Monthly Meteor*, vol. V, 1 July 1809.

War Office, *A Collection of Orders, Regulations, and Instructions for the Army* (London: T. Egerton, 1807).

War Office, *A List of the Officers of the Army and Royal Marines* (London: War Office, 1805–35).

War Office, *The Army List for January 1826, July 1829, January 1846* (London: War Office, 1825–46).

War Office, *The Army List for July 1829* (London: War Office, 1829).

War Office, *The Half-Yearly Army List, December 1939* (London: HMSO, 1940).

Weigall, Rose, 'Dr James Barry' (letter to the editor), *The Spectator*, 2 August 1919, p. 147.

Weinreb, Ben, Christopher Hibbert, John Keay and Julia Keay, *The London Encyclopaedia*, 3rd edn (London: Macmillan, 2008).

Wellington, Arthur, 1st Duke, *Supplementary Despatches, Correspondence, and Memoranda of Field Marshal Arthur Duke of Wellington*, vol. VI (London: John Murray, 1860).

Williams, Thomas Walter, *The Whole Law Relative to the Duty and Office of a Justice of the Peace*, vol. II (London: W. Clarke and Sons, 1808).

Williamson, Thomas, *The East India Vade Mecum; or, Complete Guide to Gentlemen Intended for the Civil, Military, or Naval Service of the Hon. East India Company*, vol. 1 (London: Black, Parry and Kingsbury, 1810).

Windele, John, *Historical and Descriptive Notices of the City of Cork and Its Vicinity* (London: Longman, 1839).

Wollstonecraft, Mary, *Thoughts on the Education of Daughters: With Reflections on Female Conduct in the More Important Duties of Life* (London: J. Johnson, 1787).

Wollstonecraft, Mary, *A Vindication of the Rights of Woman: With Strictures on Political and Moral Subjects* (London: J. Johnson, 1792).

Acknowledgements

In unravelling the events, connections, causes, apparent contradictions and myths in the life of Dr James Barry, we are profoundly indebted to many individuals and organisations around the world who have enabled us to evolve a comprehensive telling of the life and times of this enigmatic character. During Michael's original research – which lasted for over a decade – many were those who set him off on other paper-trails, which in turn led to valuable and unexpected information coming to light, especially with regard to James Barry's origins, early life and whole career.

Numerous and heartfelt are our thanks to all those who have helped bring this book to fruition: countless librarians, museum curators, historians and archivists from around the world fielded queries on matters medical, military, geographic, administrative and socio-economic, relating to people and places great and humble.

The Duke of Beaufort kindly allowed us to use hitherto unpublished letters written by Lord Charles Somerset to (and about) James Barry. Dr James Barry Munnik provided personal family history and generously allowed Michael to access and photograph the miniature presented to his ancestors by Dr James Barry. Nicky and Dudley Cloete-Hopkins of Alphen, Constantia, South Africa unstintingly recounted traditional family information about the duel between Dr Barry and Captain Josias Cloete, clarified complex family history, and facilitated Michael's meeting with the late Major Philip Erskine, kinsman of the Earl of Buchan, who supplemented information personally provided by the 17th Earl.

Gloria Carnevali, Venezuelan Cultural Attaché in London, provided invaluable data on General Francisco de Miranda; Alison Reboul, document analyst, enabled Michael to conclusively prove that Margaret

Bulkley and James Barry were one and the same; the late Professor Suna Kili, of Boğaziçi University, Istanbul, facilitated a highly informative visit to Selimiye Barracks, site of Scutari Hospital; the late Dr Edward Myers made available a translated copy of James Barry's MD dissertation, and its Greek epigraph was kindly translated by Dr Emily Kearns of St Hilda's College, Oxford. Dr Astrid James, deputy editor of *The Lancet* first drew attention to Barry's carotid aneurism account.

For wide and varied technical advice, grateful thanks are due to the following: Father John Azzopardi, curator, Wignacourt Museum, Rabat, Malta; Peter Baker FRCS, consultant surgeon; Professor Peter Beighton, human geneticist; Professor Herman de Groot, obstetrician and gynaecologist; Professor Natie Finkelstein, pharmacologist; Professor Peter Folb, pharmacologist; Dr G. T. Hansmann, general practitioner, Cape Town; Nina Hochstrasser, Schweizerische Rheinhäfen, Basel, Switzerland; Dr Ravidranath Kapadia, pathologist, Manipal, India; Dr Christina Kennaway, general practitioner, Bath; Professor Graham Louw, anatomist, University of Cape Town; Andrea Ludorf, Römische-Germanische Zentralmuseum, Mainz, Germany; Roger Melvill FRCS, consultant neurosurgeon, Cape Town; Professor Alistair Millar, paediatric surgeon, Red Cross Children's Hospital, Cape Town; Dr Alan G. Morris, medical biologist; Professor Raj Ramesar, human geneticist; Dr Ashley Robins, psychiatrist, University of Cape Town; Dr Colin Saunders, consultant in industrial medicine, Zimbabwe; Dr Ivan Strausz, obstetrician and gynaecologist, New York; Professor George Sweeney, physiologist, McMaster University, Canada; Professor Vijaya Teelok, Professor of History and Political Science, University of Mauritius; Professor John Wass, Professor of Endocrinology, University of Oxford; Andy Watts, master distillér, Wellington, South Africa.

For guidance and advice in their respective fields, we are hugely appreciative of the contributions made by: Miren Basterra and Gloria Henriques, historians, Archives and Library of Columbeia, Archivo del General Francisco de Miranda, Caracas, Venezuela; Dr Kate Bethune, Assistant Curator, Furniture, Fashions and Textiles, Victoria and Albert Museum, London; Mrs G. Brewer, Curator, Department of Uniforms, Badges and Medals, National Army Museum, Chelsea; Kevin Browne, National Library of Ireland, Dublin; Clare Button, Archivist, Edinburgh University Library; 3rd Lieutenant Çam, Turkish Army, Selimiye Barracks, Istanbul; Simon Chaplin and Dr Leslie Hall,

Library of the Wellcome Institute, London; Katherine Coombs, Curator, Paintings, Victoria and Albert Museum, London; Tina Craig, Archives and Library of the Royal College of Surgeons of England; Dale Dodgen, Curator, Chavonnes Battery Museum, Cape Town; Irene Ferguson, Archivist, Edinburgh University Library; Melanie Guestyn, National Library of South Africa, Cape Town; Marlene Gouder, Archives of Malta; Natie Greeff, Curator, Military History Museum, The Castle, Cape Town; Felicity Harper, Archivist, Powderham Castle, Devon; Samantha Harris, Collections Manager, Maidstone Museum and Bentlif Art Gallery, Kent; Sally Harrower and staff, National Library of Scotland, Edinburgh; Najwa Hendrikse, National Library of South Africa, Cape Town; Ibrahim Kenny, Archives of the Western Cape, South Africa; Dr Gerald Klinghardt, Curator, Department of Anthropology, South African Museum, Cape Town; Thalia Knight, Archives and Library of the Royal College of Surgeons of England; Dr Erika le Roux, Archives of the Western Cape, South Africa; Jackie Loos, author and journalist, Cape Town; Iain Macintyre FRCS, History Editor, *Journal of the Royal College of Physicians of Edinburgh*; Laddy McKechnie, National Library of South Africa, Cape Town; Elaine Milsom and Margaret Richards, Beaufort Archives, Badminton, Gloucestershire; Peter Murray, Director, Crawford Municipal Art Gallery, Cork; Thembile Ndabeni, Archives of the Western Cape, South Africa; Blanche Parker, Darien Library, Connecticut; Mark Pomeroy, Archives of the Royal Academy, London; Margaret Powell, Lewis Walpole Library, Farmington, Connecticut; Ronel Rogers, National Library of South Africa, Cape Town; Jane Ruddell, Archivist, Mercer's Company, London; Joan Self, Archives of the Meteorological Service, Exeter, Devon; Tim Smith, Deputy Head of Tides, UK Hydrographic Office, Taunton; Ms U. Sohun, National Archives of Mauritius; Captain Peter Starling, Army Medical Services Museum, Mytchett, Surrey; John D. Stevenson, Trinity Research Services, Scottish Maritime History, Edinburgh; Jaco van der Merwe, Archives of the Western Cape, South Africa; Dr Pieter van der Merwe, MBE, National Maritime Museum, Greenwich, UK; Andree Vincent, Executive Director, St James Club, Montreal; Susan Walker, Lewis Walpole Library, Farmington, Connecticut; Diana Wall, Manager, Collections, Museum Africa, Johannesburg.

Staff of the following libraries have been unfailingly helpful: Benson Village, Oxfordshire; Wellcome Library, London; British Library, Euston

Road and Colindale, London; National Library of South Africa, Cape Town; University of Cape Town Medical School; National Art Library, Victoria and Albert Museum, London; London School of Economics, London; Lewis Walpole Library, Farmington, Connecticut; as have the staff of the following archives and museums: National Archives, Kew, London; Archives of the Royal College of Physicians of London; Archives of St Thomas's, Guy's and King's College Hospitals, London; Cumbrian Archive Service, Whitehaven, Cumbria; St Thomas's Old Operating Theatre Museum, London; Florence Nightingale Museum, Claydon House, Buckinghamshire.

Michael received valued feedback on early drafts from: Dr Derrick Burns, consultant physician; Professor Emeritus A. A. Forder, bacteriologist; Dr John Gardiner, consultant neurologist, Cape Town; Professor J. P. de V. van Niekerk, editor of the *South African Medical Journal*; Professor Martin Shelton, obstetrician and gynaecologist, University of Cape Town.

This work could not have been realised without the valuable assistance of: Dr Sam Alberti, Head, Hunterian Museum, Royal College of Surgeons of England; Fanie Bekker, artist; John Carr, photographer, Communications Department, Royal College of Surgeons of England; Allen Crosbie, Cobh Genealogical Project, Merville, Cork, Ireland; Dr Lyndall Gordon, biographer and Senior Research Fellow of St Hilda's College, Oxford; Barry Gormley and Roger Ingle, antique firearms enthusiasts, South Africa; Professor Jeanne Heywood, Department of English, University of Cape Town; Ricardo Jameson and Rufus Rhode, IT specialists; Matt Jones, Friends of St Andrew's Church, Hove; Dr Emily Kearns, Senior Research Fellow in Classics, St Hilda's College, Oxford; Zephney Kennedy, educationalist and feminist, Cape Town; Professor Lars Kröger, Otto-Friedrich-Universität, Bamberg, Germany; Judith Mitchell, Royal College of Surgeons of England; Sarah Pearson, Curator, Hunterian Museum, Royal College of Surgeons of England; Dr N. M. Pettit, Headmaster, Devonport High School for Boys, Plymouth; Cynthia Rosers, 'Jamerican' researcher, Jamaica; Sue Simpson, Archivist, James Lock & Co. Hatters, London; the late Barry Smith, trustee, Friends of Kensal Green Cemetery, London; Peter Tilley, Archivist at Gieves & Hawkes, Military Tailors, London; Thandikhaya Tsondwa, Chavonnes Museum, Cape Town.

Grateful thanks are due for the generous help given by the following authors and experts: Professor W. L. Pressly, Department of Art

Index

References to illustrations are in *italics*; references to notes are indicated by n.

Abdülmecid I, Sultan 329, 330
Aberdeen, Earl of 330
Acho 274–5
Acts of Insolvency (1813) 21
Acts of Union (1800) 6
Afghanistan 291, 330
Albemarle, George Keppel, Lord
   152–3, 380–1
alcoholism 289–91, 355, 429 n. 34
Alexander, Gen Thomas 353, 364,
   365
Alexandria (ship) 31
amputation 84, 89, 107–8, 416 n. 52
anaesthetic 305
anatomy 53, 66, 68, 69–74
Anderson, James 370
Anderson, Dr Robert 76, 90–1, 92
Anderson, Lt Col Robert 279, 280
Andrews, Sarah 33, 34–5
Anglo-Spanish War 32
Antigua 285–7
Armstrong, Dr Daniel 310, 311, 321
Army Medical Board 95, 96, 97, 100
Army Medical Department 102–3,
   222, 231, 350–1

Arthur, Dr John 205, 206, 220, 221
Augustus Frederick, Prince 29
Austria 327

Bailey, Samuel 190
Bairnsfather, Nicolette 383
Barbados 284–5
Barclay, Dr John 74
Barnes, George 268–70
Barry, Dr James 4, 5–6, 11–12, 22,
   50–1, 151–4
  and Africans 160–1
  and aneurysms 227–8
  and the Army 93, 100–1, 102–4,
    111–12, 359–62, 363–6
  and arrest 268–71, 282
  and Barry, James (uncle) 13–14, 15,
    16–21
  and caesareans 213–16, 217–18
  and Canada 352–9
  and Cape tour 129–30, 131, 133,
    135, 136
  and Cape Town 119, 120, 122–3,
    140–5, 223
  and cholera 162, 163–4

Barry, Dr James (*cont.*)
  and Cloete 155–9, 368–9
  and Colonial Medical Officer
    167–72, 204–6, 207–9
  and Cooper 87–8
  and Corfu 320–3, 331–2
  and Crimean War 333–4, 335,
    336–7, 338, 341–2, 343–5
  and daughter 7–8, 57
  and death xi–xiii, 373–4, 375–8
  and delirium tremens 290–1
  and education 29–30
  and exposure 378–81, 390–1
  and finances 91–2
  and governess 43–5
  and Halford 235, 236–7
  and Helps 275–6
  and illness 293–5, 371, 372
  and Jamaica 246, 247, 248, 249,
    250, 251–2
  and Las Cases 125, 126–7, 139–40
  and leprosy 173, 174–6
  and Liesching 188–91
  and London 323–4, 369–70
  and Lonsdale 299–300, 324–5
  and male identity 58–62, 66–7,
    259–60, 422 n. 10
  and Malta 301, 302–5, 307–9,
    310–13, 315–16, 317–18
  and Mauritius 224–7
  and medicine 52–3, 55
  and mental illness 176–7
  and Miranda 33–4, 35, 38, 39–41,
    80
  and mother 256–7
  and myths 383–5
  and Nightingale 339–41
  and photograph 366–7
  and physical examination 387–9
  and prison inspection 179–81,
    191–3, 194–7, 198–202
  and RCS 95–6, 97–100
  and Redmond 42–3
  and rumours 75–7, 150–1, 182–7

and St Helena 264, 265–8, 273–5,
  276–81
and St Thomas's Hospital 81–2, 83,
  85, 86, 89
and St Vincent 284
and Sanitary Commission 350, 351
and Somerset 145–8, 149, 166,
  211, 212, 229–31, 232, 233, 239,
  240–1
and Stoke Damerel 105–6
and university 63–4, 65–6, 68–70,
  71–5, 77–8
and venereal disease 219–21
and voyage 115–17, 118
and West Indies 284–5, 286,
  287–9, 292–3
Barry, James (uncle) 5, 9, 11–12,
  14–16, 17–21, 22
  and artworks 35–7, 46–7, 55–6
  and Blue Stocking movement 52
  and Buchan 66
  and death 23–5, 26, 27, 34
  and Miranda 40–1
Barry, Patrick (uncle) 8, 9, 16
Barry, Redmond (uncle) 8–9, 16,
  203–4
  and imprisonment 42–3, 48, 56, 67
  and inheritance 25–6, 27–8, 35–6,
    37–8
'Bastaards' 134, 160, 173
Bath 235–8
Bathurst, Lord 148, 208, 210,
  218–19, 248
Bazalgette, Joseph 373
Beagle, HMS 263, 268
Bellerophon, HMS 3, 4, 94, 110–11,
  317
Bellingham, Sydney 356–7
Belmore, Somerset Lowry-Corry, 2nd
  Earl of 247
Bethune, Rev John 358–9
Bianchi, L. J. 171–2
Bigge, John 197, 199, 200
Bird, Lt Col Christopher 128, 198, 199

Birth of Pandora, The (Barry) 19, 28, 36–7, 75, 91, 402 n. 25

Bishop, Sophia xii, 370, 374, 375–6, 390, 391

Black Sea 329–31, 345

Blackwell, Elizabeth 385–6

Blizard, Sir William 99

Blue Stocking movement 52

Bolívar, Simon 79, 80

Bonaparte, Joseph 47

Bone, Dr Hugh 288

Bonomi, Joseph 24, 25, 26, 27

botany 130, 219–20, 221, 287

Bourke, Maj Gen Richard 210–11

Bradford, Edward 251–2, 291–2

Brenton, Lady Isabella 140–1

Brenton, Vice Adm Sir Jaheel 140, 141, 161

Britain, *see* Great Britain

British Army 96–7, 232–3, 321
  and 56th Foot 163, 164
  and 56th (West Essex) Reg 251–2
  and 84th Reg 249, 250
  and 91st Reg 279–81
  and agents 352–3
  and alcoholism 289–90
  and Cape Colony 135–6
  and Crimean War 331–6, 337, 342–5
  and flogging 286–7
  and Jamaica 246, 247, 248
  and Malta 301–2, 304, 315–16
  and physical examination 387–9
  and Royal York Rangers 49, 51
  and St Helena 265
  and wounded 101–2
  see also Army Medical Board; Army Medical Department; York Hospital

British Empire 4, 30

British Medical Association 386

Brougham, Henry 209, 230, 239–40

Brownrigg, Elizabeth 98

Buchan, David Steuart Erskine, 11th Earl of 19, 60, 64–5, 120, 228
  and Barry 66–7, 76–7, 104, 105
  and women 30, 78–9

Bulkley, Jeremiah (father) 4–7, 9–10, 12, 17, 57
  and imprisonment 21–2, 27

Bulkley, John (brother) 5, 7, 9–11, 12, 17, 28
  and army 48–51

Bulkley, Juliana (daughter) 7–8, 11, 57, 218, 406 n. 56

Bulkley, Margaret Anne, *see* Barry, Dr James

Bulkley, Mary Anne (mother) 5, 9, 10–11, 12, 22, 43
  and brother 16, 17, 19–21, 27–8, 29
  and death 350
  and finances 62–3, 75, 77, 90–1
  and inheritance 35–7, 55–6
  and James (Margaret) 59, 101
  and publications 46–7
  and workhouse 254–7

Burke, Edmund 52

Burnett, Bishop 185, 186, 230

Burns, Robert 64

Burrell, William 333

Cahill, Lt David 303–4

Canada 95, 352, 354–9, 365–6, 381–2

Cape of Good Hope 118–19, 121, 128–37, 260
  and Africans 160–1, 165
  and map *114*

Cape Town 119–20, 258–9

Captivity, HMS 48, 56

Cardwell, Edward 388–9

Carlisle, Anthony 23, 24, 28, 53, 398 n. 3

Carnall, John 192, 195

Castlereagh, Viscount 39

Catholics 4, 6–7, 300, 303, 329, 399 n. 25

Chandler, George 98, 99
Charlemagne (ship) 329
Charles IV of Spain, King 47
Chelsea 101–2
Chetcuti, Dr 307, 308, 309, 310
cholera 162–4, 307–17, 333, 334, 372, 373
Christie, James 28, 35, 36
Clanricarde, Marquess of 330
Clerke, Capt Shadwell 369
Cleugh, Rev John 302, 303
Cline, Henry 82, 83, 88, 98, 99–100
Cloete, Capt Josias 154–9, 164–5, 368–9, 383
Cloete, Mrs 143–5
Codrington, Sir William 337
Cole, Lt Col Arthur Lowry 360, 361
Colebrooke, Maj William Macbean 199, 200, 286
Collier, Charles 225
Collings, Dr 307, 309
Colonial Medical Officer 166, 167–72, 204–5, 207–8
Colville, Lt Gen Sir Charles 224–5, 226
Conyers, Maj Gen Charles 321
Cooper, Astley 53, 82, 83, 86–90, 92, 227
Corfu 319–21, 322–3, 331–6, 345–6
Cork 3–5, 6, 7, 255–6
Cornwallis, Cubah 248
Cotton, Maj Gen Sir Willoughby 234, 247, 249, 250
Cradock, Sir John 134
Crimean War 330–1, 332–45, 350–1
Cruikshank, George 99
Cumming, Dr Alexander 341
Curran, William Henry 16

Dance-Holland, Sir Nathaniel 36
Danzer (manservant) 172–3, 222, 223
Darwin, Charles 263, 268

Davies-Colley, Eleanor 386
Davis, Philip 28
Deane, Thomas Kift 181–2, 206
delirium tremens 196, 290–1
Denny, Lt Col William 331–3, 344–5
Denyssen, Daniel 180, 183–4, 207
and Tronk report 190, 193, 195–6, 197–8, 200–2
Dickens, Charles 42, 231, 282, 352, 384
and layers-out 390, 391
Dillon, Capt William 141
Disraeli, Benjamin 300, 330
doctresses 248
Donkin, Sir Rufane 161–2, 164, 165, 166, 230
Doughty, Edward 313
Dr James Barry (play) 384–5
Draper, Thomas 247, 288
duels 156–8, 423 n. 22
Dunne, Charles 96
D'Urban, Lt Gen Sir Benjamin 260
dysentery 146, 147–8, 225

East India Company 119–20, 252–3, 265
Eastern Orthodox Church 329
Eddie, William Cruickshank 265, 279
Edinburgh 60, 64, 65–6
Edwards, William 184–5, 186, 192
Ellice, Lt Gen Robert 310, 316, 317
Equator ritual 117–18
ether 305
Ewart, James 102
Eyre, Lt Gen Sir William 358–9, 360, 361–2

Fenton, Elizabeth (Bessie) 225–7
fever 247–8, 321
Findlay, Capt John 182
Fitzroy, Lady Mary 240–1
food 84

France 3, 6, 13, 109, 329–30
  and Revolution 31, 32
  and Spain 95
  and West Indies 47, 51
  see also Napoleon Bonaparte
Fryer, Dr Edward 28–30, 33, 38,
    40–1, 46–7
  and medicine 52, 53
Fyfe, Andrew 68, 69–70, 71, 72

Garrett Anderson, Elizabeth 385–6
Gebhard, William 169–70, 171
George, Duke of Cambridge 362
George III, King 132
Germany 327
Gibney, William 103, 104
Gibson, Dr James Brown 365, 375
Glenelg, Lord 265–6, 267, 269, 271
Godwin, William 52
Gorta Mór (Great Hunger) 306
Government of India Act (1833)
    252–3
Great Britain 6, 299, 330–1
  and Spain 32, 33, 39, 47
  see also British Empire;
    British Army
Green, Joseph 184
Greig, George 184, 185, 186
Griffon, HMS 123
Guy's Hospital 82–3, 86, 87, 88

Halford, Sir Henry 234–6, 237
Hall, Dr John 333, 334, 341, 350–1,
    353
Helps, Rev William 275–6
Hemel en Aarde (Heaven and Earth)
    173, 174–6, 209
Henderson, Dr James 339
Hermes 161
Hertzog, James Barry 217, 431 n. 9
Hopkins, Dr Richard 264, 265, 267,
    281
Hottentots Holland mountains
    129–30, 172, 173

House of Industry 255–6
Hudson, Samuel Eusebius 183
hygiene 88, 217, 315, 412 n. 27
Hyperion, HMS 164–5, 166

India 162, 252–3, 299, 300, 330
  and mutiny 353
Ireland 3–4, 6, 306, 379–80

Jamaica 234, 245–52, 283–4,
    366–7
Jefferson, Thomas 32
Jenner, Dr Edward 142
Jobson, John 75
John (manservant) 252, 253, 318,
    366, 367, 373
John Bull (ship) 365–6, 381–2
Johnson, Samuel 52
Joris 169–71
Journal of Dr James Barry, The (book)
    385

Kekewich, George 179, 180, 197,
    198–9
Keppel, George, see Albemarle, Lord
Khoikhoi people 133, 134, 135, 160
King, Margaret 54, 82
Kinnis, Dr John 163, 320
Knowles, Gen Francis Edward 269,
    270–1, 272

Lancet, The (magazine) 232, 235
Las Cases, Emmanuel, Comte de
    123–7, 138–40
layers-out xii–xiii, 375–6, 378–9,
    390–1
Lear, Edward 322
leg ulcers 289
leprosy 173–6, 426 n. 25
Liesching, Karl Friedrich 188–91
Liesching, Dr Karl Wilhelm 180, 194,
    195
Locher, Dr 214–17
Lockyer, Lt Col 334

London 13–14, 17–18, 229, 369–70,
  371–2
  and poverty 60–1
  and sewage system 372–3
London School of Medicine for
  Women 386
Longfield, Col Mountifort 6–7, 51
Longmore, Thomas 295
Lonsdale, William Lowther, 2nd
  Earl of 299–300, 301, 303, 323,
  324–5, 349, 370
Lord Cathcart (ship) 115–18, 119
Lord William Bentinck (ship) 257–9
Lovelace, William King-Noel, Earl
  of 284
Lowe, Gen Sir Hudson 124, 149
Lowry, Capt Robert 294–5, 331
Lys, William Henry 142, 206

McGregor, James 303, 304
McGrigor, Sir James 231, 253, 266–7,
  290, 320
  and Malta 302, 317
Macintosh, Maj Gen Alexander Fisher
  335–7
McKinnon, David Reid 369, 372,
  373, 375, 376
  and revelation 378–9, 381, 390
Macleod, Col Sir H. G. 289
M'Crindle 367–8
Madison, James 32
Maitland, Capt William 110
malaria 247, 293
Malta 301–5, 307–14, 315–17, 318
Margate 46
Martin Chuzzlewit (Dickens) 391
Marx, Clare 386
matrons 266
Mauritius 162–4, 222, 224–5
Maximilian, Archduke 345–6
measles 273
medicine 53–4, 84, 171–2
  and veneral disease 219–20
  and women 385–6

mental illness 176
Methuen, Lord 336
Middlemore, Maj Gen George 264,
  265–6, 269, 271–2
  and Barry 276–7, 278, 280, 281
Middlesex Hospital 53
Millar, Dr Andrew 308
Miranda, Gen Don Francisco de
  31–3, 34, 38–41, 47–8, 61, 112
  and emancipation 54–5
  and Venezuela 79–80
Miranda, Leander 33, 34–5
Molini, Tómas 39
Monro, Dr Alexander 66, 68–9, 74
Montanaro, Dr 310
Montgomery, Mr 227–8
Montreal 356, 357–8
More O'Ferrall, Richard 308, 312, 317
mosquitoes 247, 293
Mosse, Charles Benjamin 366, 367
Munnik, James Barry 260–1
Munnik, Thomas 213, 214, 217
Munnik, Wilhelmina 213, 214, 215,
  216, 217

Napoleon Bonaparte 6, 39, 47, 94, 95
  and exile 124, 263
  and imprisonment 110–11
  and Las Cases 138–9
  and Waterloo 106–7
Napoleon III, Emperor 329
Navy, see Royal Navy
Ndlambe, Chief 134, 135, 136, 137,
  160
Ngqika, Chief 134, 135, 136–7
Nicholas I, Tsar 329–30
Nightingale, Florence 335, 338–41,
  345, 350, 351, 353, 391

O'Connor, Dr Nicholas 293–5
Ottoman Empire 329–30

Paine, Thomas 32
Palestine 329–30

Palmerston, Henry John Temple, Lord 97, 330
Parker, Vice Adm Sir William 308
Pasteur, Louis 372
patient care 83–6
Peel, Sir Robert 26
Penrose, Cooper 17, 21, 35
Penrose, William Edward 27
Perceval, Dudley 210
piracy 32
Placard scandal 182–7, 189, 192–3
plantocracy 249, 284
Plasket, Sir Richard 191, 195, 198–200, 201–2, 209–10
  and Supreme Medical Committee 205–6, 208
Plymouth 104–5, 109–11
pneumonia 143–4
Polemann, Pieter Heinrich 190
Portugal 95
potato famine 306
prisoners of war 109

rabies 305
Rae, Isobel 388
Raglan, FitzRoy Somerset, Lord 231–2, 234, 235, 271–2, 280, 302
  and Crimean War 330–1, 332, 333–4, 336–7, 345
  and India 299, 300
  and Vienna 325, 326–8
Reade, George 321
Reardon, Daniel 26–7, 28, 30, 33–4, 35, 55
  and Barry 44–5
  and finances 62–3, 67
Reed, Mr 276–8, 281–2
resurrectionists 10, 70–1, 409 n. 9
Rex, George 132–3
Richardson, Dr William 311, 312
Riky, Lt Col Benjamin 344
Robb, Dr John 166, 167, 169
Roberts, Frederic 344
Rogers, Col Ebenezer 368, 384

Rollo, Col Robert 359–61
Rose, June 388
Royal Academy 5, 11, 14, 15, 52
  and women 405 n. 38
Royal College of Surgeons (RCS) 95–6, 97–100, 386
Royal Navy 8, 96, 249
Russia 95, 329–30, 333, 343, 345
Rutherford, Col Nathaniel John Crawford 383–4, 387–8
Ruttledge, Maj Thomas Ormsby 360, 361

sack-'em-up gangs 70–1
St Helena 111, 124, 125, 252–3, 263–8, 273
St Thomas's Hospital 81–6, 88–9
St Vincent, Viscount 283–4
Salter, Thomas 305, 318, 322
San people 133, 134, 160–1
Savery, Rev Servington 81
Schooles, Dr Henry 290, 304
Scott, Sir Walter 64, 66, 79
Scutari 334–5, 338, 339
Seacole, Mary 248
Sevastopol 342–3
Shand, Dr Robert 170
Shanks, Dr 224–5, 226
Sharpe, Samuel 'Daddy' 246, 249, 251
Sheridan, Capt Thomas 128–9
Sir Charles McGrigor & Co 353, 377, 378
Skey, Dr Joseph 105
slavery 133, 160, 169–71, 264, 285
  and Jamaica 245–6, 248–51, 283–4
Slavery Abolition Act (1833) 251
smallpox 142, 258–9, 273, 289
Smith, Aaron 193–6, 198, 200, 201
Smith, Andrew 320, 333, 334, 340, 353
Snow, John 314–15
Society of Arts 23, 24, 29
Society of United Irishmen 6

Somerset, Lt Gen Lord Charles
    Henry 120–3, 124, 125–6, 127,
    239–41
  and Barry 152–3, 154, 182–7,
    205–6, 376
  and Cape tour 128, 130, 133,
    134–5, 136–7
  and Cloete 155
  and departure 161, 164, 209,
    210–12
  and illness 145–9, 228, 229–31,
    232, 233, 235–9
  and Las Cases 139, 140
  and leprosy 173–4
  and Liesching 190, 191
  and marriage 165, 166
  and Tronk report 195, 196, 197–8,
    200–2
Somerset, Charlotte 122, 123, 126,
    128
Somerset, Lord Edward 234
Somerset, Maj Gen Lord FitzRoy, see
    Raglan, Lord
Somerset, Georgiana 122–3, 128
Somerset, Lady Mary 165, 166, 178,
    181, 183
Somerset Hospital 176–7, 209
Somerville, Mary 29
Southey, Robert 14–15, 16, 19, 23
Spain 31, 32, 47, 95
Spanish America 30, 31–2, 33, 47–8
Stafford, Rev Dr 21–2
stethoscopes 225
Stockenström, Andries 257
Stoke Damerel Military Hospital 104,
    105
Stuart, Lt Gen Sir Patrick 301, 303,
    306
Suffolk, HMS 25–6
Supreme Medical Committee 205–7
surgery 74, 78, 83, 89–90, 96, 97
  and amputation 84, 89, 107–8, 416
    n. 52
  and anaesthetic 305

and aneurysms 227–8, 232
  and caesareans 214–17
Sutherland, Dr John 351

Tardieu, Dr 170–1
Thorndike, Sybil 384–5
Thornhill, Capt John 279
Trafalgar, Battle of 33
Tredgold, John Harfield 190
Trinidad 32, 33, 288–90, 291–2
Tronk prison 179–81, 191–6,
    198–202
tuberculosis 289
tumours 305–6
typhus 146, 147–8, 310–11

United States of America 32, 33,
    95

Vaccine Institution 142, 166
venereal disease 220–1, 225, 265–6
Venezuela 31–2, 39, 55, 79–80,
    288
Victoria, Queen 283, 299, 326, 352
Vienna 326–8

Wall, Capt Joseph 98
war 94–5
Ward, Sir Henry George 319, 335–6
Ward, William 359, 360
Wardrop, James 227, 232, 235
Washington, George 32
Waterloo, Battle of 94, 106–7, 108
Wellington, Sir Arthur Wellesley,
    Duke of 39, 47, 95, 167, 318
  and death 324, 325–6
  and Waterloo 106–7
West Indies 47, 49, 51; see also
    Antigua; Jamaica; Windward and
    Leeward Islands
Westmorland, Lord 326–7, 328
Whitefoord, Caleb 26
Whitfield, Richard 82, 85
wildlife 130, 131–2

William IV, King 233–4
Windward and Leeward Islands
  287–8, 368–9
Wollstonecraft, Mary 45–6, 52, 79
women 52, 371
  and alcoholism 355
  and education 29, 30, 78–9
  and employment 45–6
  and hospital 86
  and layers-out 390–1

and medicine 53, 385–6
  and venereal disease 265, 266
workhouses 255–6, 315

Xhosa tribes 133–5, 136–7, 165, 260

yellow fever 247, 295
York Hospital 101–4
Yorke, Maj Gen Sir Charles 361–2